Pharmaceuticals for Targeting Coronaviruses

Edited by

Luciana Scotti

&

Marcus T. Scotti

Laboratory of Cheminformatics
Program of Natural and Synthetic Bioactive Products
(PgPNSB)
Health Sciences Center, Federal University of Paraíba
João Pessoa-PB, Brazil

Pharmaceuticals for Targeting Coronaviruses

Editors: Luciana Scotti & Marcus T. Scotti

ISBN (Online): 978-981-5051-30-8

ISBN (Print): 978-981-5051-31-5

ISBN (Paperback): 978-981-5051-32-2

Published by Bentham Science Publishers Pte. Ltd. Singapore. All Rights Reserved.

need for a court order if at any point you breach any terms of this License Agreement. In no event will any delay or failure by Bentham Science Publishers in enforcing your compliance with this License Agreement constitute a waiver of any of its rights.

3. You acknowledge that you have read this License Agreement, and agree to be bound by its terms and conditions. To the extent that any other terms and conditions presented on any website of Bentham Science Publishers conflict with, or are inconsistent with, the terms and conditions set out in this License Agreement, you acknowledge that the terms and conditions set out in this License Agreement shall prevail.

Bentham Science Publishers Pte. Ltd.
80 Robinson Road #02-00
Singapore 068898
Singapore
Email: subscriptions@benthamscience.net

BENTHAM SCIENCE

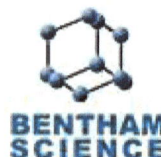

CONTENTS

PREFACE

The new coronavirus (2019-nCoV) is part of the group of viruses in a format similar to a crown (Corona), more specifically belonging to the species Betocoronavirus, such as Middle East respiratory syndrome coronavirus (MERS-CoV) and acute respiratory syndrome (SARS). The outbreak was first reported in Wuhan, China, in December 2019, where several cases similar to pneumonia and SARS started to appear with symptoms of fever, cough, and severe respiratory difficulties [1 - 4]. Its origin is still unknown. Some works suggest mutations of the virus in bats or snakes, animals commercialized in the Wuhan market, which have infected humans. The homology similar to the 2019 - nCoV than to your Sequences of Bat SARS-like coronavirus supports the hypothesis that the transmission chain began from the bat and reached the human [5, 6]. It was what happened to the infectious agent that caused COVID-19.

The improvement of drug discovery techniques is fundamental in searching for new therapies that could be selective and effective to combat SARS-CoV-2. Drug discovery approaches are based on ligands (Ligand-Based Drug Design - LBDD) or structures (Structure-Based Drug Discovery - SBDD). Concerning SBDD, it is the main and most evolved technique used for discovering new drugs. The application of SBDD techniques has been improved the pharmacological arsenal against diverse diseases, which allowed to discover innovative treatments, such as inhibitors of HIV-1 proteases. In chapter I, main SBDD techniques (*i.e.*, homology modeling; molecular dynamics and docking; de novo drug discovery; pharmacophore modeling; fragment-based drug discovery; and virtual high-throughput screenings) applied to discover new hit compounds SARS-CoV-2 (COVID-19) will be discussed in detail.

Medicinal plants with a wide range of bioactive compounds, which are exhibiting antiviral activities, are able to provide possible benefits as a preventive and treatment for COVID-19. Rockrose (*Cistus* spp.), lemon balm (*Melissa officinalis* L.), rosemary (*Rosmarinus officinalis* L.), licorice root (*Glyrrhiza glabra* L.), olive leaf (*Olea europea* L.), peppermint (*Mentha piperita* L.), basil (*Ocimum bacilicum* L.), sumac (*Rhus coriaria* L.) and different species of thyme (*Origanum, Thymus,* and *Thymbra*) are important medicinal plants having antiviral activities. Chapter II provides an overview of published scientific information on the development of plant-based antiviral therapeutic agents based on the extensive literature survey. Researchers from all over the world are dedicating themselves to several studies in an attempt to find the best treatment and prevention against the coronavirus. Chapter III addresses the main characteristics of SARS, the main targets and drugs that have achieved excellent results in clinical trials.

With increasing COVID-19 cases globally, it would be too difficult to provide proper treatment even for the severe cases in hospitals. Therefore, the general public is advised to wear the mask, maintain social distancing and use sanitizers. The COVID-19 mild infected patients may be isolated at home and can be taken care of by natural medicines. In chapter IV, an attempt has been made to repurpose all potential natural drugs and natural Ayurvedic formulations that may be beneficial to combat viruses like the SARS-CoV-2 due to their antiviral and immune-modulator properties available under Indian traditional medicine and Chinese traditional medicine system for the effective treatment or prevention of COVID-19.

Peptidomimetics have emerged as a potential class for designing new effective drugs against COVID-19, in addition to lopinavir/ritonavir, in which these drugs are currently being investigated in clinical trials. In chapter V, the authors describe peptidomimetic and peptide-derived inhibitors of 3CL^{pro} from SARS-CoV-2, and also SARS- and MERS-CoV viruses, summarizing all relevant studies based on warhead groups utilization and SAR analysis for all of them to contribute to the development of compounds more selective, effective, and low-costs to combat these emerging viruses.

Luciana Scotti

&

Marcus T. Scotti
Laboratory of Cheminformatics
Program of Natural and Synthetic Bioactive Products (PgPNSB)
Health Sciences Center, Federal University of Paraíba
João Pessoa-PB, Brazil

REFERENCES

[1] Benvenuto D, Giovanetti M, Ciccozzi A, Spoto S, Angeletti S, Ciccozzi M. The 2019-new coronavirus epidemic: Evidence for virus evolution. J Med Virol 2020; 92(4): 455-9.
[http://dx.doi.org/10.1002/jmv.25688] [PMID: 31994738]

[2] Zaher NH, Mostafa MI, Altaher AY. Design, synthesis and molecular docking of novel triazole derivatives as potential CoV helicase inhibitors. Acta Pharm 2020; 70(2): 145-59.
[http://dx.doi.org/10.2478/acph-2020-0024] [PMID: 31955138]

[3] Phan T. Novel coronavirus: From discovery to clinical diagnostics. Infect Genet Evol 2020; 79: 104211.
[http://dx.doi.org/10.1016/j.meegid.2020.104211] [PMID: 32007627]

[4] Li G, Fan Y, Lai Y, *et al.* Coronavirus infections and immune responses. J Med Virol 2020; 92(4): 424-32.
[http://dx.doi.org/10.1002/jmv.25685] [PMID: 31981224]

[5] Mahase E. Coronavirus: doctor who faced backlash from police after warning of outbreak dies. Bmj-British Medical Journal 2020; 368
[http://dx.doi.org/10.1136/bmj.m528]

[6] Mowbray H. In Beijing, coronavirus 2019-nCoV has created a siege mentality. Bmj-British Medical Journal 2020.
[http://dx.doi.org/10.1136/bmj.m516]

[7] York A. Novel coronavirus takes flight from bats? Nat Rev Microbiol 2020; 18(4): 191.
[http://dx.doi.org/10.1038/s41579-020-0336-9] [PMID: 32051570]

List of Contributors

Anil Kumar Saxena	Global Institute of Pharmaceutical Education and Research, Kashipur-244713, Uttarakhand, India
Edeildo Ferreira da Silva-Júnior	Chemistry and Biotechnology Institute, Federal University of Alagoas, Maceió, Brazil Laboratory of Medicinal Chemistry, Pharmaceutical Sciences Institute, Federal University of Alagoas, Maceió, Brazil
Herbert Igor Rodrigues de Medeiros	Laboratory of Cheminformatics, Program of Natural and Synthetic Bioactive Products (PgPNSB), Health Sciences Center, Federal University of Paraíba, João Pessoa-PB, Brazil
Igor José dos Santos Nascimento	Chemistry and Biotechnology Institute, Federal University of Alagoas, Maceió, Brazil
João Xavier de Araújo-Júnior	Laboratory of Medicinal Chemistry, Pharmaceutical Sciences Institute, Federal University of Alagoas, Maceió, Brazil
Luciana Scotti	Laboratory of Cheminformatics, Program of Natural and Synthetic Bioactive Products (PgPNSB), Health Sciences Center, Federal University of Paraíba, João Pessoa-PB, Brazil
Marcus Tullius Scotti	Laboratory of Cheminformatics, Program of Natural and Synthetic Bioactive Products (PgPNSB), Health Sciences Center, Federal University of Paraíba, João Pessoa-PB, Brazil
Mayank Kumar Khede	Care Support and Treatment Division, Chhattishgarh State Aids Control Society, Department of Health and Family Welfare, Chhattisgarh, India
Mayara dos Santos Maia	Laboratory of Cheminformatics, Program of Natural and Synthetic Bioactive Products (PgPNSB), Health Sciences Center, Federal University of Paraíba, João Pessoa-PB, Brazil
Nazim Sekeroglu	Department of Horticulture, Faculty of Agriculture, Kilis 7 Aralik University, 79000 Kilis, Turkey Advanced Technology Application and Research Center (ATARC), Kilis 7 Aralik University, 79000 Kilis, Turkey
Paulo Fernando da Silva Santos-Júnior	Chemistry and Biotechnology Institute, Federal University of Alagoas, Maceió, Brazil
Sevgi Gezici	Advanced Technology Application and Research Center (ATARC), Kilis 7 Aralik University, 79000 Kilis, Turkey Department of Molecular Biology and Genetics, Faculty of Science and Literature, Kilis 7 Aralik University, 79000 Kilis, Turkey
Sisir Nandi	Global Institute of Pharmaceutical Education and Research, Kashipur-244713, Uttarakhand, India
Thiago Mendonça de Aquino	Chemistry and Biotechnology Institute, Federal University of Alagoas, Maceió, Brazil

CHAPTER 1

Structure-Based Drug Discovery Approaches Applied to SARS-CoV-2 (COVID-19)

Igor José dos Santos Nascimento[1], Thiago Mendonça de Aquino[1] and Edeildo Ferreira da Silva-Júnior[1,2,*]

[1] *Chemistry and Biotechnology Institute, Federal University of Alagoas, Maceió, Brazil*

[2] *Laboratory of Medicinal Chemistry, Pharmaceutical Sciences Institute, Federal University of Alagoas, Maceió, Brazil*

Abstract: Viral diseases have caused millions of deaths around the world. In the past, health organizations and pharmaceutical industries have neglected these diseases for years, mainly because they affected a small geographic population. In contrast, since 2016, several viral outbreaks have been reported worldwide, such as those caused by Ebola, Zika, and SARS-CoV2 (COVID-19). Thus, these have received more attention, leading to increased efforts to search for new antiviral drugs. The SARS-CoV-2 pandemic, already responsible for more than 1,254,567 deaths worldwide, is the greatest example of a virus that has always been present in our society, responsible for small outbreaks in Asian and Arabic countries in 2004 and 2012. But, investments in research to identify/discover new drugs and vaccines were only intensified in 2020, in which only the remdesivir (an FDA-approved drug) was developed to addressCOVID-19 until today. Nonetheless, it has been used in hospitals in the United States and Japan, in emergency cases. Indeed, it justifies greater investments in discovering new alternatives that could save thousands of people. In this context, improving drug discovery techniques is fundamental in searching for new therapies that could be selective and effective to combat SARS-CoV-2. Drug discovery approaches are based on ligands (Ligand-Based Drug Design - LBDD) or structures (Structure-Based Drug Discovery - SBDD). Concerning SBDD, it is the main and most evolved technique used for discovering new drugs. The application of SBDD techniques has improved the pharmacological arsenal against diverse diseases, which allowed the discovery of innovative treatments, such as inhibitors of HIV-1 proteases. In this chapter, main SBDD techniques (*i.e.* homology modeling; molecular dynamics and docking; *de novo* drug discovery; pharmacophore modeling; fragment-based drug discovery; and virtual high-throughput screenings) applied to discover new *hit* compounds SARS-CoV-2 (COVID-19) will be discussed in details.

* **Corresponding author Edeildo Ferreira da Silva-Júnior:** Chemistry and Biotechnology Institute, Federal University of Alagoas, Maceió, Brazil and Laboratory of Medicinal Chemistry, Pharmaceutical Sciences Institute, Federal University of Alagoas, Maceió, Brazil; Tel: +55-87-9-9610-8311; E-mail: edeildo.junior@iqb.ufal.br

Keywords: Drug discovery, Dynamics simulations, Molecular modeling, SARS-CoV-2, Structure-Based Drug Discovery, TMPRSS2, Virtual screening.

1. INTRODUCTION

On December 31st, 2019, an outbreak of pneumonia was reported caused by an unknown etiologic agent in Wuhan, a province of Hubei in China. Thus, with the sporadic number of cases, on January 9th, 2020, the new coronavirus was recognized as the causative agent by the Chinese Center for Disease Control and Prevention (CDC). When it started spreading at an alarming pace to other countries in the world, the new coronavirus (SARS-CoV-2, or COVID-19) was declared a pandemic by the world health organization (WHO) on March 11th, 2020 [1 - 3].

Since its discovery, SARS-CoV-2 has been responsible for several victims worldwide. To date (09/11/2020), there are already 50,266,033 confirmed cases with 1,254,567 deaths [4]. The main symptoms are fever, cough, fatigue, myalgia, and dyspnea. Its transmission occurs mainly through coughing, sneezing, and respiratory droplets [5]. These alarming statistics make research groups from around the world focus on discovering new therapies against this pandemic virus [6]. Advances in drug developments resulted in the repurposing of remdesivir in the United States. However, this drug still does not show the best effectiveness. So, a molecule that could be effective in eliminating SARS-CoV2 from the body is an unmet needed [6, 7].

Currently, biological targets guide the process of discovering new drugs. Then, the structure of a macromolecule is fundamental for this process [8]. Such structures provide valuable information on mechanisms of action and their correlation with biological activity [9]. In addition, information about the biological target and the availability of three-dimensional structures for these therapeutically attractive targets have resulted in several advances in the identification of inhibitors, as well as potential binding sites, contributing to the basis of structure-based drug discovery strategies (SBDD) [10].

In addition, *in silico* methods are increasingly gaining more visibility in the drug development field. These methods are used in SBDD and are related to higher chances of success with less financial cost and less time-consuming [11, 12].

In this context, this chapter will be addressed to the main SBDD techniques (homology modeling; molecular docking and dynamic; pharmacophore modeling; virtual screening and virtual high-throughput screening; fragment-based drug design; and *de novo* drug design) applied for the discovery of new promising compounds against SARS-CoV2.

2. CORONAVIRUSES: HISTORY AND STRUCTURE

Coronaviridae is a family of several groups of viruses responsible for the infection of both animals and humans. From this family, there are seven viruses that can infect humans, being: Severe Acute Respiratory Syndrome Coronavirus (SARS-CoV); Middle East Respiratory Syndrome Coronavirus (MERS-CoV); Severe Acute Respiratory Syndrome Coronavirus 2 (SARS-CoV-2); HCoV-OC43; HCoV-KHU1; HCoV-NL63; HCoV-229E [13]. Among these, the first three belong to the genus *Betacoronavirus*, and all of them display high potential for mutability, leading to plasticity and genetic variability, which contributes to their adaptation to different types of hosts [13, 14].

The first discovery of SARS-CoV was around the 1960s [15]. This pathogen is related to flu-like symptoms. However, its progress generates respiratory failure and, in many cases, death since it presents a higher mortality rate [16]. The SARS-CoV is a virus from animal reservoirs (in this case, bats) that can spread to other animals and humans, initially reported in Guangdong (China), in 2002 [16 - 18]. One year later, it spread to Asia and America, affecting 26 nations and causing 8,000 deaths. After its control, other reports were associated with laboratory accidents or transmission from animals to humans [16].

Concerning MERS-CoV, the main reservoir is dromedary camels and bats. These pathogens can infect bat cells through the receptor dipeptidyl peptidase-4 (DPP4), which is similar to the human receptor. The MERS-CoV exhibited widespread exposure in the Middle East and North, as well as in East Africa [17]. This disease was initially identified in 2012, in Saudi Arabia, and it has spread to about 20 countries. Since then, MERS-CoV has been detected in Europe, the Gulf region, and Korea. Since 2016, it is estimated that were infected approximately 1,638 people, of which around 35% were fatal victims [16].

As mentioned in the introduction, a new CoV variant was detected in Wuhan, China (December 2019), giving rise to one of the most significant outbreaks of unknown viral pneumonia. The new SARS-CoV (SARS-CoV-2) is more genetically similar to the SARS-CoV than MERS-CoV. Thus, it could be used information from SARS- and also MERS-CoV to discover new therapies [19, 20].

Deeming the knowledge about the structure and function of the virus, it is possible to model drugs with a focus on each target. In this context, the structure of SARS-CoV-2 is composed of structural and non-structural proteins, being used frequently for the design of new inhibitors. The structural proteins are spike (S) glycoprotein, membrane (M), envelope (E), and nucleocapsid (N) proteins. Among these, S protein is one of the most promising targets in drug discovery for SARS-CoV-2. This protein is related to viral entry by recognition of the membrane receptor and membrane fusion, mainly interacting with the Angiotensin-Converting Enzyme-2 (ACE-2) [21, 22]. In Fig. (**1**), it is shown the structural proteins from the SARS-CoV-2.

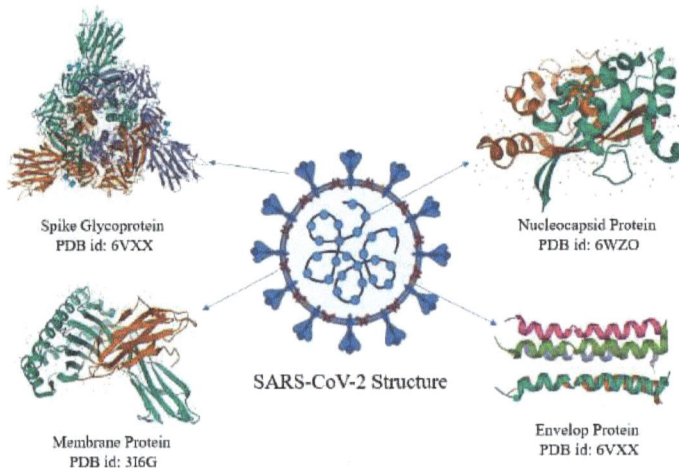

Fig. (1). Structural proteins from SAR-CoV-2.

In total, SARS-CoV-2 has 16 non-structural proteins with different functions. These proteins are the main protease (3CL^{pro} or CL^{pro} or M^{pro} or nsp5) papain-like protease (PL^{pro} ou nsp3), RNA-dependent RNA polymerase (RdRp ou nsp12), complex nsp7_nsp8, methyltransferase stimulating factor complex nsp16_nsp10; complex nspP10_nsp16, binding proteins nsp9; and endoribonuclease nsp15 [21]. Among these, the 3CL^{pro} seems to be the most attractive target for drug discovery against the SARS-CoV-2 since it is responsible for cleaving polypeptide sequences after the glutamine residue. Moreover, there are no human proteases with similar structures or functions, making 3CL^{pro} an ideal target for designing new drugs [23].

3. DRUG DISCOVERY PROCESS

Developing a new drug is a costly and time-consuming procedure [24, 25]. The estimated time to discover a drug is about 12-14 years, costing approximately US$ 1 billion [26, 27]. Before the substance reaches clinical trials, several steps are needed, which include evaluation and its effectiveness, adverse effects, pharmacokinetics, and other parameters. Additionally, combinatorial chemistry and high-throughput screening (HTS) has become quite common in drug development groups. However, there is a need for methods that reduce the financial cost related to research, making drug discovery enter in "*big data era*", which refers to a large amount of data using mainly the field of information technology [24].

The drug discovery process is divided into 4 stages being 1) Selection and validation of the biological target; 2) Screening of compounds in a database and *lead* optimization; 3) preclinical studies; and 4) Clinical studies. In this context, *in silico* studies are widely used in steps one and two, in order to decrease the number of candidates in biological tests and increase the possibility of obtaining new *hits* [28].

In this context, computer-aided drug design (CADD) methods emerged to reduce the time (approximately 50%) and costs associated with the search for new therapeutic agents. Two approaches are more common within CADD methods, namely SBDD and ligand-based drug design (LBDD) [26, 29].

SBDD is a strategy based on information about the 3D-structures of targets Thus, the 3D-structure normally refers to the crystalline structure of a target complexed with a ligand. These structures can be used in the screening of large libraries of compounds. The screening can be rationally guided, showing the ligand's complementarity at the binding site, improving the potency and selectivity of molecules [26, 30]. Molecular docking is the main technique used in SBDD protocols, which provides conformations and interactions of a ligand with a macromolecule. Pharmacophore models are also widely used to guide virtual screenings and designing new active ligands [30]. In cases where there are no 3D-structures for the target, homology modeling can be used to solve this problem by building a target from 3D-based template with high similarity *via* alignment with other targets (from the same organism or other organisms) [30].

LBDD strategy is usually applied when there is no crystal structure for targets. In sense, LBDD is performed based on ligands, which represent a set of inhibitors with well-known activity. Still, utilizing pharmacophore groups, the analysis of the similarity between ligands, or the development of Quantitative Structure-Activity Relationship (QSAR) models, results in successful strategies in drug design [26, 30]. In Fig. (**2**), is presented the main techniques comprised of LBDD and SBDD approaches.

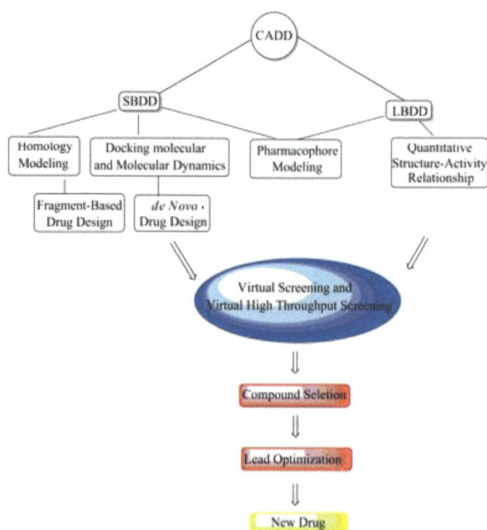

Fig. (2). Main techniques used in CADD.

4. SBDD STRATEGIES AND DISCOVERY OF *HITS* AGAINST CORONAVIRUSES

4.1. Homology Modeling

The main factor related to success in an SBDD approach is to obtain the 3D-structure of the targeted macromolecule [31]. The main database for obtaining 3D-protein structures is the Research Collaboratory for Structural Bioinformatics Protein Data Bank (RCSB PDB), which contains thousands of experimentally obtained structures. Additionally, the National Center for Biotechnology Information (NCBI) database is one of the main servers for obtaining protein sequences and performing amino acids' alignments and contains millions of deposited sequences. Furthermore, it is clear that the number of deposited sequences is higher than 3D-structures' number [32].

Given the fact that there are more sequences deposited than 3D-structures of proteins, the prediction of these structures made through computational techniques has been considered promising. Thus, when there is no a 3D-model of a targeted protein, homology modeling can fill that gap by using its amino acid sequence (normally in FASTA format). Therefore, homologous protein sequences with known 3D-structures models are used and thus generate a 3D-structure for the intended target, in which it has not been experimentally characterized [33, 34].

For a model to be considered homologous should present over a 30% similarity index between the template and retrieved sequences. A convenient homology procedure is based on the following steps: 1) Identification of a known 3D-structure that could serve as a model for building a hypothetical model; 2) Alignment of the template and model proteins' sequences; 3) Building 3D-models from the alignments; 4) Validation of the best built homologous model. For the refinement, these steps should be repeated as many times as necessary until obtaining the ideal model validated [35] (Fig. **3**). All these steps can be performed using the SWISS-MODEL web server, which is one of the most used tools for building homology models [36].

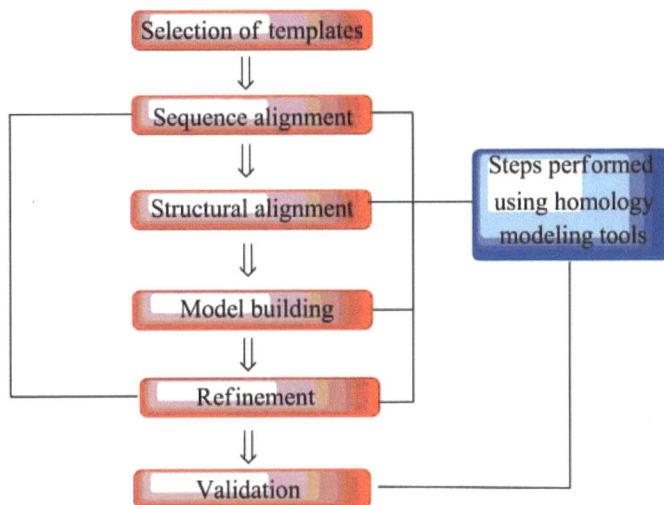

Fig. (3). Typical homology modeling procedures.

A study performed by Dong and colleagues (2020) was carried out to build homologous models using amino acid sequences of structural and non-structural proteins from SARS-CoV2 obtained at the NCBI. They used the BLAST server to identify the best models and perform homology modeling [37]. As a result, it was demonstrated that the ORS1ab protein from SARS-CoV2 is highly similar to that one from SARS- and MERS-CoV, with similarity indexes of 90% and 60%, respectively. Moreover, the authors showed that non-structural proteins could be built using homology models, such as 3CL^{pro}, which exhibited a similarity index of 94%, in comparison with known templates. Also, it was verified that the structural S, E, and N proteins could be built using the SARS-CoV structures as a template. Finally, this study may be useful for the virtual screening of new compounds against SARS-CoV-2. Similarly, Grifoni *et al* (2020) showed that SARS-CoV is the most similar to SARS-CoV-2 in phylogenetic and sequence identity analyses. By bioinformatic techniques, it was possible to identify B and T cell epitopes from SARS-CoV-2 that could be effectively recognized by the human immune response and thus could be promising targets for discovering new vaccines against this virus [38]. Regarding the identification of epitopes, Tilocca *et al.* (2020) carried out a homology study involving the main epitopes from coronaviruses N proteins [39]. Then, they showed a high-similarity index between SARS-CoV-2 N protein and RaTG13 (99%), while for SARS-CoV *vs* SARS-CoV-2 N protein was 90%; and 88% for SARS-CoV-2 *vs* pangolin. Also, epitope mapping by homology showed a potential immunogenic value in low identity sequences with SARS-CoV-2 N proteins. Finally, these observations may help in the discovery of new drugs for the treatment and prevention against SARS-Co--2.

Still focused on demonstrating the similarity between SARS-CoVs, Uddin and colleagues (2020) carried out homology studies to investigate the origin of SARS-CoV-2, as well as similarities between its structural proteins [40]. Thus, there was a high similarity index between these SARS-CoV-2 proteins with those from SARS-CoV, in which S, N, M, and E proteins showed 36-95% coverage and similarity indexes ranging from 40 to 90%.

Bai and coworkers (2020) performed calculations to determine binding free energy values from SARS-CoV-2 and SARS-CoV during their interaction with the ACE2 receptor [41]. Initially, it was necessary to build a model by homology modeling. The authors have built models for ACE2/SARS-CoV-2 and m396 (antybody)/SAR-CoV-2 complexes. They showed that residues outside the binding domain were the main ones related to the most potent binding with SARS-CoV-2. The essential SARS-CoV-2 evolution occurs in the binding domain from the trimeric body of S protein, which facilitates conformational alterations and infection process by virus binding in ACE2. In addition, its connection with the m396 antibody shows the lowest energy contribution, which explains the lack of cross-reactivity with the antibody.

Wu and colleagues (2020) performed a homology modeling study of proteins encoded by SARS-CoV-2 against the proteins from other coronaviruses. Also, they built 19 homology models and performed their virtual screening in three databases, being FDA-approved drugs from the ZINC; compounds from traditional Chinese medicine; and 78 antiviral compounds commonly used in virtual screening for coronaviruses [42]. Still, human proteins ACE2 and TMPRSS2 were also built by homology modeling and used in their virtual screening protocol. Thus, the authors proposed several compounds that could be experimentally screened in order to verify their effectiveness against SARS-Co--2, comprising antivirals (valganciclovir (**1**), ribavirin (**2**), and thymidine (**3**)); antimicrobials (phenethicillin (**4**), oxytetracycline (**5**), cefpiramide (**6**), sulfasalazine (**7**), doxycycline (**8**), demeclocycline (**9**), lymecycline (**10**), and tigecycline (**11**)); antiasthmatics (fenoterol (**12**), montelukast (**13**), and reproterol (**14**)), and among others (Fig. 4). Additionally, the authors proposed that Nsp3b,

Nsp3c, Nsp7-Nsp8 complex, Nsp14, Nsp15, 3CL^{pro}, PL^{pro}, E-channel, RdRp, helicase, ACE2, and S proteins are the most favorable targets for these drugs. Finally, they demonstrated that remdesivir triphosphate binds strongly to RdRp, inhibiting RNA synthesis, with affinity energy of -112.8 kcal/mol. In addition, it binds strongly to TMPRSS2. The drugs lopinavir/ritonavir had no affinity for the 3CL^{pro}, PL^{pro}, RdRp, and others. Thus, the authors suggested that these drugs are not suitable to treat SARS-CoV-2 symptoms. In conclusion, through homology and virtual screening methods, the authors provided essential information for repurposing drugs for SARS-CoV-2.

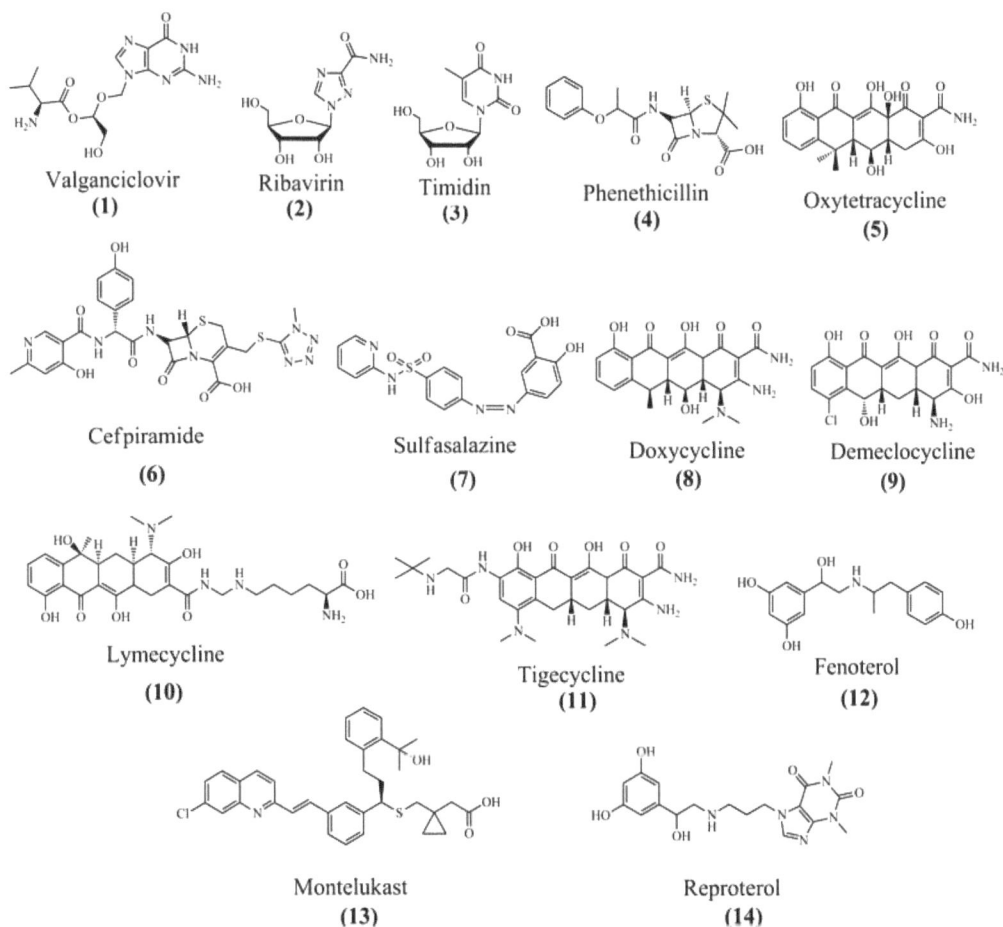

Fig. (4). Chemical structures of drugs identified by Wu and colleagues (2020) as promising compounds against SARS-CoV-2.

Hall and coworkers (2020) used homology modeling to build SARS-CoV S protein, in order to perform a virtual screening using 3,447 FDA-approved drugs

[43]. They built a 3D-structure of the intended target by using the S protein from the SARS-CoV as a sequence template. Docking studies of the compound **(15)** (-7,234 kcal/mol) towards S protein and **(16)** (-11,016 kcal/mol) (Fig. **5**) towards 3CL^{pro}.

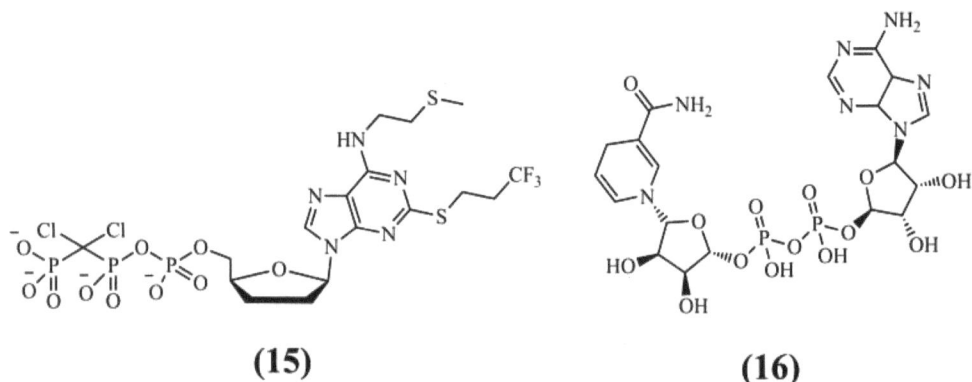

(15)   **(16)**

Fig. (5). Chemical structures of compounds identified by Hall and coworkers (2020).

Similar to previous studies, Feng and colleagues (2020) performed a homology study by using structural proteins from SARS- and SARS-CoV-2. In addition, the authors performed a virtual screening in a library of 1,234 FDA-approved drugs towards S protein [44]. There was observed a high similarity between all proteins in this study. Then, the screening was carried out with 13 hits (dactinomycin **(17)**, glycyrrhizic acid **(18)**, eltrombopag **(19)**, azilsartan medoxomil **(20)**, bictegravir **(21)**, temsirolimus **(22)**, dolutegravir **(23)**, elbasvir **(24)**, irbesartan **(25)**, gliquidone **(26)**, tasosartan **(27)** lanreotide **(28)**, and velpatasvir **(29)**) (Fig. **6**), displaying affinity energies ranging from -9.3 to -12.3 kcal/mol, and interactions with the main amino acid residues, as well.

4.2. Pharmacophore Modeling

A pharmacophore group shows molecular characteristics or structural elements responsible for the biological activity of specific molecules [45, 46]. This term has gained more prominence in recent years since it is related to the discovery of new drugs, being useful in the pharmacophore-based virtual screening protocols for identifying *hits* and *leads* compounds [45].

Although the concept of pharmacophore is older than the discovery of computers, it has become essential in CADD, including mainly the molecular docking technique [45, 47]. Each atom has its characteristics of molecular recognition, such as H-bond donors or acceptors, cations, anions, hydrophobic, aromatics, or any combination which helps in molecular recognition [45, 48].

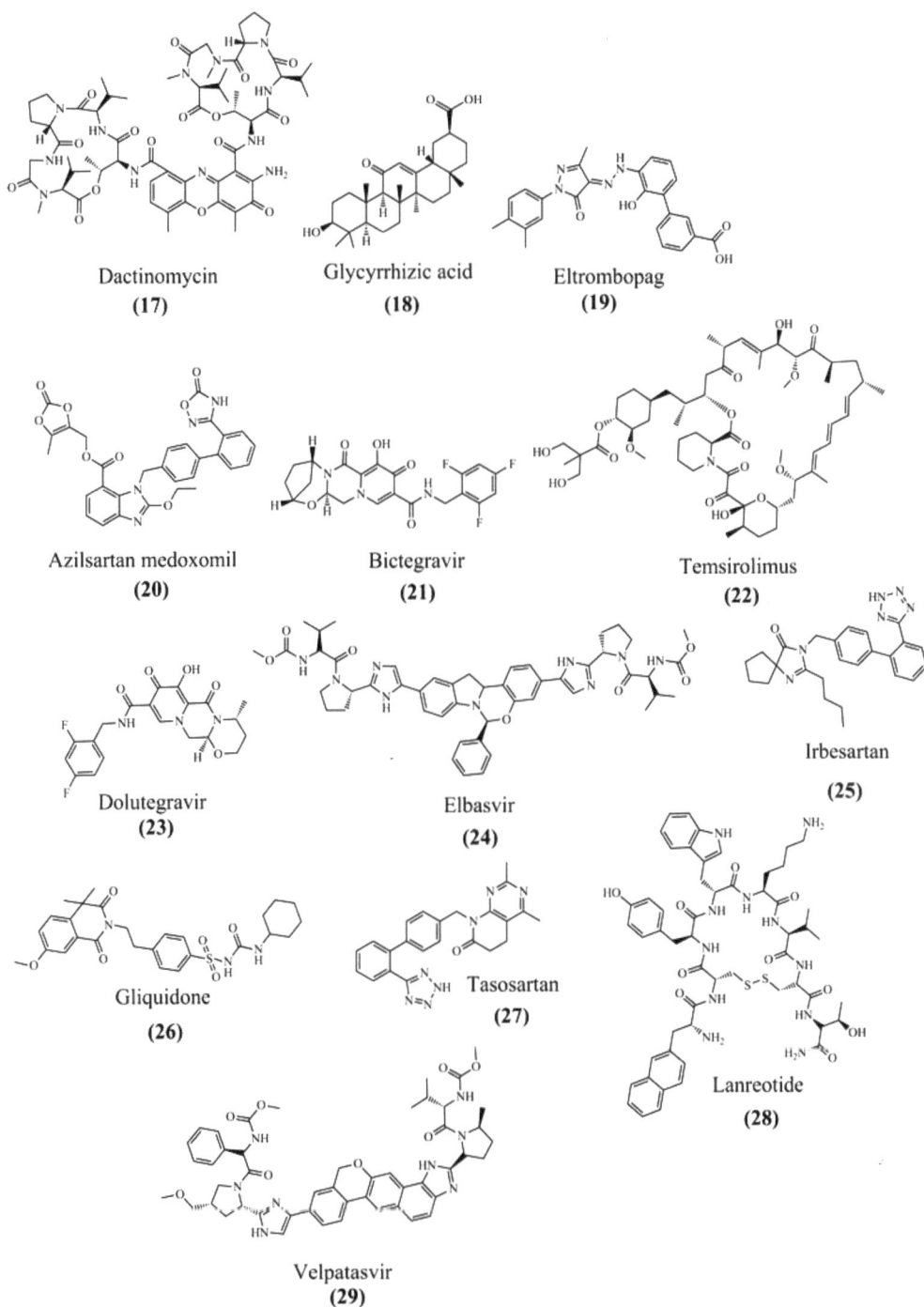

Dactinomycin
(17)

Glycyrrhizic acid
(18)

Eltrombopag
(19)

Azilsartan medoxomil
(20)

Bictegravir
(21)

Temsirolimus
(22)

Dolutegravir
(23)

Elbasvir
(24)

Irbesartan
(25)

Gliquidone
(26)

Tasosartan
(27)

Lanreotide
(28)

Velpatasvir
(29)

Fig. (6). Chemical structures of compounds identified by Feng and colleagues (2020).

Pharmacophore models can be either ligand-based, where active molecules are superimposed, in which the essential structural characteristics for the maintenance or increase of biological activity are extracted, or [46]. In general, pharmacophore modeling provides an initial modulation of the ligand structure to improve its interaction with the receptor and, as a consequence, the biological activity [49]. Fig. (7) displays the pharmacophore modeling procedure and applications.

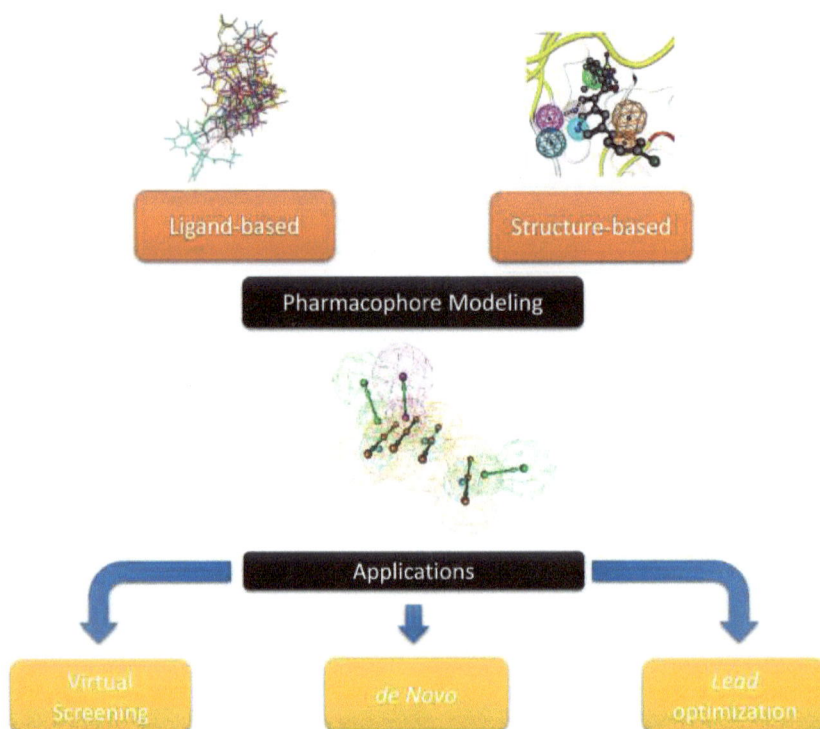

Fig. (7). Pharmacophore modeling procedure and applications (based on Yang and coworkers 2010).

Since the SARS-CoV 2002 outbreak, pharmacophore modeling has been employed to discover new potentially active compounds. This fact is shown in the study performed by Sirois and colleagues (2004) [50]. They applied pharmacophore modeling based on the KZ7088 **(30)** in complex with SARS-CoV M^{pro}, followed by a virtual screening to identify other drug candidates. The study showed that from 3.6 million screened compounds, only 0.07% had interactions with five of six points present in the interaction of KZ7088 **(30)** (Fig. **8**). The druggability of the compounds was evaluated based on physical, structural, and chemical properties. So, the authors concluded that 0.03% of the compounds are worthy of being tested biologically. Finally, the authors point out that the model generated may be useful in the discovery of anti-SARS-CoV compounds.

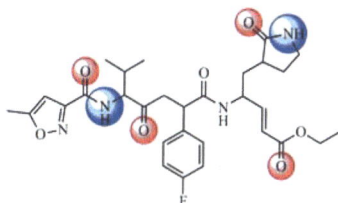

KZ7088 **(30)**

Fig. (8). Pharmacophore model for KZ7088 (30). In red: H-bond acceptors; blue: H-bond donors).

Using pharmacophore modeling and virtual screening, Radwan and colleagues (2018) searched for new MERS-CoV 3CL^{pro} inhibitors [51]. Initially, the Lipinski rule of five was applied to the NCI database, resulting in the selection of 3,120 molecules. Thus, the pharmacophore model was generated from the MERS-CoV 3CL^{pro} crystal structure (PDB: 4YLU), in which the pharmacophore groups were defined (Fig. **9**). Based on this model, 109 compounds were chosen for the docking simulations, among which the compounds **(31)**, **(32)**, **(33)**, **(34)**, and **(35)** (Fig. **9**) presented higher scores than the crystallized compound. Finally, the authors conclude that molecules could be used in biological tests to demonstrate their possible effectiveness.

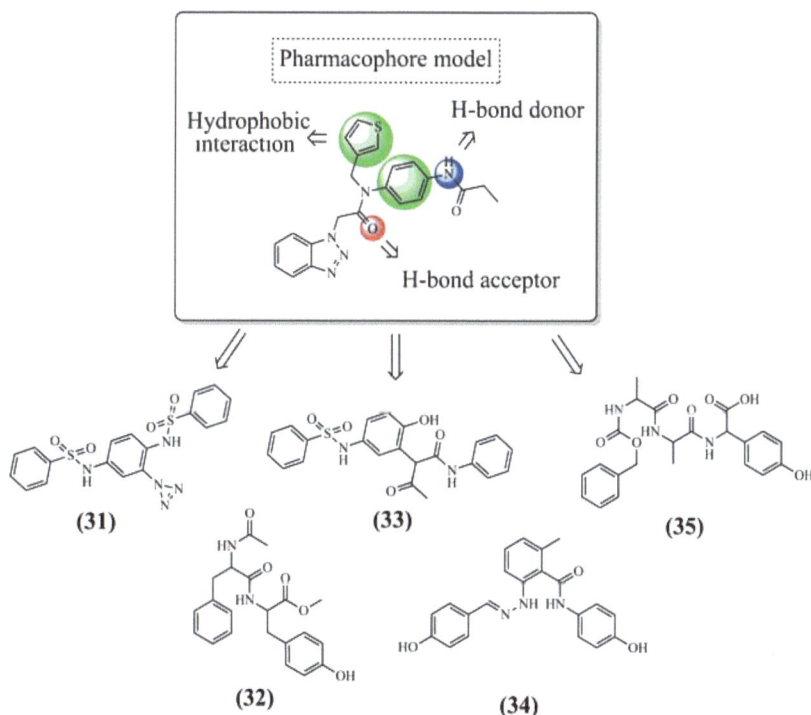

Fig. (9). Pharmacophore model and compounds discovered by Radwan and colleagues (2018).

Dhankhar and colleagues (2020) created a pharmacophore model and performed a virtual screening on the SARS-CoV-2 NTD-N-protein, using compounds from the ZINC database [52]. The pharmacophore model showed the five most important points, being three H-bond acceptors, the presence of aromatic rings, and hydrophobic interactions (Fig. **10**), at a distance of 1 Å. By using this model and the Lipinski rule as filters, 4,576 compounds were selected. Finally, compounds **(36)**, **(37)**, and **(38)** (Fig. **10**) showed better results in molecular docking studies, as well as excellent predictions *in silico* pharmacokinetic properties. Finally, studies involving molecular dynamics and MMPBSA showed that these compounds bind efficiently to the enzyme, forming stable complexes.

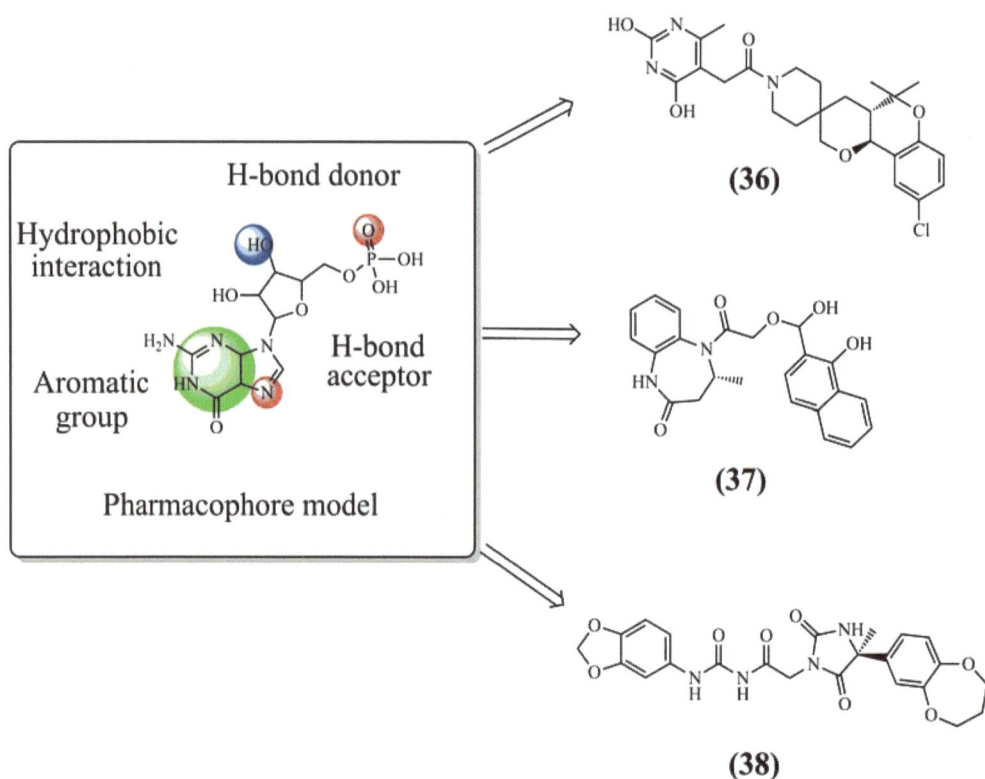

Fig. (10). Pharmacophore model and compounds identified by Dhankhar and colleagues (2020).

To obtain new compounds against SARS- and SARS-CoV-2, Idris and colleagues (2020) developed a pharmacophore model based on active compounds against these viruses, followed by a virtual screening on the TMPRSS2 protein using compounds from the ZINC database [53]. Initially, the authors built the structure of TMPRSS2, and then it was generated a pharmacophore model (Fig. **11**) based on six drugs with promising activity upon this target, being camostat **(39)**, nafamostat **(40)**, pefabloc SC **(41)**, baricitinib **(42)**, phenylmethylsulfonyl fluoride **(43)**, and ruxolitinib **(44)** (Fig. **11**). The model obtained was used in the initial screening in the ZINC database, resulting in 3,000 promising compounds. These molecules were used in the built model for TMPRSS2, obtaining 33 compounds. Finally, it was revalidated by docking and ADME studies, resulting in the compounds **(45)** and **(46)** that were evaluated in dynamics simulations and also in the MMPBSA method. Lastly, it was verified the good stability at the active site and interactions with His^{296}, Ser^{441}, Gln^{438}, Gly^{439}, Lys^{340}, and Val^{280} Residues.

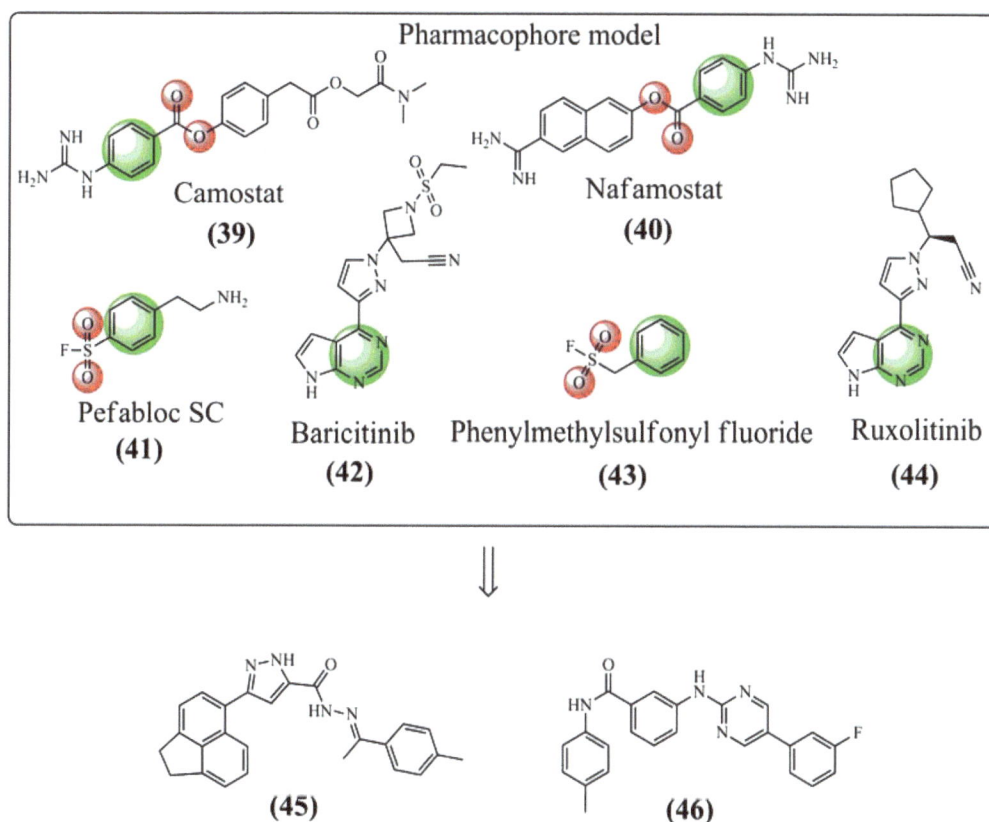

Fig. (11). Pharmacophore model and compounds (45 and 46) identified by Idris and colleagues (2020).

Arun and colleagues (2020) performed a virtual drug repurposing based on a pharmacophore hypothesis created from the imidazole derivative in complex with the enzyme 3CL^{pro} [54]. The authors determined the pharmacophore model as containing three aromatic rings and two H-bond acceptors (Fig. **12**). Subsequently, they applied this model in the SuperDRUG2 database (4,600 compounds), in which 1,000 ligands were by molecular docking. Then, 40 compounds showed excellent affinity (lower than -8,243 kcal/mol). Finally, affinity energy calculations by MMGBSA identified drugs such as binifibrate (48) (-69.04 kcal/mol), macimorelin (49) (-64.25 kcal/mol), bamifylline (50) (-63.19 kcal/mol), rilmazafone (51) (-61.37 kcal/mol), afatinib (52) (-60.89 kcal/mol), and ezetimibe (53) (-60.21 kcal/mol) (Fig. 12) as the most promising ligands.

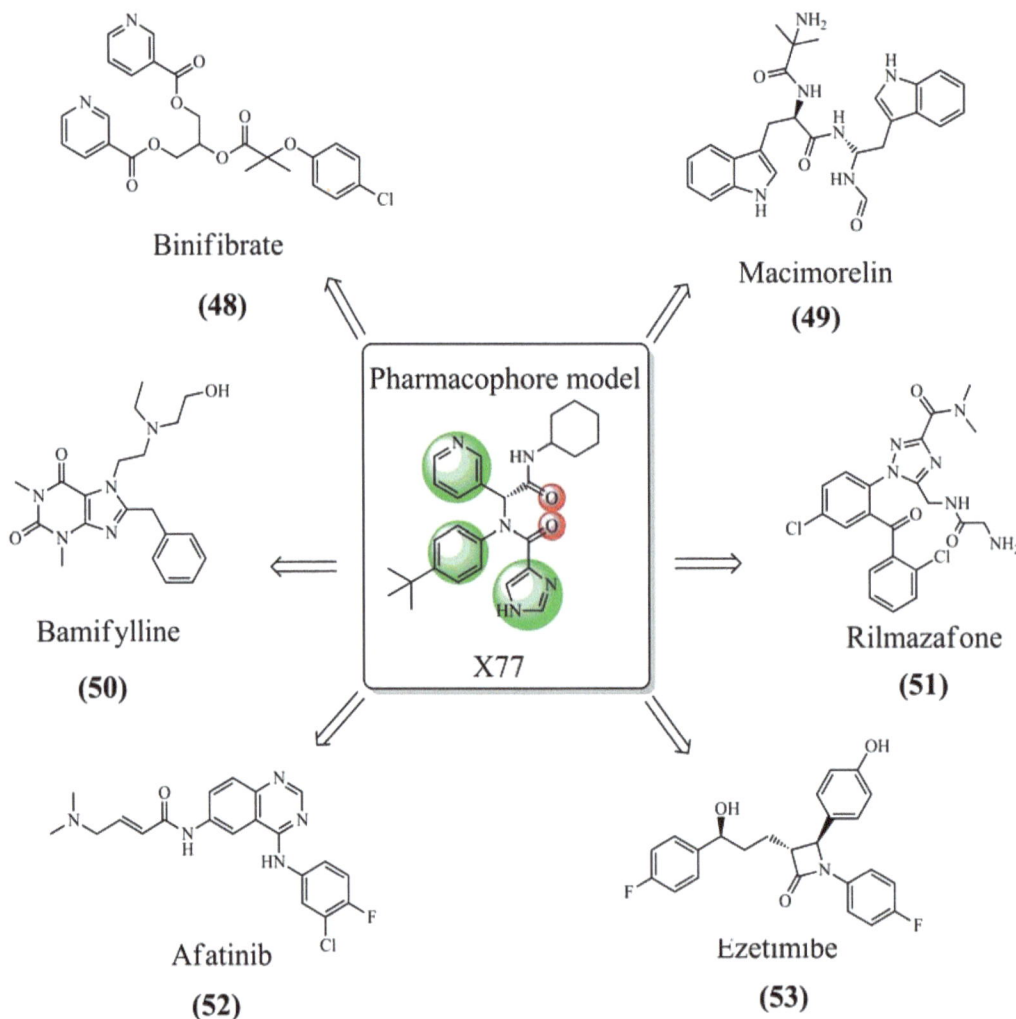

Fig. (12). Pharmacophore model and drugs repurposed by Arun and colleagues (2020).

Yoshino and colleagues (2020) mapped the main interactions responsible for the inhibitory activity upon SARS-CoV2 3CL^{pro} [55]. The alignment of two ligands co-crystallized with the enzyme (compounds (54) and (55)) was carried out, revealing that there are two donor atoms and two H-bond acceptors, allowing interactions with His[41], Gln[189], Gln[143], Ser[144], Cys[145], and Glu[166] residues (Fig. **13**). Finally, simulations of molecular dynamics suggest that hydrogen bonding interactions with Gly[166], the interaction of the thiol from the Cys[145] with the 2OP9 ligand, and hydrogen bonding and π-stacking interactions with His[41] are crucial for the design of more potent inhibitors.

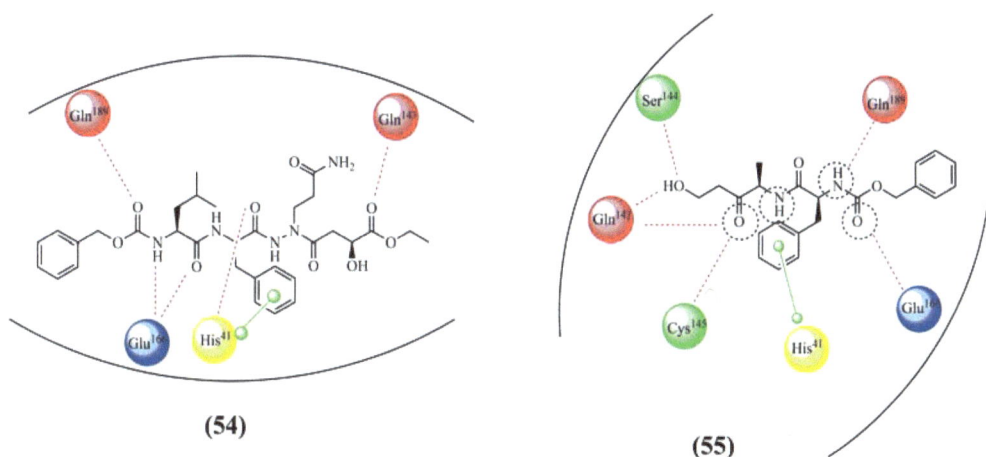

(54)   **(55)**

Fig. (13). Pharmacophore models and interactions (H-bond in red and π-stacking in green) proposed by Yoshino and colleagues (2020).

Andrade and colleagues (2020) carried out computational studies to propose a new compound against SARS-CoV2 3CL^{pro} [56]. The authors built a pharmacophore model based on the structure of OEW, remdesivir, hydroxychloroquine, and N3, followed by virtual screening among 50,000 compounds contained in the ZINC database. After defining the pharmacophores of each ligand applied to an ADMET filter, the compounds were screened upon the target. In total, 40 best pharmacophore-like ligands were selected, being compounds **(56)**, **(57)**, **(58)**, **(59)**, **(60)**, **(61)**, **(62)**, **(63)**, **(64)**, **(65)**, and **(66)** (Fig. **14**) with the best affinities. Moreover, it was verified that beta-carboline, alkaloid, and polyflavonoid derivatives interact with the catalytic dyad residues, Cys[145] and His[41]. Thus, the authors concluded that these compounds might be promising against SARS-CoV-2.

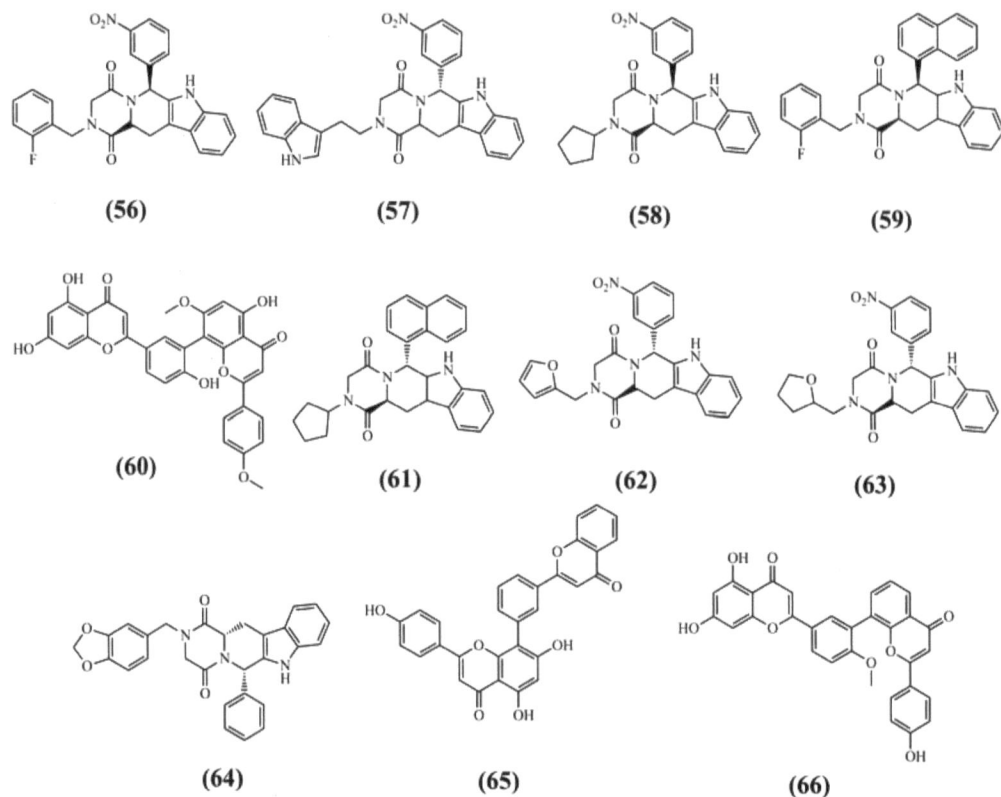

Fig. (14). Chemical structures of compounds identified by Andrade and colleagues (2020).

By analyzing HIV protease inhibitors, Jain and colleagues (2020) used such compounds against determined SARS-CoV-2 3CL^{pro} to propose the main interactions at the active site [57]. In this context, it was shown that the OH groups carry out hydrogen bonds with Cys^{145} e His^{164}; sulfonyl oxygen with Gly^{143}, and the carbonyl oxygen with Glu^{166} and Glu^{189}, in addition to van der Waals interactions with His^{41}, Thr^{25}, Thr^{26}, Gly^{143}, Asn^{142}, Gln^{189}, and Met^{165} residues. This pharmacophore model was used for screening in the ZINC database, resulting in 25 ligands. Among these compounds, compound **(67)** (Fig. **15**) showed higher affinity (-308,427 kcal/mol) and hydrogen bonding interactions with Thr^{25}, His^{41}, Ser^{144}, Thr^{45}, and Ser^{46} residues, in addition to steric interactions with Thr^{24}, Cys^{145}, Leu^{141}, Glu^{166}, and Thr^{45} residues.

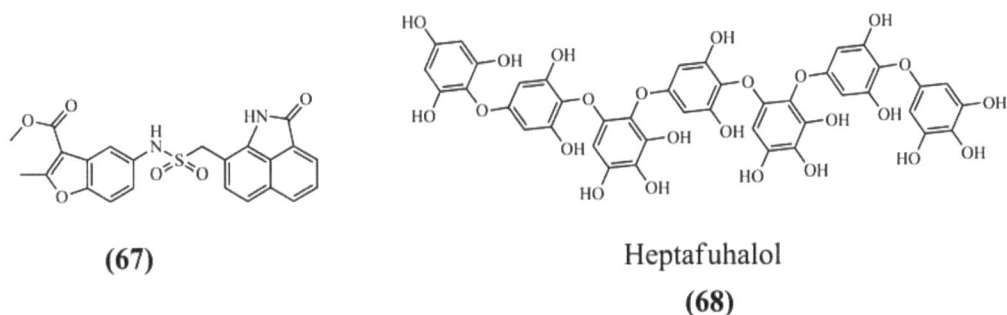

(67)

Heptafuhalol

(68)

Fig. (15). Chemical structures of compounds (67) and heptafuhalol (68).

Similar to this study, Gentile and coworkers (2020) built a pharmacophore model based on the SARS-CoV2 3CL^{pro} to perform a virtual screening in the Marine Natural Products (MNP) library, involving approximately 14,064 compounds [58]. The proposed pharmacophore model was based on three amide nitrogens (H-bond donors); two negatively charged oxygen, such as carbonyls (H-bond acceptors), and an isopropyl group for hydrophobic centers. So, it was revealed that it is possible to donate hydrogen bonds to Thr^{190}, Glu^{166}, Gnl^{189}, and His^{164}, while Glu^{166} could accept H-bonds. Then, 180 molecules were selected by using molecular docking, in which heptafuhalol **(68)** (Fig. **15**) was identified as the best ligand (-14.60 kcal/mol). Finally, it was observed that its hydroxyl group performs H-bonding interactions with His^{41} residues, as verified after 10 ns dynamics simulation.

Beura and colleagues (2020) studied the interactions of chloroquine with SARS-CoV-2 3CL^{pro} using *in silico* methods [59]. The authors developed 20 pharmacophore models, in which the best contained H-bond donors, three hydrophobic regions, and two aromatic systems. It allowed to identify of three chloroquine analogs (**(69)**, **(70)**, and **(71)**) as promising ligands (Fig. **16**). Such compounds showed an affinity toward the enzyme, with values of -6.17, -5.14, and -4.19 kcal/mol, respectively. Lastly, these analogs showed good stability in molecular dynamics simulations.

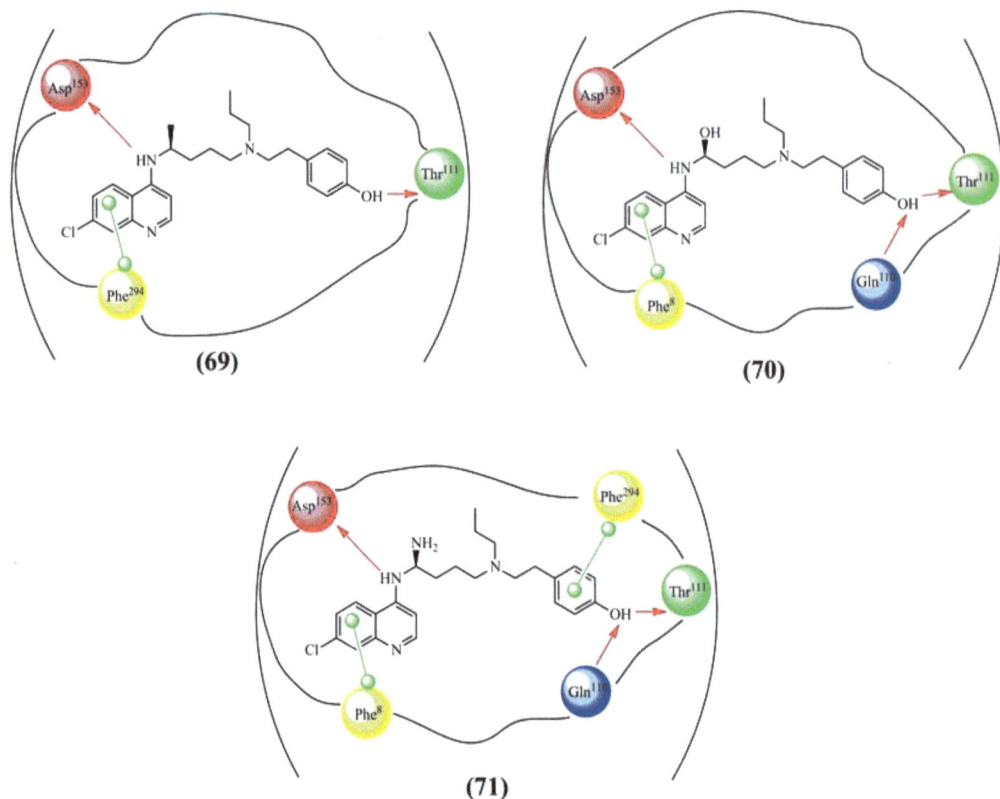

Fig. (16). Chemical structures and interactions of compounds identified by Beura and coworkers (2020). In red: H-bonds; green: π-stacking interactions.

Pharmacophore modeling against SARS-CoV2 3CL^{pro} was used in the study by Karaman (2020) [60]. Based on residues His^{41}, Glu^{166}, and Cys^{145}, the model was created, containing two H-bond acceptors, three H-bond donors, and two aromatic rings. After validating this model, the authors performed molecular docking of the reported inhibitors, showing that the presence of H-bond donors or acceptors close to the aromatic ring is essential for the enzyme inhibition, providing critical information for designing drugs.

Based on the structure of the ligand co-crystallized with SARS-CoV-2 3CL^{pro}, Haider and coworkers (2020) developed a pharmacophore model followed by virtual screening [61]. They identified that the main characteristics form the presence of a hydrophobic pharmacophore, an aromatic ring, as well as H-bond acceptor and donor groups. Such pharmacophore features were used to screen compounds in the ZINC database, resulting in 700 compounds after the application of the Lipinski filters. Then, the compounds were analyzed by docking, in which 200 ligands showed higher affinity than the reference inhibitor (lower than -8.1190 kcal/mol). Finally, after ADMET studies and visual inspection of the complexes, compounds **(72)**, **(73)**, and **(74)** (Fig. **17**) showed the best results and strong interactions with Val[3], Leu[4], Thr[24], Thr[26], His[41], Cys[44], Thr[45], Ser[46], Met[49], and Gln[189] residues.

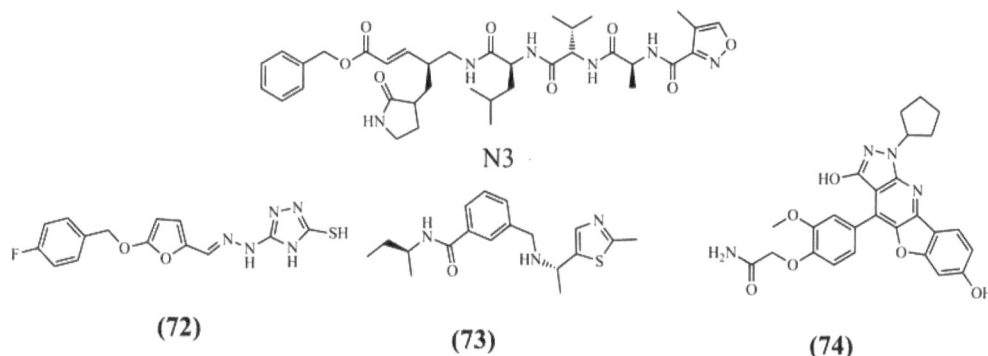

Fig. (17). Chemical structures of compounds identified by Haider and colleagues (2020).

Abhithaj and colleagues (2020) performed a virtual screening on the DrugBank database based on a pharmacophore model developed from the non-covalent inhibitor present in the SARS-CoV2 3CL[pro] [62]. The model showed that two H-bond acceptors and three aromatic rings are essential. In sense, the model was applied to the DrugBank database so that 1,000 compounds were selected for further analysis. The authors performed molecular docking, in which 30 compounds showed better affinity than the crystallographic inhibitor (-4.5 kcal/mol). Among these, seven molecules were approved-drugs or under experimental investigation (ezetimibe **(53)** (see **12**), larotrectinib **(75)**, simeprevir **(76)**, cobicistat **(77)**, alogliptin, and capmatinib). Finally, MMGBSA calculations revealed that eight ligands ((**78**), (**79**), (**80**), (**81**), and (**82**)) (Fig. **18**) have energy comparable to the co-crystalized inhibitor (-80 kcal/mol).

4.3. Molecular Docking and Dynamics Simulations

Docking and molecular dynamics simulations are two essential tools for any drug discovery and development protocol. These tools are mainly related to the rational design of new drugs, as well as the modeling of biochemical processes. Thus, assisting in perceptions about conformations and mechanisms, helping researchers to characterize the ligand's interactions with its receptor. Such methods are related to identifying potential drugs *in silico* among large libraries of compounds, even before obtaining or synthesizing the molecule [63, 64].

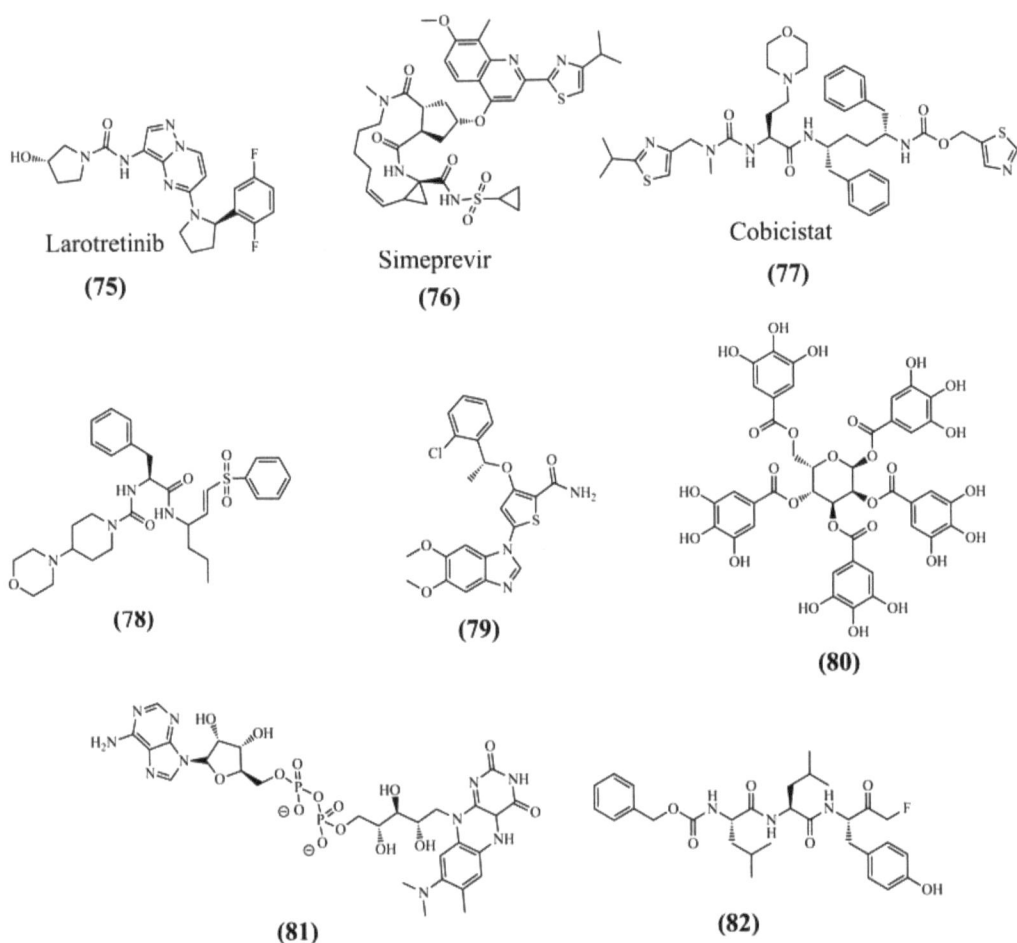

Fig. (18). Chemical structures of compounds identified by Abhithaj and colleagues (2020).

Molecular docking is a technique that aims to predict the best way to bind a ligand to a receptor (or binding site). Several conformations (binding modes or poses) are generated for one ligand. In this context, the availability of the target 3D-structure is fundamental for this approach. This technique is based on two stages: 1) Generation of poses for the ligand at the active site; 2) Raking of predicted conformations, leading to the choice of the pose with the highest affinity for the binding site [65].

Molecular dynamics simulations are essential since these take into account the flexibility of proteins and ligands. Another critical point is to estimate the binding energy of a ligand at the binding site using the molecular mechanics/Poisson-Boltzmann and surface area (MMPBSA) method [66].

Currently, the key-lock model to explain the interactions of a ligand with its receptor site has fallen into disuse since it is known that there is a flexibility factor in the ligand interactions with its biological target. In this context, the conformation of the receptor is fundamental for flexibility, so that several studies highlight the importance of the conformation that the receptor adopts in docking analysis. Thus, it is essential to observe the flexibility of the receptor before the docking procedure, allowing conformational changes in the docking process. This process reduces the possibility of improper conformation. In this context, simulations of molecular dynamics prove to be useful tools in estimating the flexibility of the receptor. In this context, molecular dynamics are essential to perform a conformational analysis of the receptor, using the most relaxed conformation, representing the system in native state [67]. In Fig. (**19**) is shown the functions of molecular docking and dynamics simulations.

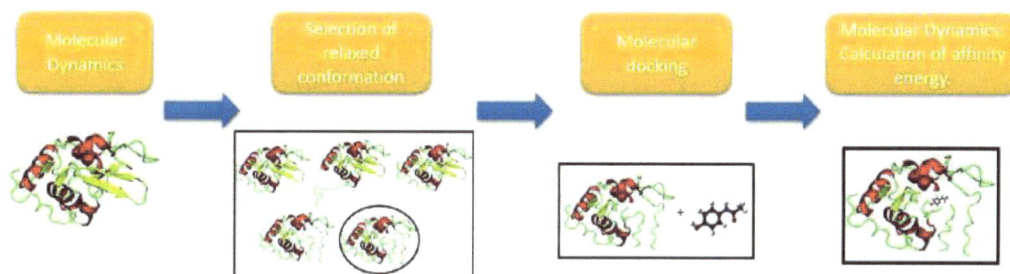

Fig. (19). Graphical representation of molecular docking and dynamics in drug discovery.

Studying protein-protein interactions by using computational techniques, Amin and colleagues (2020) performed an analysis at the binding mode between SARS-CoV-2 S protein and ACE2 receptor, using molecular dynamics and Monte Carlos sampling [68]. The authors showed that in the ACE2 surface, the binding domain receptor (RBD) binds to the S protein from SARS- and SARS-CoV-2, since there is a negative (ACE2) and positive (SARS- and SARS-CoV-2) electrostatic potential. On the other hand, interactions with SARS-CoV-2 were more relevant for presenting higher binding energy. The main interactions observed were saline bridges between Arg[426] from SARS-CoV and Glu[329] from ACE2, whereas, for SARS-CoV-2, interactions were observed between Lys[417] and Asp[40] residues from ACE2.

Similar to the previous study, Spinello and colleagues (2020) investigated the molecular properties that allow a higher affinity between ACE2 and S protein from SARS- and SARS-CoV-2. The authors showed by molecular dynamics that the SARS-CoV-2 greatest transmissibility is mainly due to the presence of a Gly[482], which makes the L3 loop longer and more structured, allowing interactions of Gly[485] with Cys[488], and also Gln[474] with Gly[476]. This amino acid allows for a tighter bond and stronger interactions between ACE2 and SARS-CoV-2. In addition, the SARS-CoV-2/ACE2 adduct has a higher number of hydrogen bonding interactions and even more favorable free Gibbs energy (ΔG= 20.8 kcal/mol, calculated by MMGBSA method) than the SARS-CoV/ACE2 adduct. The authors further suggest that ACE2 may be a potential target in the discovery of new compounds against SARS-CoV-2.

Given the evidence that the HR1 and HR2 regions from the S protein are responsible for fusion in host cells, Ling and coworkers (2020) designed two peptides that could bind to these regions and prevent the virus from fusing in the cell [69]. It was shown that ΔG values of -33.4 kcal/mol for the HR2-like peptide and -21.8 kcal/mol for the HR1-like peptide were obtained by molecular dynamics. In addition, HR2-P showed to be more effective for inhibiting viral infection, and still showing competitive inhibition of HR2 to HR1, blocking viral fusion. Although, HR1-P was less efficient in inhibiting such binding. Finally, the results demonstrated that the design of peptide inhibitors that are similar to the HR2 domain could be is an interesting alternative for discovering new compounds against SARS-CoV-2.

Souza and colleagues (2020) carried out a molecular docking and dynamics study involving eight peptide derivatives against SARS-CoV-2 S protein [70]. Before their *in silico* studies, all compounds were tested for their antiviral activity. Hence, the chosen compounds showed an inhibitory percentage between 70-85%. By using molecular docking and dynamics, the authors showed that all peptides interact with S protein, which induce conformational changes in the S protein structure that prevent the interaction with the ACE2 enzyme. Therefore, such compounds could prevent SARS-CoV-2 infection in cells.

Bai colleagues (2020) investigated the activity of DNA aptamer against the RBD from the SARS-CoV-2 S protein by using machine learning and molecular dynamics. Thus, the sequences CoV2-RBD-1 and CoV2-RBD-4 were optimized, generating high-affinity values (K_d= 5.8 nM for CoV2-RBD-1C, and 19.9 nM for CoV2-RBD-4). Then, molecular dynamics simulations showed the binding protein-protein interactions. Finally, the authors concluded that such aptamers could be promising against SARS-CoV-2.

Molecular dynamics simulations can also be used to propose catalytic mechanisms of proteases. Thus, Paasche and colleagues (2020) used molecular dynamics simulations to obtain information from the SARS-CoV-2 3CL^{pro} catalytic system that leads to the Cys$^-$/His$^+$ ion-pair, generating useful information for the design of new inhibitors [71]. Initially, simulations involving free and complex enzymes were performed. As a result, the results showed that the catalytic dyad (Cys^{145} and His^{41}) has a neutral state, and His^{164} is discharged. In this context, with the protonation state identified, proton transfer within the active site was evaluated, with the enzyme-free, complexed with an inhibitor, and complexed with a substrate. The results showed that the ion-pair formation is more favorable in the substrate presence. In this context, it generates energy decrease between the neutral and zwitterionic states, which indicates the binding of the dyad to the substrate, thus contributing to its proteolysis. The authors suggested that proteins entering a catalytic site interact differently from natural substrates; therefore, they are not able to decrease such energy, preventing the reaction. Finally, the authors concluded that compounds that mimic natural substrates might be an alternative in the design of SARS-CoV-2 $3CL^{pro}$ inhibitors.

Molecular dynamics simulations can also be used to study conformational changes in the enzyme and produce results that aid in drug discovery. Thus, Suarez and coworkers (2020) investigated the structure and flexibility of SARS-CoV2 $3CL^{pro}$ in 2 μs molecular dynamics simulations [72]. The authors used several enzyme structures deposited in the PDB and performed electrostatic calculations of pKa, considering the enzyme unbound and in a non-covalent complex with the peptide Ace-Ala-Val-Leu-Gln-Ser-Nme, similar to polyproteins recognized naturally at the active site. In addition, the homodimeric and monomeric configurations for each configuration were evaluated. The results showed that in the absence of a substrate, the monomeric form does not present stability. However, in the presence of a substrate, the monomeric form has more stability. Although, the orientation of the peptide bond with the catalytic dyad is not favorable.

Thuy and colleagues (2020) used CG-MS method for the identification of natural compounds from essential garlic oil and molecular docking to verify their effectiveness against SARS-CoV-2 [73]. The authors identified 18 active compounds in garlic essential oil. Among these compounds, 17 ligands **(83-100)** (Fig. **20**) were organosulfur derivatives. Then, molecular docking studies were carried out to verify *in silico* efficacy of the isolated compounds against ACE2. In sense, the authors showed that the compounds might have inhibitory activity against ACE2 and SARS-CoV-2 $3CL^{pro}$, with score values ranging from -14.06 to -7.89 kcal/mol for ACE2; and -15.32 to -11.68 kcal/mol for $3CL^{pro}$. Such results also suggest that the 17 substances have a synergistic effect against both proteins

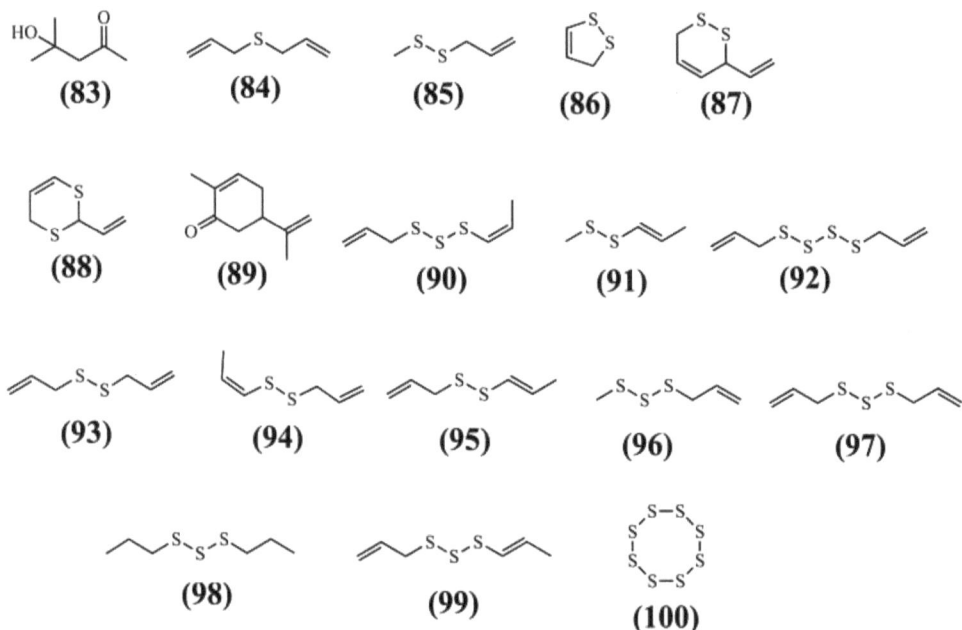

Fig. (20). Chemical structures of compounds identified by Thuy and coworkers (2020).

Molecular docking studies were also carried out by Vardhan and colleagues (2020) involving four SARS-CoV-2 targets (3CL^{pro}; PL^{pro}; SGp-RBD (spike glycoprotein-receptor binding domain); an RdRp) and 154 natural substances from limonoids and triterpenoids classes [74]. The results showed that maslinic acid **(101)**, glycyrrhizic acid **(18)**, 7-deacetyl-7-benzoylgedunin **(102)**, limonine **(103)**, corosolic acid **(104)**, obacunone **(105)**, and ursolic acid **(106)** (Fig. **21**) presented comparable dock score values, ranging from -7.8 to -9.9 kcal/mol. Finally, these compounds have interactions with the main amino acid residues from each target.

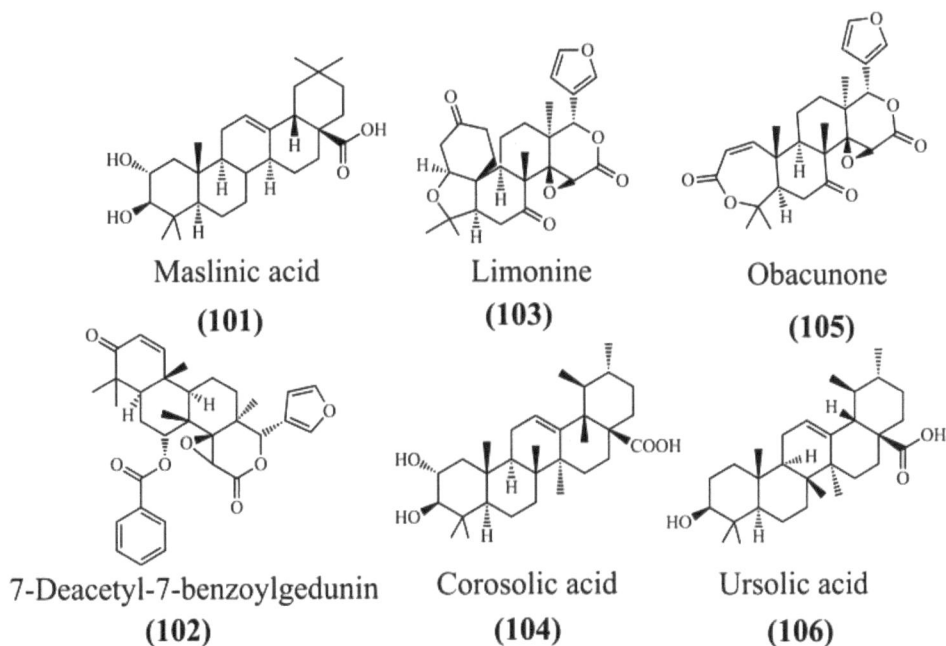

Fig. (21). Chemical structures of compounds identified by Vardhan colleagues (2020).

Still working with compounds from natural sources, Kiran and coworkers (2020) carried out computational studies of molecular docking using the SARS-CoV-2 S protein to verify the effectiveness of the chemical constituents from the *Siddha official* formulation *Kabasura Kudineer,* and the herbal preparation (JACOM) [75]. Thus, 37 compounds were docked, in which 9 were classified as the best drug candidates for presenting better Gibbs free energy ($\Delta G_{binding}$) and good synthetic accessibility. The authors stated that the compounds chrysoeriol (**107**) (-11.39 kcal/mol), quercetin (**108**) (-11.47kcal/mol), magnoflorine (**109**) (-9.76 kcal/mol), 6-methoxygenkwanin (**110**) (-9.293 kcal/mol), 5-hydroxy-7-8-dimethoxyflavanone (**111**) (-9.03 kcal/mol), tinosponone (**112**) (-8.14 kcal/mol), cirsimaritin (**113**) (-9.22 kcal/mol), vasicinone (**114**) (-8.16 kcal/mol), and luteolin (**115**) (-11.15 kcal/mol) (Fig. **22**) could be explored in biological assays.

Given the evidence that *Aloe vera* compounds can be promising against SARS-CoV-2, Mpiana and colleagues (2020) conducted a molecular docking study involving 10 compounds against SARS-CoV-2 3CL^{pro} [76]. In this sense, the results showed that compounds (**116**), (**117**), and (**118**) (Fig. **22**) could be promising since these presented docking score values of -7.9; -7.7; -7.7 kcal/mol, respectively. Also, hydrogen bonding interactions at the active site and no violations of the Lipinski rule were observed.

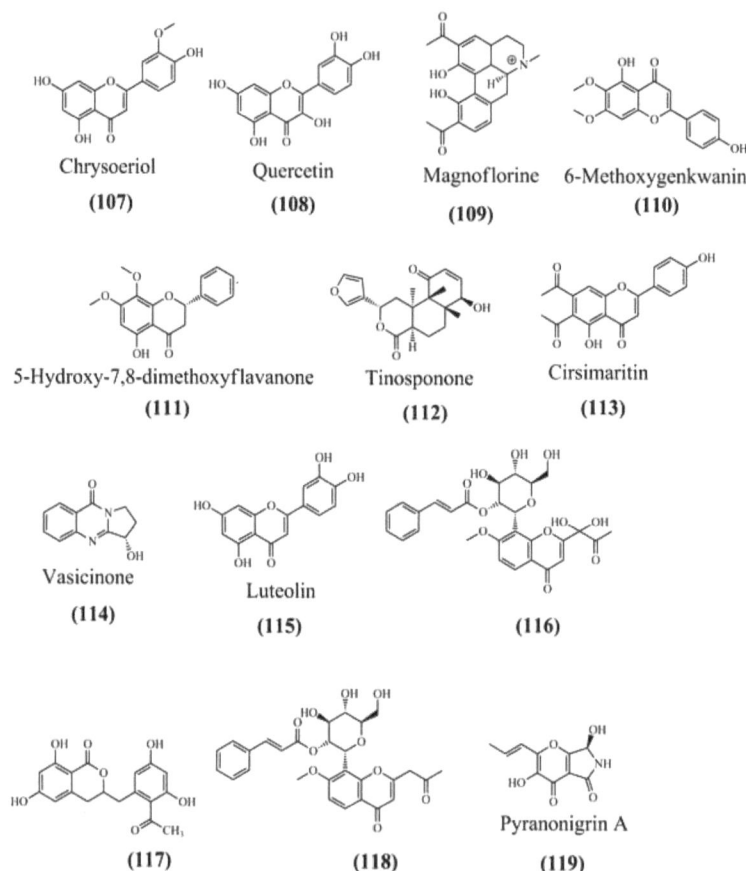

Chrysoeriol
(107)

Quercetin
(108)

Magnoflorine
(109)

6-Methoxygenkwanin
(110)

5-Hydroxy-7,8-dimethoxyflavanone
(111)

Tinosponone
(112)

Cirsimaritin
(113)

Vasicinone
(114)

Luteolin
(115)

(116)

(117)

(118)

Pyranonigrin A
(119)

Fig. (22). Chemical structures of natural compounds identified by *in silico* studies against SARS-CoV-2.

Compounds from fungi also play an essential role in the discovery of antiviral drugs. In this context, Rao and coworkers (2020) carried out a molecular docking study on approximately 100 secondary fungi metabolites against 3CL^{pro} using the crystallized N3 inhibitor as a reference [77]. After docking, it was shown that the metabolite Pyranonigrin A **(119)** (Fig. **22**) was shown to be more promising, as it presents hydrogen bonding interactions similar to the N3 inhibitor at the active site from 3CL^{pro}. Additionally, the authors carried out a study by using molecular dynamics to analyze the N3 and pyranonigrin A complex, showing the stability at the active sites by analyzing the RMSD (Root Mean Square Deviation) and RMSF (Root-Mean-Square Fluctuation) ranges, having less number of hydrogen bonding interactions.

Drug repurposing also proves to be an exciting approach in the search for new alternatives against SARS-CoV-2. Thus, to repurpose tetracyclines with known antiviral activity, the study by Bharadwaj and colleagues (2020) was based on *in silico* simulations of four antibiotics against SARS-CoV-2 3CL^{pro} [78]. Thus, molecular docking showed that tetracycline **(120)**, minocycline **(121)**, doxycycline **(122)**, and demeclocycline **(123)** (Fig. **23**) showed higher affinity in the enzyme than the N3 (less than -7 kcal/mol) and also interactions with the catalytic dyad, composed of Cys^{145} and His^{41}. Additionally, the study of molecular dynamics proved the stability of the compounds compared to the co-crystallized inhibitor (N3). Finally, the authors conclude that drugs minocycline and doxycycline **(122)** may be the most potent compound.

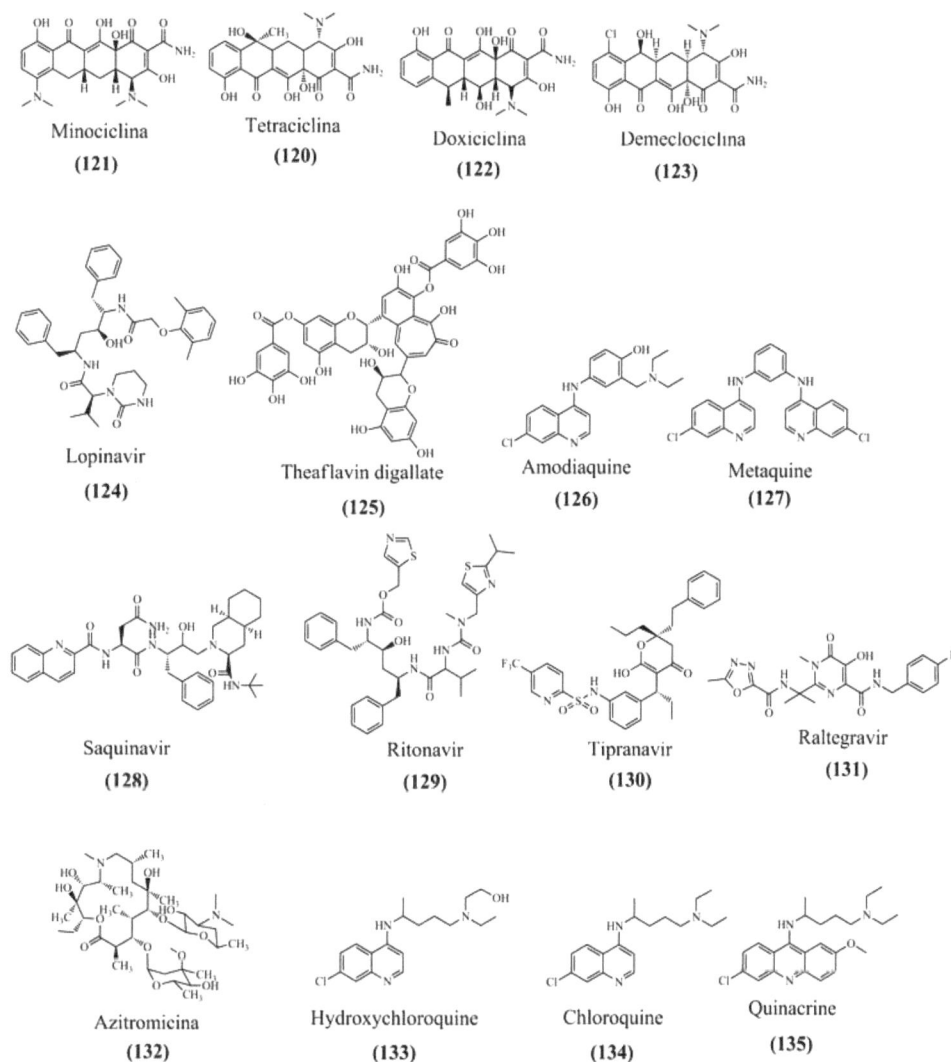

Fig. (23). Chemical structures of potential compound repurposed against SARS-CoV-2.

Peele and colleagues (2020) used docking and molecular dynamics studies on 62 FDA-approved drugs against SARS-CoV-2 3CL[pro] [79]. Initially, for each ligand, 32 conformations were generated, and the compounds with the highest score were found to be lopinavir (124) (docking score= -9.918kcal/mol; glide score= -9.918 kcal/mol; glide e-model= -101.59kcal/mol), theaflavin digallate (125) (docking score= -10,574 kcal/mol; glide score= -10,722 kcal/mol; glide e-model= -135,584 kcal/mol), and amodiaquine (126) (docking score= -7,429 kcal/mol; glide score= -8,023 kcal/mol; glide e-model= -76.898kcal/mol) (Fig. 23). Thus, these compounds were chosen for molecular dynamics studies and presented RMSD values of 0.23, 0.25, and 0.22 nm, respectively. In addition, the RMSF values were found to be 0.15, 0.17, and 0.2 nm, for amodiaquine (126), lopinavir (124), and theaflavin digallate (125), respectively (Fig. 23). In addition, the authors showed that all inhibitors performed hydrogen bonding interactions with His[41]. Finally, the authors emphasize that biological assays are necessary to confirm the potential of these molecules.

Barros and colleagues (2020) conducted a docking study on 24 compounds against four SARS-CoV-2 targets (Nsp9, 3CL[pro], Nsp15 endoribonuclease, and S protein) [80]. Thus, the results indicated metaquina (127) and saquinavir (128) (Fig. 23) are the most promising compounds since these interact with all the targets tested and in the main amino acid residues of each enzyme, (Nsp9: Asn[28], Thr[78], and Lys[85]; 3CL[pro]: Cys[145], and His[41]; Nsp5: Ser[294], and His[250]; and S protein: Asn[33], Glu[37], Phe[390], and Lys[417]) representing new compounds that could be further explored against SARS-CoV-2.

Kumar and colleagues (2020) carried out *in silico* studies involving 75 FDA-approved drugs against SARS-CoV-2 3CL[pro] [81]. Thus, a re-docking was performed to validate the procedure, exhibiting an RMSD value of 0.51 Å. Then, the molecular docking was performed, identifying the 4 top *hits*, being lopinavir (124), ritonavir (129), tipranavir (130), and raltegravir (131) (Fig. 23), with a better score value than the co-crystallized ligand. In this context, three compounds were subjected to molecular dynamics, in which their conformational stability at the active site was demonstrated by RMSD and RMSF analyzes. Finally, the authors concluded that these compounds could be evaluated in humans to demonstrate their effectiveness.

Drugs commercially available and with known activity against SAR-CoV-2 were used in the study by Marinho and coworkers (2020), employing molecular docking to characterize their interactions with SAR-CoV-2 3CL[pro] [82]. The authors tested azithromycin (132), hydroxychloroquine (133), chloroquine (134), quinacrine (135) (Fig. 23), baricitinib (43), and ruxolitinib (44) (see 11), in which was showed that these all compounds have a greater affinity for domain III from the enzyme, while the co-crystallized inhibitor (N3) interacts with domains I and II. Additionally, the authors point out that azithromycin **(132)**, baricitinib **(43)**, quinacrine **(135)**, and ruxolitinib **(44)** present free binding energies according to the literature.

Given the evidence of the promising potential of α-ketoamide **(136)** against SARS-CoV-2 3CL^{pro} (IC$_{50}$ of 0.67 ± 0.18 μM), Liang and colleagues (2020) carried out docking and molecular dynamics studies to investigate the interactions of this compound in the active site of SARS-CoV-2 3CL^{pro} and also compare them with the antibiotic amoxicillin **(137)** (Fig. **24**) [83]. Thus, the results showed that α-ketoamide **(136)** (Fig. **24**) has a higher affinity with the active site, exhibiting score values of -8.7 and -9.2 kcal/mol for protomer A and B, respectively; when compared to amoxicillin (-5.0 and -4.8 kcal/mol). In addition, molecular dynamics studies showed the stability of α-ketoamide **(136)**, ΔG values of -25.2, and -22.3 kcal/mol for protomers A and B, respectively. In contrast, amoxicillin showed unfavorable interaction energy, with ΔG of +32.8 kcal/mol, being detached from the active site during some moments of the simulation. Finally, the authors highlighted the importance of using α-ketoamide in the search for new inhibitors against SARS-CoV-2.

Bhowmik and colleagues (2020) used *in silico* techniques to identify potential compounds against SARS-CoV-2 in a library of 548 compounds upon the main structural proteins as targets, being E, M, and N proteins [84]. Thus, the docking results showed that flavonoid rutin **(138)** and doxycycline **(122)** present the most favorable affinity toward E protein; caffeic acid **(139)** and ferulic acid **(140)** toward M protein, simeprevir **(76)** and grazoprevir **(141)** (Fig. **24**) toward N protein. In addition, the compounds had excellent pharmacokinetic properties, as well as stability at the site of action during molecular dynamics simulations.

Kumar and colleagues (2020) carried out docking and molecular dynamics studies for discovering new SARS-CoV-2 3CL^{pro} inhibitors [85]. Initially, the docking of 13 antiviral compounds resulted in indinavir **(142)** (Fig. **24**) as compounds with better docking score values (-8.824 kcal/mol), and also XP Gscore (-9.466 kcal/mol). The authors observed that the compound has a vital pharmacophore, hydroxyethylamine (HEA). In this sense, approximately 2,500 compounds were docked in this group, resulting in 25 *hits* with better score values than indinavir **(142)**. Among these compounds, ligand **(143)** (Fig. **24**) was found to be the most promising molecule, as it had an affinity for domains I and II due to hydrophobic interactions, π-π interactions, and hydrogen bonding interactions. In addition, molecular dynamics studies for indinavir **(142)** and compound **(143)** have shown stability in the active site on both RMSD and RMSF analyzes.

Alpha-cetoamida
(136)

Amoxillin
(137)

Rutin
(138)

Caffeic acid
(139)

Ferulic acid
(140)

Grazoprevir
(141)

Indinavir
(142)

(143)

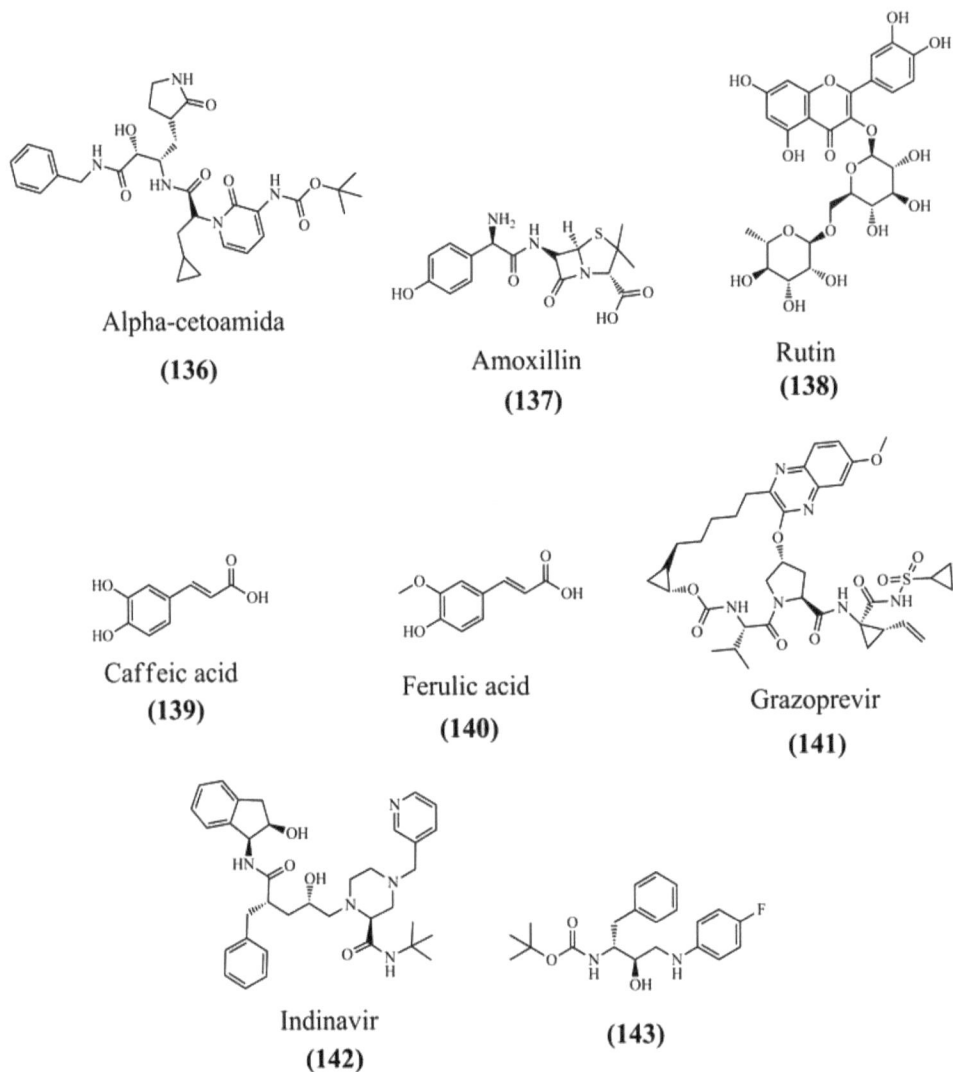

Fig. (24). Chemical structures of compounds identified by Liang and colleagues (2020), Bhowmik and colleagues (2020), and Kumar and colleagues (2020).

4.4. Fragment-Based Drug Discovery

The fragment-based drug discovery strategy (FBDD) has the main objective of identifying starting chemical structures and optimizing them based on a specific target [86, 87]. This strategy was first presented in 1996 by Fesik and co-workers (Abbott Laboratories) and its concept was proposed by Hol and co-workers in the 90s [86]. Since its discovery to the present time, FBDD has been associated with several successful cases, in which other methods were not enough [86, 87].

An FBDD procedure begins with the construction of a library of fragments, low molecular weight molecules designed for a specific target [88]. These fragments should be of sufficient size and a small degree of complexity to attractively interact with the target and also to avoid unfavorable interactions [87, 88]. In this context, the initial focus is to identify active fragments and then optimize them. The fragments have a weak binding affinity in the range mM e μM [87]. In this way, the desired power for the fragments is obtained through the strategies of fusion, linking, and growing, which are the main approaches used when applying an FBDD protocol [87, 88].

The preferred approach by researchers for optimizing compound leads is fragment growing [86]. This approach is based on the placement of a fragment with significant interactions, followed by the addition of other fragments that complement a specific active site to improve pharmacological activity [86]. This process can be performed through the X-ray structure by using molecular docking or even by NMR as a guide for replacing or adding fragments [86, 87]. During this process, the most crucial consideration is to maintain the interactions of the initial fragment during the formation of the optimized compound [86].

Although less used, the fragment linking approach shows versatility in binding fragments at adjacent protein locations, being a powerful optimization tool [86]. This approach is based on adding fragments in the target's pocket and then linking them to form a single compound [86, 89]. This approach is more challenging, as it requires optimal identification of linking between fragments [89]. Fig. (**25**) exemplified the process of linking and growing in fragment-based drug discovery.

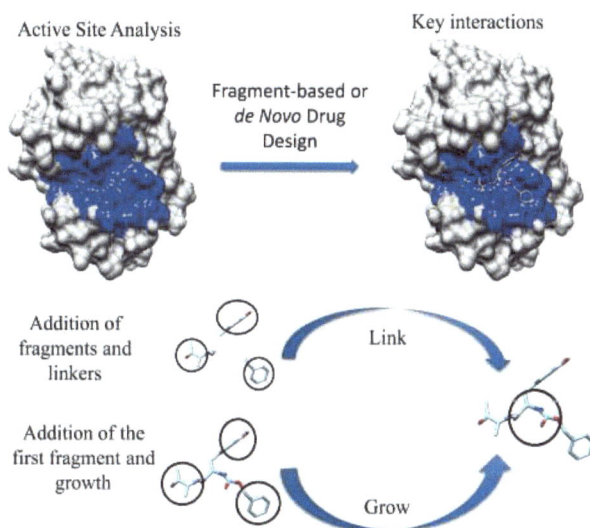

Fig. (25). Process of linking and growing in fragment-based drug discovery.

Inspired to identify a new compound against SARS-CoV-2 3CL^{pro}, Tang and coworkers (2020) used the FBDD strategy for the discovery of new *lead* compounds [90]. By using an advanced deep Q-learning network with the fragment-based drug discovery (ADQN-FBDD), a database of 4,922 structures was generated with the possibility of forming covalent bonds with the target. Then, the compounds were docked in the target, in which 47 fragments were selected based on their scores. Among these compounds, ligand **(144)** (Fig. **26**) attracted the researchers' attention, as it had the best covalent docking score and had an aldehyde function. Thus, this molecule was optimized, generating compounds **(145)**, **(146)**, and **(147)** (Fig. **26**). Finally, these analogs presented essential interactions with the target and could be explored in biological assays against SARS-CoV-2.

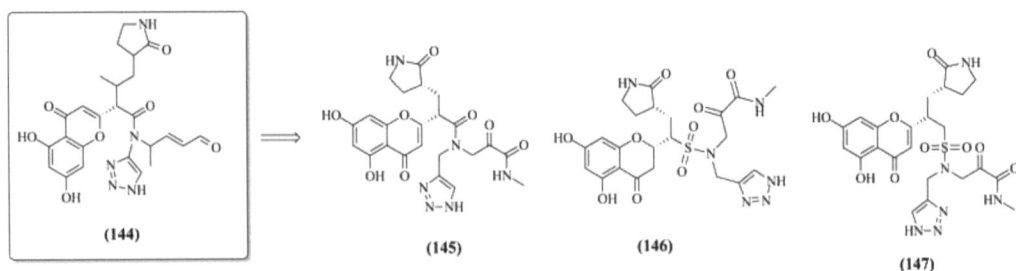

Fig. (26). Chemical structures of compounds identified by Tang and colleagues (2020).

Virtual screenings using fragment libraries are the most common approaches in FBDD. Thus, Gao and colleagues (2020), in the search for new compounds against SARS-CoV-2 3CL^{pro} carried out the fragment screening approach for the identification of low molecular weight molecules containing pharmacophore groups [91]. Initially, the authors compared 3,508 in a fragment library with drugs reused from virtual screenings. Thus, it was compared if the pharmacophores bind to the receptor. Therefore, a total of 38 compounds/pharmacophores were selected and an STD-NMR analysis was performed, in which three hits were identified, being niacin **(148)**, compounds **(149)** and **(150)** (Fig. **27**). The first two compounds inhibit 3CL^{pro} by binding to the catalytic pocket. Then, the authors searched for compounds similar to niacin **(148)** and ligand **(149)**. Thus, carmofur **(151)**, bendamustine **(152)**, triclabendazole **(153)**, emedastine **(154)**, and omeprazole **(155)** were identified, presenting IC$_{50}$ against 3CL^{pro} of 2.8 ± 0.2; 26 ± 1.0; 82 ± 7 and 283 ± 24 μM. In addition, omeprazole **(155)** is the only drug that binds to the *C*-terminal domain from the enzyme. Finally, the authors concluded that carmofur **(151)**, bendamustine **(152)** could be more promising, and triclabendazole **(153)**, emedastine **(154)**, and omeprazole **(155)**, despite these results, could be used in the early stages.

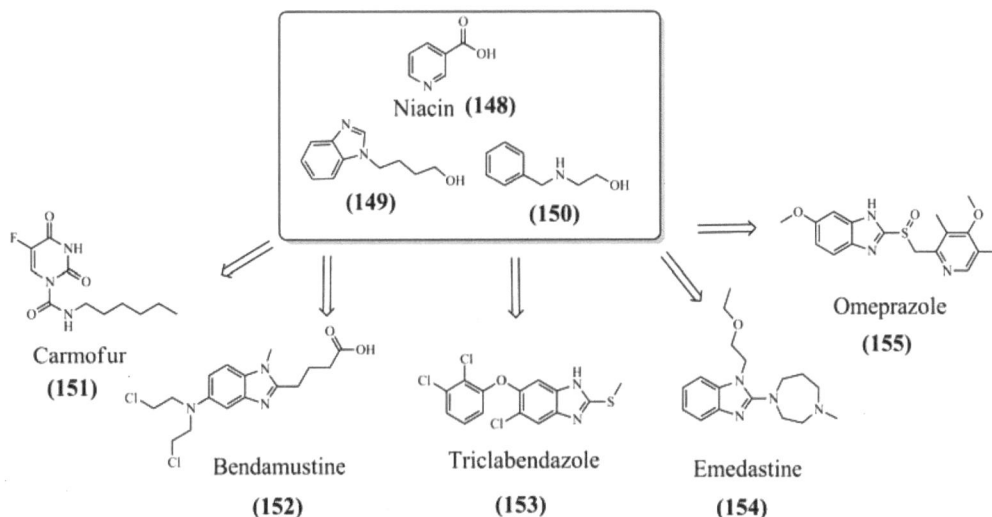

Fig. (27). Chemical structures of compounds identified by Gao and colleagues (2020).

Choudhury (2020), designed molecular fragments with action on the active site of SARS-CoV-2 3CL^{pro} [92]. Thus, a database was built with about 191,678 molecular fragments and adapted to generate new molecules. Therefore, 1,974 fragments were selected and utilized to generate 487 molecules, in which molecular docking was carried out, obtaining 142 molecules with a docking score better than -10 kcal/mol. Then, ADMET filters were applied to select 83 compounds with satisfactory pharmacokinetic properties. ΔG_{bind} calculations were performed by using the MMGBSA method, obtaining 17 molecules with values between -70.0 to -80.97 kcal/mol. Finally, molecular dynamics simulations were carried out, in which 15 compounds **(156-170)** (Fig. **28**) showed stability at the active site, in addition to hydrogen bonding interactions, saline bridge, and hydrophobic contacts with the main amino acid residues.

Verma and coworkers (2020), using the structure of SARS-CoV-2 3CL^{pro}, performed an ADQN-FBDD protocol for the discovery of new compounds [93]. Thus, the authors identified 10 compounds **(171-180)** (Fig. **29**) with similarity to the inhibitors found in the literature. Finally, such compounds could be explored in biological assays against SARS-CoV-2.

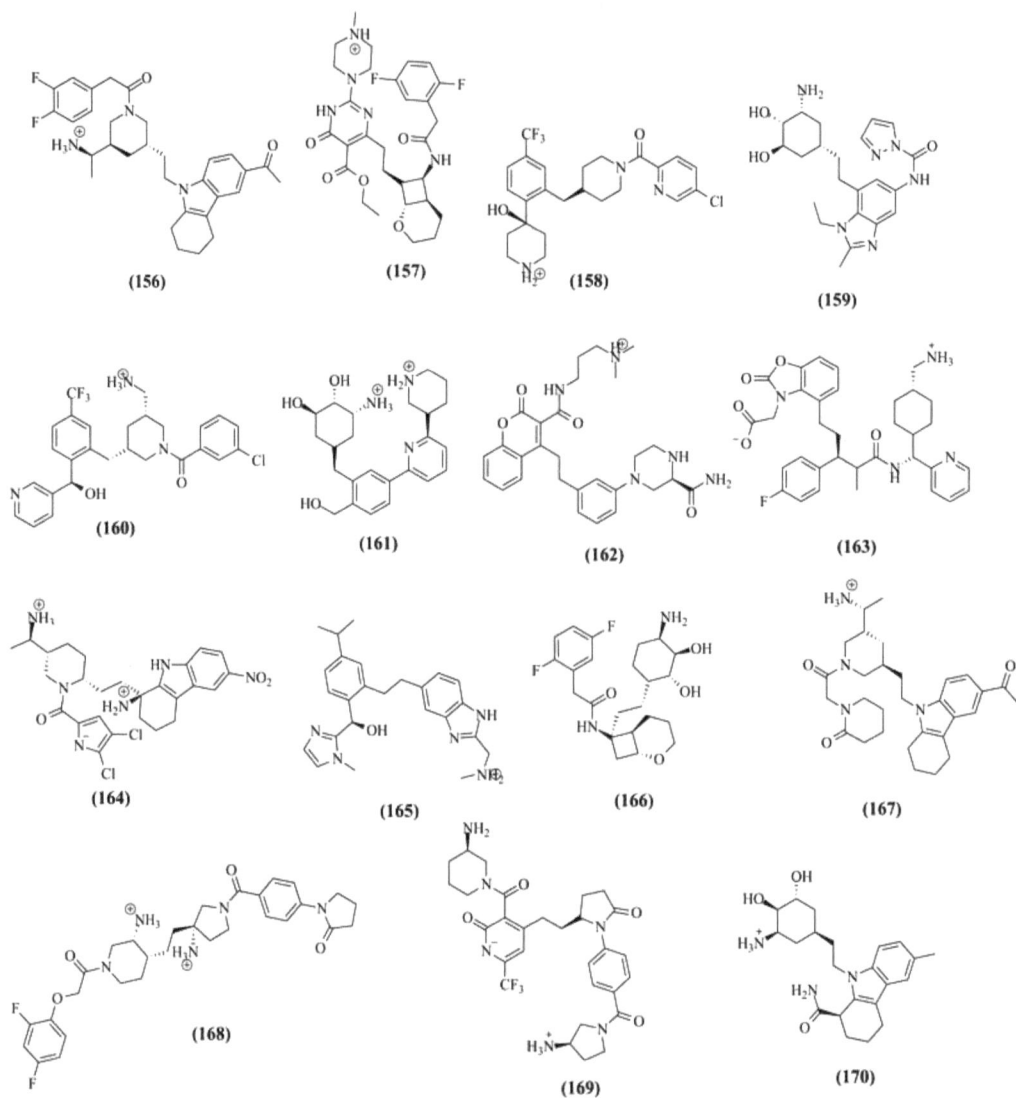

Fig. (28). Chemical structures of compounds identified by Choudhury (2020).

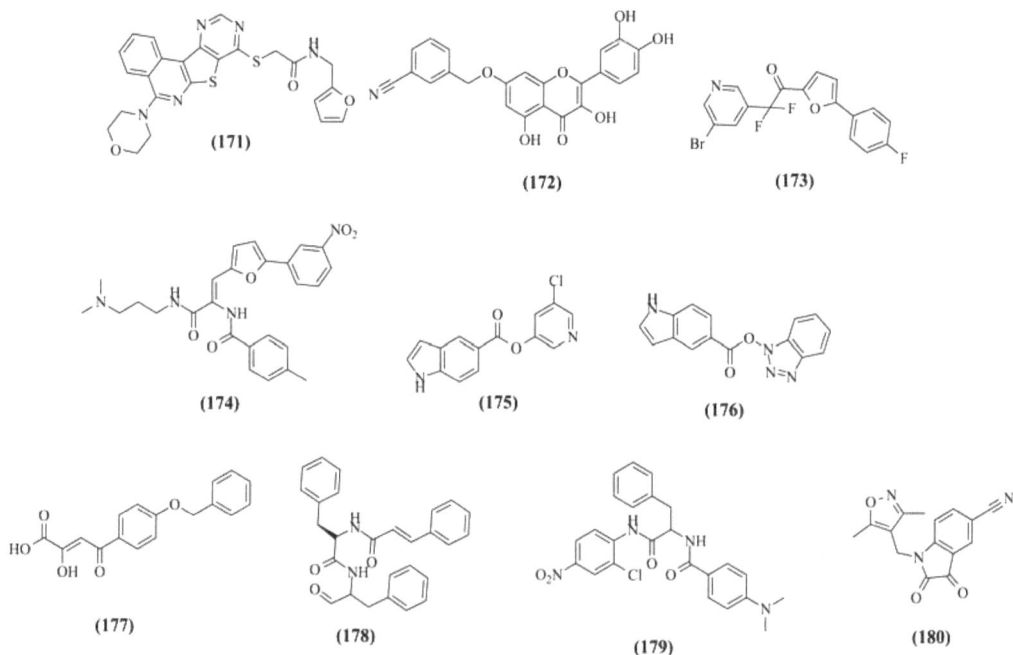

Fig. (29). Structures of compounds identified by Verma and coworkers (2020).

4.5. *De Novo* **Drug Discovery**

De novo drug discovery is a drug design strategy based on the 3D-structure of both receptor and pharmacophore groups present in the ligand [94]. It is a strategy that promotes building new *lead* compounds from scratches. The objective of this technique is to design new chemical structures with the best adaptation at the binding site from a specific target [95]. Thus, it can be performed in two ways: outside-in method (also known as linking), in which the main interactions at the active site are analyzed, and the drugs are designed to perform these interactions. The second is inside-out (also known as growing), in which the molecular fragment addition and the molecule is built inside the active site to carry out the main interactions with the receptor [95].

Note that the concepts of *de novo* and FBDD are similar. In fact, the difference between the two techniques is rarely addressed in the literature, and in many cases, the concepts are confused. One of the factors pointed out as differences between these methods is in the building blocks, so that *de novo* drug design starts with smaller building blocks. However, there is no clear definition regarding the size scale. Thus, strategy definition between *de novo*, or FBDD, is left to the authors of the works, given this gap in the literature [96].

Similarly, to current drug design techniques, *de novo* is also carried out by computer-aided protocol. As an example, the Caveat and SPROUT software could be cited, which perform the placement of fragments using the outside-in method. Another exciting software is LUDI, which fits the fragments inside-out [95]. Recently, LigBuilder V3 software has been developed and it has become a fundamental tool in *de novo* design [97].

Using a *de novo* drug design strategy, Bung and colleagues (2020) used predictive models and deep neural network-based generative as the basis for their design of new SARS-CoV-2 3CL^{pro} inhibitors [98]. The authors used the ChEMBL database (1.6 million compounds), in which protease inhibitor molecules were selected and ranked, resulting in 2,515 promising molecules. To these molecules, a transfer and reinforcement learning model was applied to obtain molecules with desired properties. Then, small molecules were generated by AI (artificial intelligence) and docked to the 3CL^{pro}. The model was used in a chemical dataset containing 50,000 molecules, which after applying synthetic viability and drug-likeness filters, resulted in 3,960 best molecules. Among these, 1,333 ligands had an affinity better than -7 kcal/mol in their virtual screening procedure. Finally, 31 molecules were considered to be promising against SARS-CoV-2, being the compounds **(181)** and **(182)** (Fig. **30**) similar to auratiamide **(183)** (Fig. **30**), a natural product with antiviral activity.

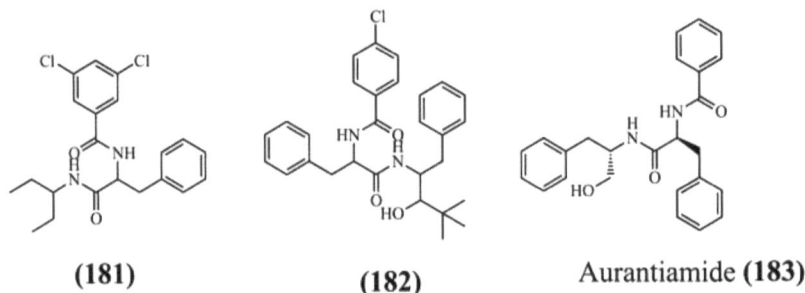

(181)   **(182)**   Aurantiamide **(183)**

Fig. (30). Chemical structures of compounds identified by Bung and colleagues (2020).

4.5. Virtual Screening (VS) and Virtual High-throughput screening (vHTS)

One of the main problems from drug design methodologies is related to the synthesis of high yields of compounds, being a process with higher financial and laboratory costs, and that in many cases, there are no guarantees of success in obtaining promising molecules [99]. HTS, despite performing thousands of tests *per* minute, this technique consumes a substantial financial cost and time, which led researchers to adopt other strategies for a fast screening of compounds [100]. In this context, the search for screening techniques and rational drug design has evolved to use *in silico* strategies, based on the utilization of computers has become essential in medicinal chemistry research [101].

VS techniques are increasingly helping in the search for new drugs. The first proposal of virtual screening is the selection of potential molecules from a library of compounds, using structural descriptors that interact with the receptor and which are related to biological activity [102, 103]. In contrast, *v*HTS performs a large screening of thousands or millions of molecules on a biological target, and these are ranked according to their score (evaluation). Thus, VS techniques select the best compounds, reducing the number of molecules to be tested in biological assays [103].

Most researchers who use VS in their research programs use molecular docking software [103]. However, the idea is to test several algorithms and observe which one could perform the docking in a mode closer to the experimental co-crystallized ligand. When checking all poses and identifying the one that most reproduces the behavior of the original ligand and if it has the highest score, it means that the algorithm could be used in the VS procedure. Otherwise, the simulations should be redone. After this validation, it is advisable to carry out a small VS on ligands with a well-known activity to verify the fit/score and ensure the accuracy of the results obtained. Finally, the software mainly used in these procedures is Autodock, Autodock Vina, Glide, and GOLD [103]. Fig. (**31**) presents the general process for a VS.

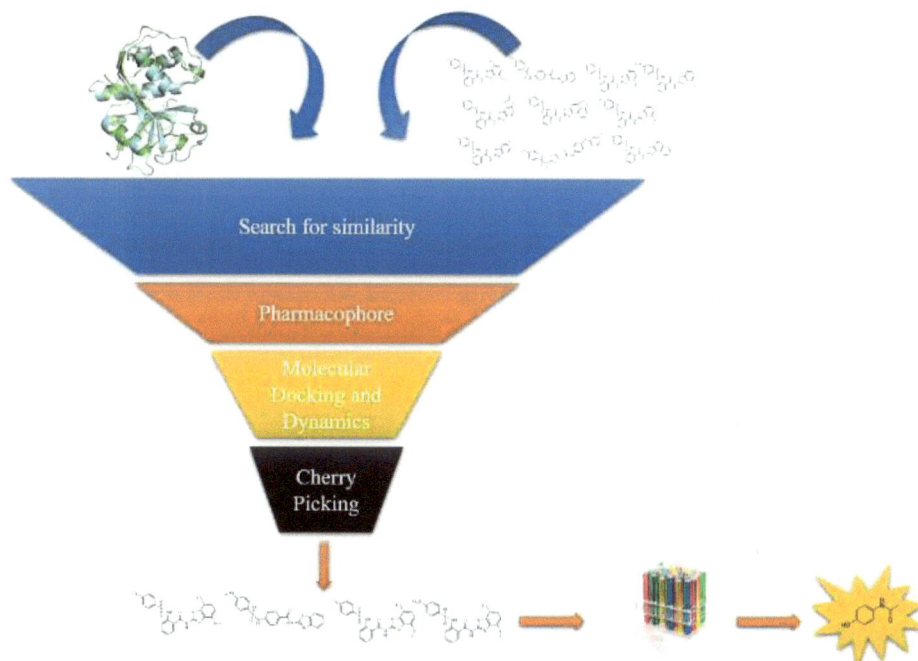

Fig. (31). General procedure for virtual screening.

Sharma and colleagues (2020) used VS to discover new 2'-*O*-methyltransferase (2'OMTase) inhibitors, aiming to identify new active compounds against SARS-CoV-2 [104]. Initially, the structure of 2'OMTase was built by comparative modeling and, subsequently, a vHTS was performed on a library containing 3,000 FDA-approved drugs. In total, 20 ligands presented the best score values, ranging from -10.0 to -8.7 kcal/mol. Posteriorly, a second docking analysis was carried out, which allowed selecting sinefungin **(184)**, digitoxin **(185)**, dihydroergotamine **(186)**, irinotecan **(187)**, and teniposide **(188)** (Fig. **32**). These drugs demonstrated interactions with Asp[130], Lys[170], and Glu[203] residues, which are related to the catalytic site of the enzyme. Finally, molecular dynamics studies showed that all compounds, except for irinotecan **(187)**, showed both good stability and affinity at the active site. Lastly, the authors concluded that these drugs could be explored *in vivo* to discover new alternatives against SARS-CoV-2.

Wang (2020) performed a VS on 2,201 approved drugs and others from clinical trials obtained from the DrugBank database in order to identify potential SARS-CoV-2 3CL[pro] inhibitors [105]. After the docking score calculations (better than -8.5 kcal/mol), 39 top hits were selected for further analysis. In addition to the top *hits*, MMPBSA-WSAS calculations were performed, in which the top 5 compounds (carfilzomib **(189)**, eravacycline **(190)**, valrubicin **(191)** (Fig. **32**), lopinavir **(124)**, and elbasvir **(24)**) were found to present $\Delta G_{bind} \leq -5.0$ kcal/mol. All these drugs were submitted to molecular dynamics simulations, where it was observed good stability at the active site for them. In addition, the author highlighted the importance of His[41] amino acid residue for designing new inhibitors against 3CL[pro] since it is essential in stabilizing ligand-protein complex by π-π stacking interactions.

Iftikhar and colleagues (2020) performed an *in silico* screening using three important SARS-CoV-2 enzymes (RdRp, 3CL[pro], and helicase) and a library of 4,574 FDA-approved drugs [106]. Thus, these compounds were docked into the targets, in which those with the highest score and binding site complementarity were selected for further studies. In this context, rimantadine **(192)**, casopitant **(193)**, meclonazepam **(194)**, and oxiphenisatin **(195)** (Fig. **32**) were selected as top hits from this study that could be tested in biological tests. In order to avoid false-positive results, the authors utilized molecular docking to analyze rimantadine **(192)** upon another 100 enzymes, thus ruling out nonspecific drug binding to 3CL[pro].

Still using drug repurposing methods, Cavasotto and colleagues (2020) conducted a VS towards S; 3CL[pro], and PL[pro] proteins and a library of 11,552 FDA-approved drugs [107]. Thus, the compounds were ranked considering the value of QM docking score. The authors concluded the compounds sovaprevir **(196)**, anatibant

(197), and pralatrexate **(198)** (Fig. **32**) could be further experimentally studied against 3CL^{pro}, and PL^{pro}, and S proteins, respectively.

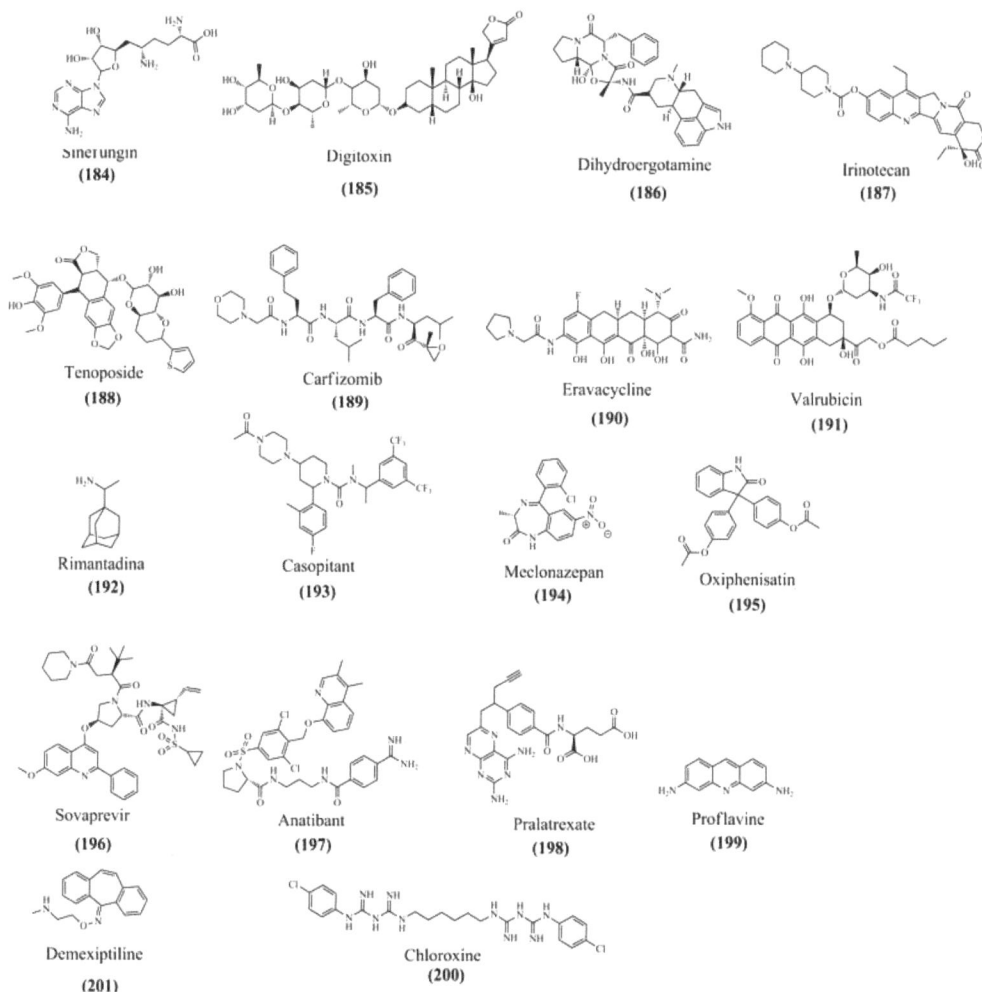

Fig. (32). Promising anti-SARS-CoV-2 compounds repurposed by Sharma and colleagues (2020), Wang (2020), Iftikhar and colleagues (2020), Cavasotto and colleagues (2020), and Gao colleagues (2020).

Gao and colleagues (2020) performed a VS against 3CL^{pro} in two libraries from DrugBank, one comprising 1,553 and another with 7,012 FDA-approved drugs or under investigation [108]. Then, the authors identified 20 drugs potentially active against SARS-CoV-2, being proflavine **(199)** (-8.37 kcal/mol), chloroxine **(200)** (-8.24 kcal/mol), and demexiptiline **(201)** (-8.14 kcal/mol) (Fig. **32**). Additionally, the authors predicted their IC$_{50}$ values (pIC$_{50}$) using the derivation where IC$_{50}$ = 10$^{x/1.3633}$ x 10^{-6}, where X is their affinities values. Finally, proflavine **(199)** was found to be the most promising candidate, with a pIC$_{50}$ value of 0.77 μM, followed by chloroxine **(200)** (pIC$_{50}$ of 0.89 μM), and demexiptiline **(201)** (pIC$_{50}$ of 1.06 μM).

Also, using the drug repurposing approach, Gurung and colleagues (2020), working on the discovery of new compounds against SARS-CoV-2 3CL^{pro}, performed a VS on a database of 75 FDA-approved drugs and 263 phytochemical compounds from different classes [109]. Initially, the phytochemical compounds were filtered according to the Lipinski and Veber filters. So, only 46 compounds remained that could be non-toxic and with good oral bioavailability. Then, 46 phytochemical compounds and 75 FDA-approved drugs were studied against 3CL^{pro} from SARS-, MERS-, and SARS-CoV2. The authors identified that the drugs glecaprevir **(202)**, daclatasvir **(203)** are able to inhibit this enzyme from SARS- and SARS-CoV-2, while paritaprevir **(204)** inhibits SARS- and MERS-CoV, and then atazanavir **(205)** inhibits SARS-CoV-2 and MERS-CoV. On the other hand, from the phytochemical compounds, vincapusine **(206)**, allyohimbine **(207)**, and gummadiol **(208)** presented inhibitory potential against the targets from three organisms.

In another study, Gurung and coworkers (2020) performed a VS on plant antiviral compounds against MERS-CoV, SARS-, and SARS-CoV-2 3CL^{pro} [110]. The authors selected 38 compounds, in which 10 molecules fitted to the Lipinski rule of five. Thus, molecular docking simulations were performed, where it was verified that bonducellpin D had the most promising result, with a docking score of −9.28 kcal/mol and an inhibition constant of 156.75 nM (Calculated by the equation K$_i$ = exponential (ΔG/RT)). In addition, this molecule performs hydrogen bonding interactions with Glu^{166} and Thr^{190} and hydrophobic interactions with Met^{49}, His^{164}, Met^{165}, Pro^{168}, Asp^{187}, Arg^{188}, Gln^{189}, and Gln^{192}. In addition, this compound showed a high affinity for SARS-CoV (-8.66 kcal/mol) and MERS-CoV (-8.93 kcal/mol) 3CL^{pro}. Finally, compound **(209)** and caesalmin B **(210)** showed similar results, representing potential leads against SARS-CoV-2 (Fig. **33**).

FDA-approved drugs were also used in a screening performed by Gahlawat and colleagues (2020) [111]. In this context, the authors initially carried out a comparative study of the amino acid sequences from SARS- and SARS-CoV-2 3CL^{pro}, as well as a VS using a natural products database; some 3CL^{pro} inhibitors found in the literature and FDA-approved drugs obtained from ZINC. Comparative modeling results showed mutations in Ser^{46} and Phe^{134} residues. For Ser^{46}, it increases the contribution of two hydrophilic residues; and for Phe^{134}, it improves the catalytic efficiency, facilitating the transfer of the proton from His^{41} to Cys^{145}. Then, 73 promising compounds were initially identified (Combo score > 2.0). However, after some additional analysis involving molecular dynamics, the best five compounds were identified, being saquinavir **(128)**, acteoside **(211)**, chebulinic acid **(212)**, delphinidin-3,5-diglucoside **(213)**, and lithospermic acid **(214)** (Fig. **34**). Finally, these compounds showed perfectly fit into the binding site and demonstrated essential interactions with His[41] and Cys[145] residues [111].

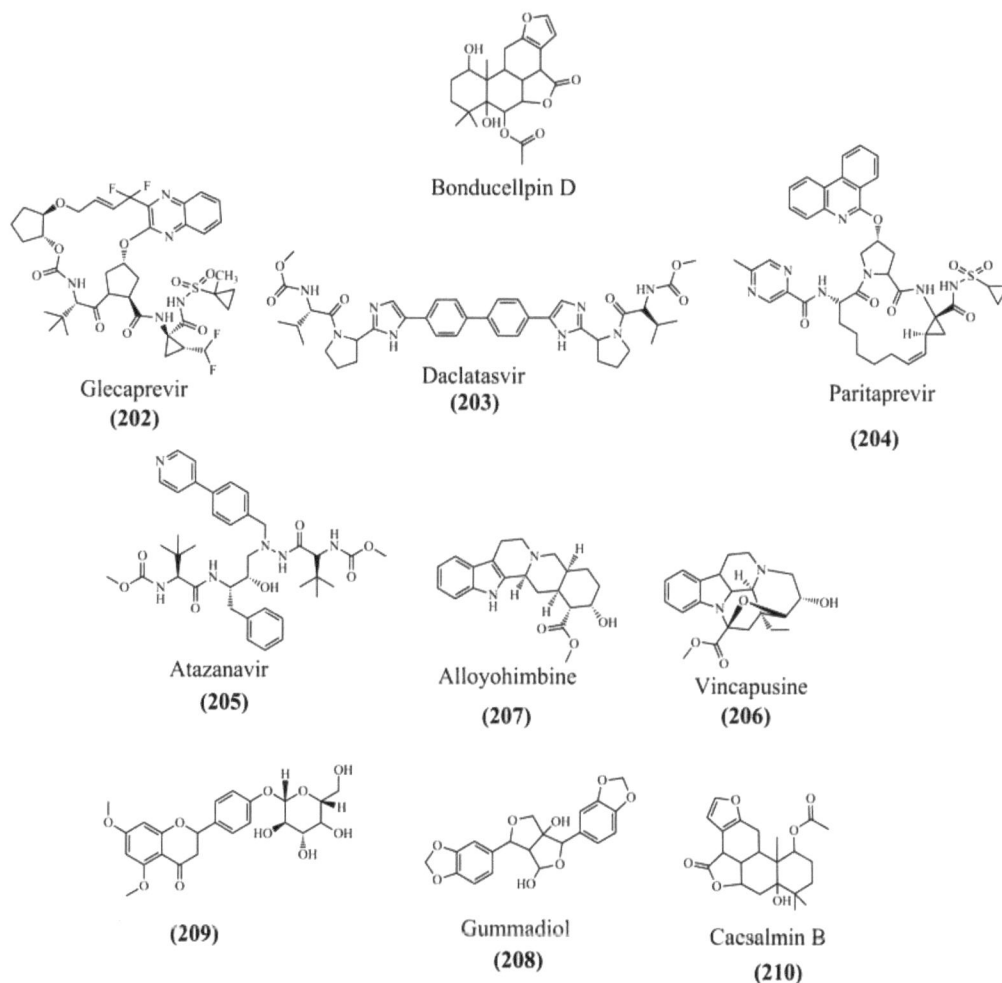

Fig. (33). Chemical structures of compounds identified by Gurung and colleagues (2020).

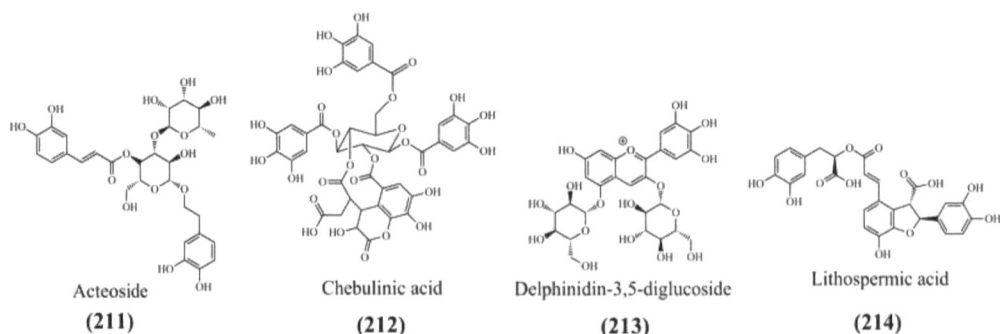

Fig. (34). Chemical structures of compounds identified by Gahlawat and colleagues (2020).

Interestingly, Kandeel and colleagues (2020) highlighted that their work was the first to present a VS on FDA-approved drugs and the first SARS-CoV-2 3CL[pro] deposited structure in Protein Data Bank (PDB id: 6LU7) [112]. In addition, an analysis of MERS-, SARS- and SARS-CoV-2 3CL[pro] sequences was performed. Thus, it was verified highly conserved sequences between SARS- and SARS-CoV2 were shown. However, it was not observed for MERS-CoV 3CL[pro], which had fewer similarities. Then, a VS was carried out on the Selleckchem Inc. database (WA, USA), using only FDA-approved drugs virtual screening. As a result, 20 top hits were initially identified, although only three compounds were found to be more promising dockscore, being ribavirin **(2)**, telbivudine **(215)**, and nicotinamide **(216)**. Further, visual inspection of these compounds showed that ribavirin **(2)** interacts *via* hydrogen-bonding interactions with Thr[25] and Gln[189] residues and telbivudine **(215)** with Ser[49] and Gln[189].

In another study, Alberto and colleagues (2020) performed a virtual screening docking-based of approximately 4,384 FDA-approved drugs against SARS-Co--2 3CL[pro] [113]. After the screening procedure, 10 compounds were selected with a docking score ranging from -9.17 to -10.25 kcal/mol. These compounds were chosen for ΔG calculations by using molecular dynamics, in which the drugs daunorubicin **(217)** (−138.8 kcal/mol), *N*-trifluoroacetyladriamycin **(218)** (−46.2 kcal/mol), ergotamine **(186)** (−119.2 kcal/mol), bromocriptine **(219)** (−116.7 kcal/mol), amrubicin **(220)** (−117.5 kcal/mol), ergoloid **(221)** (−109.1 kcal/mol), and meclocycline **(123)** (−115.1 kcal/mol) were found to be the best candidates to anti-SARS-CoV activity (Fig. **35**).

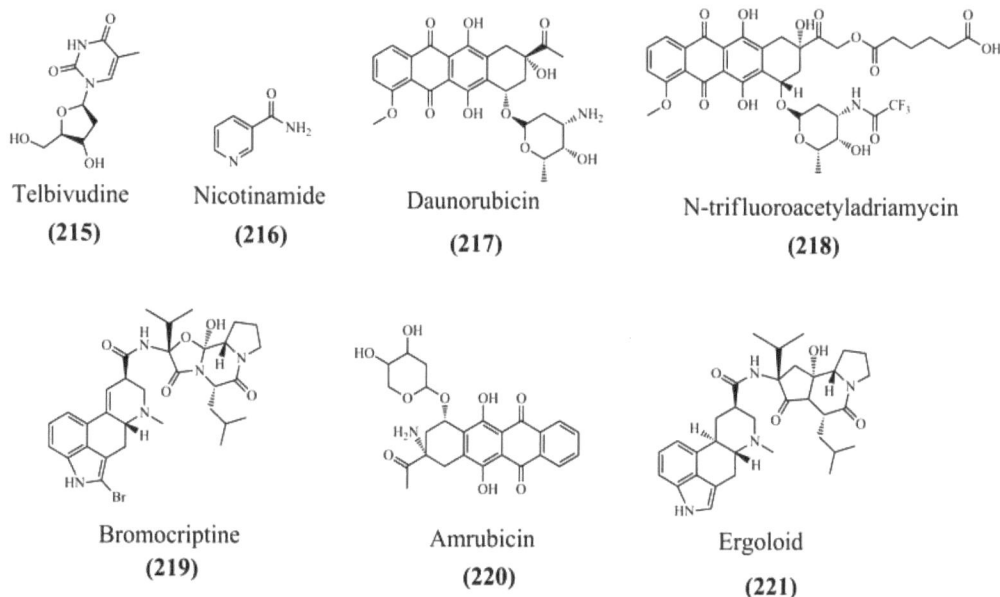

Fig. (35). Chemical structures of compounds identified by Kandeel and colleagues (2020), and Alberto and colleagues (2020).

Ngo and colleagues (2020) carried out a VS for discovering potential new SARS-CoV-2 3CL^{pro} inhibitors [114]. Initially, three previously discovered ligands were selected and their affinity energies determined. Based on these data, a VS was carried out on the Vietherb database, with approximately 4,600 natural compounds and eight anti-HIV synthetic compounds. Thus, 44 compounds were selected and submitted to the fast pulling of ligand (FPL) method, resulting in 5 compounds (darunavir **(222)**, ritonavir **(129)**, lopinavir **(124)**, cannabisina A **(223)**, and isoactoside **(224)** (Fig. **36**), which these were later validated by using the free energy perturbation (FEP) method. The authors showed that cannabisin A **(223)**, isoactoside **(224)**, and darunavir **(222)** have high-affinity energies ($-12.76 + 1.37$ kcal/mol; -9.40 ± 2.64 kcal/mol; -11.96 ± 1.99 kcal/mol, respectively). Additionally, the authors point out that H-bonds with Gly^{166} play a fundamental role in the activity of these inhibitors thus the replacement of this residue with an alanine generates a decrease in its affinity energy.

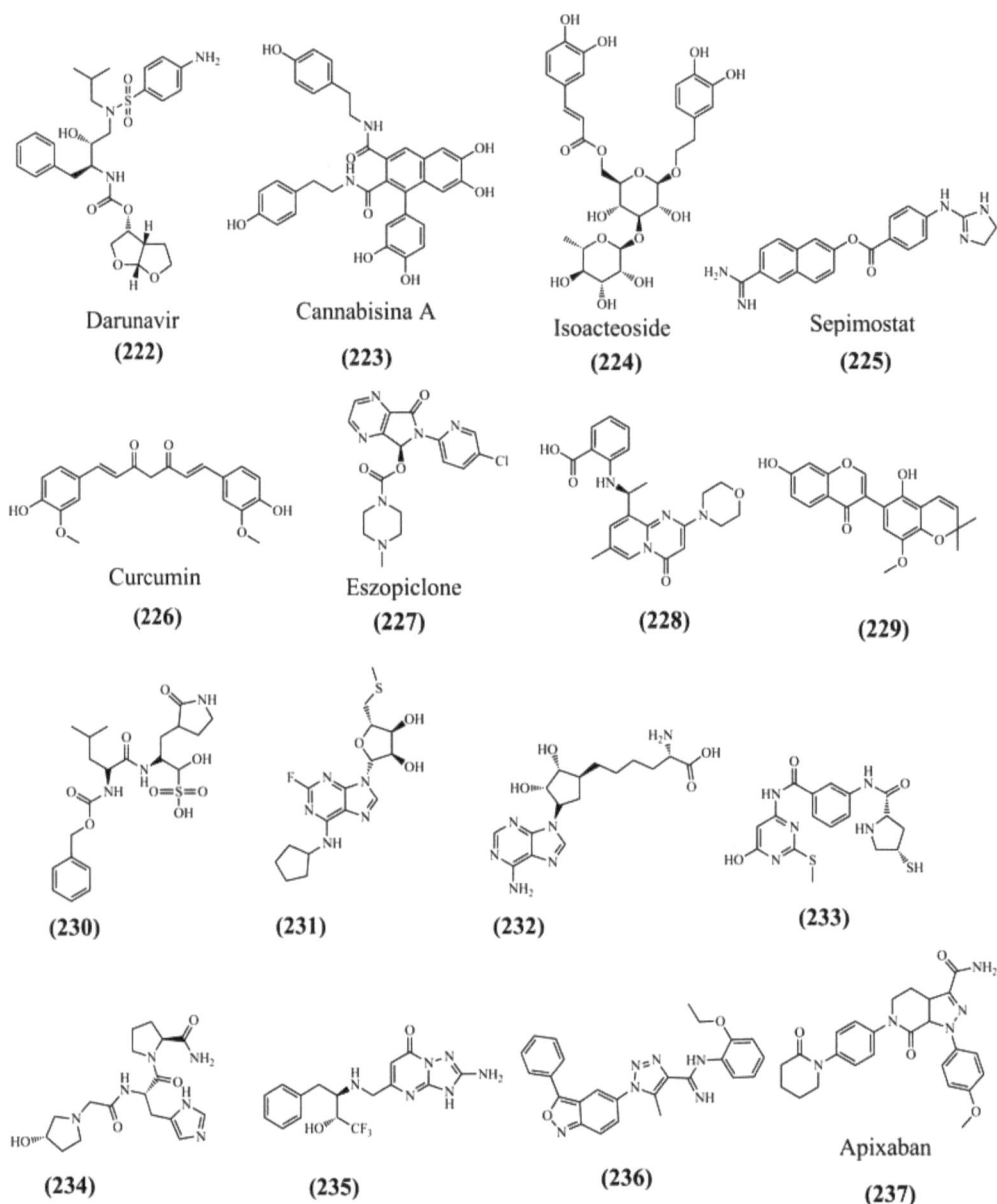

Fig. (36). Chemical structures of compounds identified by Ngo and colleagues (2020), Mohammad and coworkers (2020), Santibáñez-Morán and colleagues (2020), Tsuji (2020), and Hage-Melim and colleagues (2020).

Using SARS-CoV-2 3CL^{pro} as a target, Tsuji (2020) performed a VS on the ChEMBL database (1,485,144 compounds) [115]. The first analysis performed was the score determination, in which compounds with affinity energy greater than -50 kcal/mol were selected for further studies, resulting in the selection of 27,561 compounds. Among the best compounds, 64 molecules were potential drugs since these had already been approved or were in clinical studies. Additional docking studies were performed, allowing to classify 28 compounds as promising, being sepimostat **(225)** (-7.9 kcal/mol), curcumin **(226)** (-7.3 kcal/mol), and eszopiclone **(227)** (-10 kcal/mol) (Fig. **36**). Finally, it was verified that all of these compounds present a carbonyl group that interacts with the catalytic dyad, composed of Cys^{145} and His^{41}.

Mohammad and coworkers (2020) used several SBDD techniques to perform a VS in the PubChem database (10,433 compounds) [116]. Initially, a docking study of 121 compounds in SARS-CoV-2 $3CL^{pro}$ was performed. Thus, the authors used the top 10 compounds as scaffolds and their drug-like properties to filter compounds from the PubChem database. In this context, 4,802 compounds were selected and submitted to docking simulations, in which the top 5 compounds **(228-232)** (Fig. **36**) were analyzed for their interactions at the active site. Then, interactions with the main amino acid residues were observed, being Thr^{25}, Phe^{140}, Leu^{141}, Asn^{142}, Gly^{143}, Ser^{144}, Cys^{145}, His^{163}, His^{164}, Glu^{166}, and Gln^{189}. By using software for biological activity prediction (PASS server prediction), the authors point out that compounds **(232)** and **(230)** could be promising as antiviral agents. Finally, studies of molecular dynamics suggested that these present good stability at the active site during the entire simulation time.

Santibáñez-Morán and colleagues (2020) performed a virtual drug repurposing screening against SARS-CoV-2 $3CL^{pro}$, combining both SBDD and LBDD approaches [117]. Initially, compounds lopinavir **(124)**, ritonavir **(129)**, nelfinavir was used as a basis for the search for structural similarity in the food chemicals (22,880 compounds) and molecules in the Dark Chemical Matter (DCM) databases (139,329 compounds). The second step involved 1,052 compounds with potential reported activity against SARS-CoV and SARS-CoV-2 $3CL^{pro}$. Thus, 40 molecules were selected from the food chemicals database and 500 molecules from the DCM database. Based on the second approach, 178 food chemicals and 174 from DCM were selected, generating a total of 888 compounds for docking simulations. Then, these compounds were filtered and categorized into 4 groups, according to their 1) interactions with His^{41} and Cys^{145}; 2) commercial availability; 3) ADMETox profile, and 4) characteristic activity predicted by machine learning (ML), thus, resulting in 105 promising compounds. Finally, compounds **(233)**, **(234)**, and **(235)** (Fig. **36**) were identified as the best ones.

Hage-Melim and colleagues (2020) performed a VS in two libraries of compounds against SARS-CoV-2 $3CL^{pro}$ [118]. The top 100 hits were evaluated for their pharmacokinetic viability, compared to properties of antivirals and hydroxychloroquine. Thus, 25 molecules with a better pharmacokinetic profile were selected. The toxicological profile of these molecules was predicted, thus generating the selection of 10 compounds. The compound (236) (Fig. 36) showed interactions similar to favipiravir and hydroxychloroquine. Finally, a search for similarity with the compound (236) was carried out, in which the compound apixaban (237) (Fig. 36) was found, showing interactions with several critical amino acid residues, including the catalytic dyad (Cys[145] and His[41]).

A widely explored target in the discovery of compounds against SARS-CoV-2 is the TMPRSS2, responsible for facilitating the viral fusion to host cells. In this context, Singh and coworkers (2020) performed a VS on the Drug-lib (4,600 compounds) and AIEfd-Db (10,000 compounds) databases against TMPRSS2 [119]. Initially, the protein structure was built by homology modeling. Then, the compounds were screened, analyzed, and ranked using a consensus score (Vina scores, Vinardo scores, RFScoreVs). In this context, 156 compounds that could act on the catalytic site and 100 compounds that could fit into the serine protease domain exosite were selected. The most promising compounds found were tanogitran (238) (Vina Score: -8,785; Vinardo: -9.2743, and RF-Score-VS: 6.3581) and radotinib (239) (Vina Score: -9.310; Vinardo: -8.5883; RF-Score-VS: 6.1410) (Fig. 37).

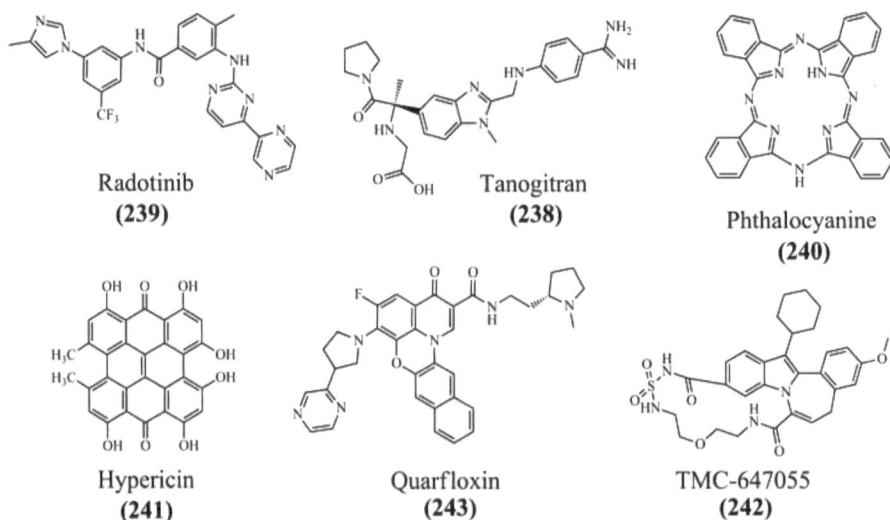

Radotinib
(239)

Tanogitran
(238)

Phthalocyanine
(240)

Hypericin
(241)

Quarfloxin
(243)

TMC-647055
(242)

Fig. (37). Chemical structures of compounds identified by Singh and colleagues (2020) and Romeo colleagues (2020).

In addition to TMPRSS2, S protein is also a promising target. Thus, Romeo and colleagues (2020) performed a VS in a library of 8,770 compounds obtained in the Drugbank database against SARS-CoV-2 S protein [120]. Initially, the 3D-structure of the S protein was built using homology modeling. The library was docked and among the top ten compounds, two of them had reported antiviral activity, being phthalocyanine **(240)** and hypericin **(241)**. These were then subjected to molecular dynamics simulations, which confirmed the main interactions shown in the docking (hydrophobic interactions in HR1) and the stability at the active site by the MMGBSA calculations. In addition, the authors showed that the presence of drugs blocks the HR1 region, preventing conformational changes and subsequent preventing SARS-CoV-2 attachment. Finally, the reweighting scoring function was applied and it was revealed that the compounds phthalocyanine **(240)**, hypericin **(241)**, TMC-647055 **(242)**, and quarfloxin **(243)** could be promising against SARS-CoV-2.

Using other well-explored targets, Naik and colleagues (2020) performed a vHTS against six SARS-CoV-2 targets (helicase, endoribonuclease, exoribonuclease, RdRp, methyltransferase, and 3CL^{pro}) using 35,032 compounds from NPASS database [121]. Initially, these targets were built by homology modeling. Then, 21 top hits were selected from docking simulations based on their core values. Among these, compounds **(244)** and **(245)** (Fig. **38**) presented interactions with three or more proteins and still good stability at the active site during molecular dynamics simulations.

Ruan and colleagues (2020) performed a VS on 7,964 compounds obtained from the ZINC database against some non-structural complexes from SARS-CoV-2 (nsp12-nsp7-nsp8) and SARS-CoV (nsp12-nsp7-nsp8) obtained from the Protein Data Bank (PDB), and also nsp12-nsp8 and nsp12-nsp7 complexes, which were built by using homology modeling [122]. Thus, 44 compounds were selected for further evaluation, and among these, 8 compounds were considered for MMGBSA calculations. The authors found tegobuvir **(246)**, olysio **(247)**, filibuvir **(248)**, and cefarantina **(249)** (Fig. **38**) as potential agents against SARS-CoV-2.

Mirza and colleagues (2020) performed a VS using compounds from the ZINC database against three SARS-CoV-2 targets: 3CL^{pro}, nsp12 polymerase, and nsp13 helicase [123]. Initially, the authors built a model for each of the targets using homology modeling. Then, ADMET properties were predicted for the removal of molecules that could present pharmacokinetic and toxicity problems. For 3CL^{pro}, a total of 13 compounds showed excellent score values and strong interactions with the catalytic dyad (His^{41} and Cys^{145}). Among these compounds, 13 ligands were submitted to molecular dynamics, where the affinity for MMGBSA was calculated. Thus, the compound **(250)** (Fig. **38**) was found to be more promising (ΔG_{tol} = -45.22 kcal/mol), in addition to presenting hydrogen bonding interactions with Ser^{144}, Cys^{145}, Met^{165}, Gln^{189}, and Gln^{192} residues. For nsp12 polymerase, 17 molecules were chosen for the MMGBSA calculations, in which compound **(251)** (Fig. **38**) showed the best ΔG_{tol} results (-41.74 kcal/mol), and also hydrogen bonds with Ser[759], Lys[798,] and Ser[814] residues. Finally, for nsp13 helicase, four molecules were chosen for MMGBSA, in which the compound **(252)** (Fig. **38**) had better ΔG_{tol} (-49.73 kcal/mol) and hydrogen bonding interactions with Ser[310], Glu[375], and Lys[288] residues.

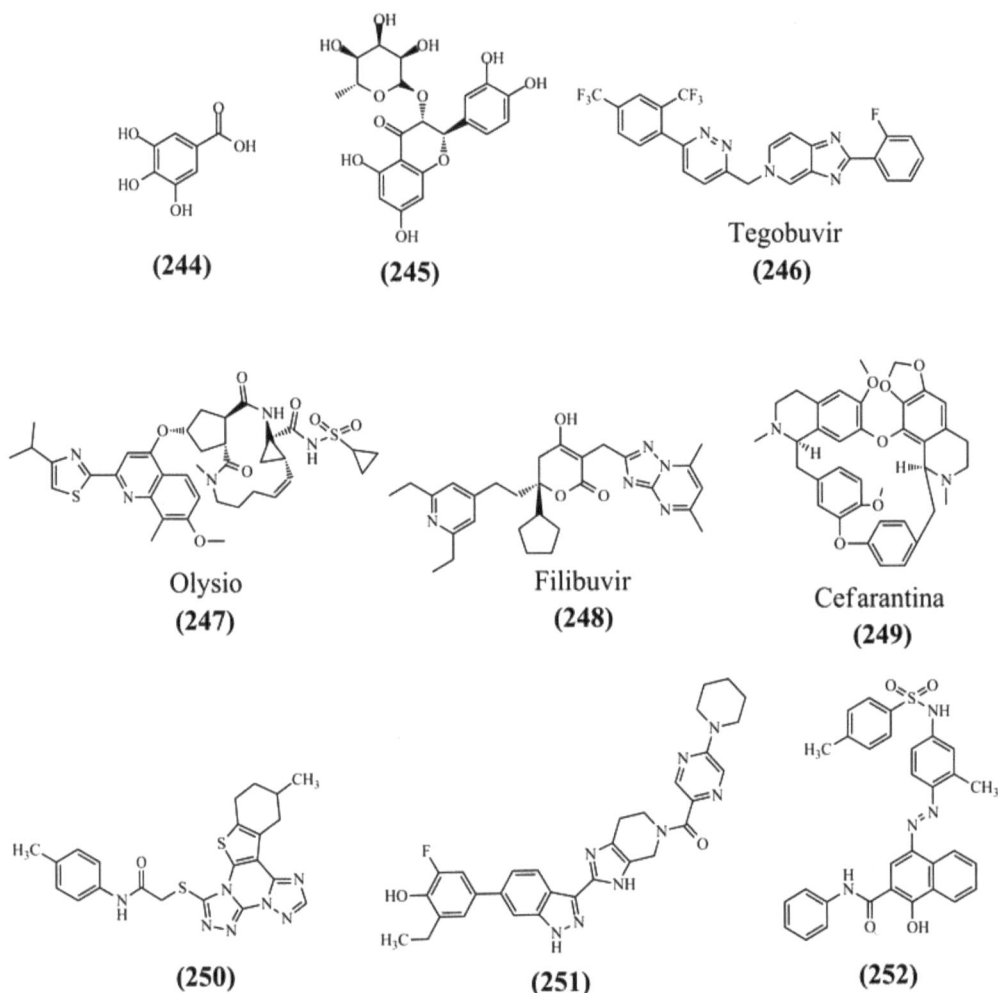

Fig. (38). Chemical structures of compounds identified by Naik and colleagues (2020), Ruan and colleagues (2020), and Mirza and colleagues (2020).

5. CHALLENGES IN SBDD FOR SARS-COV-2

The discovery of a new drug is an expensive and time-consuming process, with an estimated investment of approximately US$ 800 million. Thus, SBDD appears to reduce this monetary burden in the design of drugs. In addition, successful cases in the last decade have shown the versatility of these methods, such as the discovery of HIV-1 protease inhibitors. However, just as there are cases of success, there are failures, as in the discovery of the antidepressant/anxiolytic PRX00023, being a low-efficiency 5-HT$_{1A}$ receptor antagonist. Such failures are related to the challenges and limitations still imposed on SBDD methodologies [95].

The first limitation of SBDD approaches remains in the identification of the target. If the target has an available 3D-structure, a homology study can be performed. However, building models with similarities below 40% should use more refinement resources to obtain a quality structure, increasing the complexity of the process [95]. Also, an important limiting factor of SBDD approaches is the target's flexibility in molecular docking studies since the proteins are presented in their crystallographic structures in a static model (PDB), although in reality, proteins are structures with dynamic nature. Thus, ignoring the protein's flexibility can generate misleading or less accurate results in SBDD protocols. In this context, the utilization of flexible docking or molecular dynamics techniques can be essential to overcome such limitations [124]. Another limiting factor related to molecular docking is the choice of the appropriate algorithm and scoring functions, as no software is capable of working with all proteins and ligands. Thus, the algorithm should be able to reproduce results closer to the real one [31].

In the case of VS, existing software ignores protonation states and tautomerism, and ionization, which can result in the selection of molecules with different results than the real one. Another obstacle is the forecast of ADMET and toxicity of molecules because the software should carry out a prediction closer to the real, requiring more significant investment in the development of computer technology [31].

In the case of obtaining a *lead* compound by *de* novo design and FBDD approaches, the selection of potential compounds is carried out manually. In addition, the compounds selected in the screening are often not synthetically viable. Thus, it is necessary to have software that considers the complexity of synthesis before selecting the molecules [31, 95].

Finally, the potential resistance of SARS-CoV-2 in the face of antiviral agents is one of the main challenges to be overcome in the search for new therapies. In this sense, prolonged exposure to the drug and continuous viral replication are vital factors that lead to the development of resistance to any treatment against this disease. Thus, both factors related to the virus and the host are related to viral resistance, mainly by genomic interference mechanism that results in high rates of mutation and recombination, leading to high rates of viral replication, which is a challenge to be overcome by scientists for the discovery of new therapies [125].

CONCLUSION

The SARS-CoV-2 pandemic has reached alarming levels like never before seen in other pandemics. This virus has been responsible for thousands of deaths around the world (more than 5,004,855), causing damage to the health and economy of countries. The high rate of transmissibility, associated with the lack of drugs or vaccines useful in treatment or prevention, further worsens the statistics, showing how far we are from the end of this pandemic. In addition, this virus has always been present in our society for a long time ago. However, because it affected only specific locations and a low number of people, investment in new therapies was superficial, resulting in the state that we are living in nowadays.

In recent years, strategies in medicinal chemistry have evolved in such a way that the use of computational molecular modeling techniques in the design of new drugs has become indispensable. It is notable, both in industry and in academia, the growth in the use of SBDD techniques for the discovery of new drugs, related to several success cases, boosting research in the improvement of these molecular modeling techniques.

As shown in this chapter, the techniques in SBDD are not used separately but together. Thus, the combination of techniques associated with the validation of protocols makes the discovery process closer to the real one and reduces the chances of errors in the screening of molecules. In addition, the lower cost and time associated with the research demonstrate how much the investment in using such techniques is worth. Despite the limitations that some of them present, the previous validation of *in silico* experiments could solve these problems and improve the research to success.

Finally, here were presented the main techniques in SBDD in the discovery of new hits against SARS-CoV-2. It is hoped that this chapter will serve as an inspiration for researchers around the world to design new molecules and perhaps result in the discovery of a new therapy that could end the distressing situation that we find ourselves.

CONSENT FOR PUBLICATION

Not applicable.

CONFLICT OF INTEREST

The authors declare no conflict of interest, financial or otherwise.

ACKNOWLEDGEMENTS

The authors thank the Coordenação de Aperfeiçoamento de Pessoal de Nível Superior, Brazil (CAPES) and the National. Council for Scientific and Technological Development (CNPq), Brazil for their support to the Brazilian Post-Graduate Programs. Finally, we would like to thank the BioRender (https:// https://biorender.com/) for providing biological schemes.

REFERENCES

[1]   D'Angelo G, Palmieri F. Discovering Genomic Patterns in SARS-CoV-2 Variants. Int J Intell Syst 2020; 1-19.

[2]   Macchiagodena M, Pagliai M, Procacci P. Identification of potential binders of the main protease 3CL^{pro} of the COVID-19 *via* structure-based ligand design and molecular modeling. Chem Phys Lett 2020; 750: 137489.
       [http://dx.doi.org/10.1016/j.cplett.2020.137489] [PMID: 32313296]

[3]   Bektaş O, Çerik İB, Çerik HÖ, *et al.* The relationship between severe acute respiratory syndrome coronavirus 2 (SARS - COV - 2) pandemic and fragmented QRS. J Electrocardiol 2020; 62: 10-3.
       [http://dx.doi.org/10.1016/j.jelectrocard.2020.07.009] [PMID: 32736117]

[4]   WHO Coronavirus Disease (COVID-19) Dashboard | WHO Coronavirus Disease (COVID-19) Dashboard. https://covid19.who.int/

[5]   Bhattacharya M, Sharma AR, Patra P, *et al.* SARS-CoV-2 Vaccine Candidate: In-Silico Cloning and Validation. Informatics Med. Unlocked 2020; p. 20.

[6]   Shi Y, Zhang X, Mu K, *et al.* D3Targets-2019-nCoV: a webserver for predicting drug targets and for multi-target and multi-site based virtual screening against COVID-19. Acta Pharm Sin B 2020; 10(7): 1239-48.
       [http://dx.doi.org/10.1016/j.apsb.2020.04.006] [PMID: 32318328]

[7]   Hatada R, Okuwaki K, Mochizuki Y, *et al.* Fragment Molecular Orbital Based Interaction Analyses on COVID-19 Main Protease - Inhibitor N3 Complex (PDB ID: 6LU7). J Chem Inf Model 2020; 60(7): 3593-602.
       [http://dx.doi.org/10.1021/acs.jcim.0c00283] [PMID: 32539372]

[8]   Lounnas V, Ritschel T, Kelder J, McGuire R, Bywater RP, Foloppe N. Current progress in Structure-Based Rational Drug Design marks a new mindset in drug discovery. Comput Struct Biotechnol J 2013; 5(6): e201302011.
       [http://dx.doi.org/10.5936/csbj.201302011] [PMID: 24688704]

[9]   Hubbard RE. Structure-based drug discovery and protein targets in the CNS. Neuropharmacology 2011; 60(1): 7-23.
       [http://dx.doi.org/10.1016/j.neuropharm.2010.07.016] [PMID: 20673774]

[10]   van Montfort RLM, Workman P. Structure-based drug design: aiming for a perfect fit. Essays Biochem 2017; 61(5): 431-7.
       [http://dx.doi.org/10.1042/EBC20170052] [PMID: 29118091]

[11]   Rognan D. The impact of *in silico* screening in the discovery of novel and safer drug candidates. Pharmacol Ther 2017; 175: 47-66.
       [http://dx.doi.org/10.1016/j.pharmthera.2017.02.034] [PMID: 28223231]

[12]   dos Santos Nascimento IJ, de Aquino TM, da Silva-Júnior EF. Drug Repurposing: A Strategy for Discovering Inhibitors against Emerging Viral Infections. Curr Med Chem 2020; 27.
       [PMID: 32787752]

[13]   Ortiz-Prado E, Simbaña-Rivera K. Gómez- Barreno, L.; Rubio-Neira, M.; Guaman, L.P.; Kyriakidis, N.C.; Muslin, C.; Jaramillo, A.M.G.; Barba-Ostria, C.; Cevallos-Robalino, D.; Sanches-SanMiguel, H.; Unigarro, L.; Zalakeviciute, R.; Gadian, N.; López-Cortés, A. Clinical, Molecular, and Epidemiological Characterization of the SARS-CoV-2 Virus and the Coronavirus Disease 2019 (COVID-19), a Comprehensive Literature Review. Diagn Microbiol Infect Dis 2020; 98.

[14]   Shuai H, Chu H, Hou Y, *et al.* Differential immune activation profile of SARS-CoV-2 and SARS-CoV infection in human lung and intestinal cells: Implications for treatment with IFN-β and IFN inducer. J Infect 2020; 81(4): e1-e10.
[http://dx.doi.org/10.1016/j.jinf.2020.07.016] [PMID: 32707230]

[15]   Amirfakhryan H. safari, F. Outbreak of SARS-CoV2: Pathogenesis of Infection and Cardiovascular Involvement. Hell J Cardiol 2020.

[16]   Ezhilan M, Suresh I, Nesakumar N. SARS-CoV, MERS-CoV and SARS-CoV-2: A Diagnostic Challenge. Measurement 2021; 168: 108335.
[http://dx.doi.org/10.1016/j.measurement.2020.108335] [PMID: 33519010]

[17]   de Souza Silva GA, da Silva SP, da Costa MAS, *et al.* das C.; da Silva Melo, A.R.; de Freitas, A.C.; Lagos de Melo, C.M. SARS-CoV, MERS-CoV and SARS-CoV-2 Infections in Pregnancy and Fetal Development. J Gynecol Obstet Hum Reprod 2020; 49(10): 101846.
[http://dx.doi.org/10.1016/j.jogoh.2020.101846]

[18]   Ma C, Su S, Wang J, Wei L, Du L, Jiang S. From SARS-CoV to SARS-CoV-2: safety and broad-spectrum are important for coronavirus vaccine development. Microbes Infect 2020; 22(6-7): 245-53.
[http://dx.doi.org/10.1016/j.micinf.2020.05.004] [PMID: 32437926]

[19]   Hussain A, Hasan A, Nejadi Babadaei MM, *et al.* Targeting SARS-CoV2 Spike Protein Receptor Binding Domain by Therapeutic Antibodies. Biomed Pharmacother 2020; 130: 110559.
[http://dx.doi.org/10.1016/j.biopha.2020.110559] [PMID: 32768882]

[20]   Xie M, Chen Q. Insight into 2019 novel coronavirus - An updated interim review and lessons from SARS-CoV and MERS-CoV. Int J Infect Dis 2020; 94: 119-24.
[http://dx.doi.org/10.1016/j.ijid.2020.03.071] [PMID: 32247050]

[21]   Gil C, Ginex T, Maestro I, *et al.* COVID-19: Drug Targets and Potential Treatments. J Med Chem 2020; 63(21): 12359-86.
[http://dx.doi.org/10.1021/acs.jmedchem.0c00606] [PMID: 32511912]

[22]   Vallamkondu J, John A, Wani WY, *et al.* SARS-CoV-2 pathophysiology and assessment of coronaviruses in CNS diseases with a focus on therapeutic targets. Biochim Biophys Acta Mol Basis Dis 2020; 1866(10): 165889.
[http://dx.doi.org/10.1016/j.bbadis.2020.165889] [PMID: 32603829]

[23]   Ullrich S, Nitsche C. The SARS-CoV-2 main protease as drug target. Bioorg Med Chem Lett 2020; 30(17): 127377.
[http://dx.doi.org/10.1016/j.bmcl.2020.127377] [PMID: 32738988]

[24]   Zhao L, Ciallella HL, Aleksunes LM, Zhu H. Advancing computer-aided drug discovery (CADD) by big data and data-driven machine learning modeling. Drug Discov Today 2020; 25(9): 1624-38.
[http://dx.doi.org/10.1016/j.drudis.2020.07.005] [PMID: 32663517]

[25]   Hughes JP, Rees S, Kalindjian SB, Philpott KL. Principles of early drug discovery. Br J Pharmacol 2011; 162(6): 1239-49.
[http://dx.doi.org/10.1111/j.1476-5381.2010.01127.x] [PMID: 21091654]

[26]   Surabhi S, Singh B. COMPUTER AIDED DRUG DESIGN: AN OVERVIEW. J Drug Deliv Ther 2018; 8(5): 504-9.
[http://dx.doi.org/10.22270/jddt.v8i5.1894]

[27]   Mohs RC, Greig NH. Drug discovery and development: Role of basic biological research. Alzheimers Dement (N Y) 2017; 3(4): 651-7.

[http://dx.doi.org/10.1016/j.trci.2017.10.005] [PMID: 29255791]

[28]   Chan HCS, Shan H, Dahoun T, Vogel H, Yuan S. Advancing Drug Discovery *via* Artificial Intelligence. Trends Pharmacol Sci 2019; 40(8): 592-604.
[http://dx.doi.org/10.1016/j.tips.2019.06.004] [PMID: 31320117]

[29]   Yu W, Jr ADM. Chapter 5 Computer-Aided Drug Design Methods. Antibiot. Methods Protoc 2017; 1520: pp. 85-106.

[30]   Njogu PM, Guantai EM, Pavadai E, Chibale K. Computer-Aided Drug Discovery Approaches against the Tropical Infectious Diseases Malaria, Tuberculosis, Trypanosomiasis, and Leishmaniasis. ACS Infect Dis 2016; 2(1): 8-31.
[http://dx.doi.org/10.1021/acsinfecdis.5b00093] [PMID: 27622945]

[31]   Batool M, Ahmad B, Choi S. A Structure-Based Drug Discovery Paradigm. Int J Mol Sci 2019; 20(11): 20.
[http://dx.doi.org/10.3390/ijms20112783] [PMID: 31174387]

[32]   Muhammed MT, Aki-Yalcin E. Homology modeling in drug discovery: Overview, current applications, and future perspectives. Chem Biol Drug Des 2019; 93(1): 12-20.
[http://dx.doi.org/10.1111/cbdd.13388] [PMID: 30187647]

[33]   França TCC. Homology modeling: an important tool for the drug discovery. J Biomol Struct Dyn 2015; 33(8): 1780-93.
[http://dx.doi.org/10.1080/07391102.2014.971429] [PMID: 25266493]

[34]   Munsamy G, Soliman MES. Homology Modeling in Drug Discovery-an Update on the Last Decade. Lett Drug Des Discov 2017; 14(9): 14.
[http://dx.doi.org/10.2174/1570180814666170110122027]

[35]   Cavasotto CN, Phatak SS. Homology modeling in drug discovery: current trends and applications. Drug Discov Today 2009; 14(13-14): 676-83.
[http://dx.doi.org/10.1016/j.drudis.2009.04.006] [PMID: 19422931]

[36]   Sliwoski G, Kothiwale S, Meiler J, Lowe EW Jr. Computational methods in drug discovery. Pharmacol Rev 2013; 66(1): 334-95.
[http://dx.doi.org/10.1124/pr.112.007336] [PMID: 24381236]

[37]   Dong S, Sun J, Mao Z, Wang L, Lu YL, Li J. A guideline for homology modeling of the proteins from newly discovered betacoronavirus, 2019 novel coronavirus (2019-nCoV). J Med Virol 2020; 92(9): 1542-8.
[http://dx.doi.org/10.1002/jmv.25768] [PMID: 32181901]

[38]   Grifoni A, Sidney J, Zhang Y, Scheuermann RH, Peters B, Sette A. A Sequence Homology and Bioinformatic Approach Can Predict Candidate Targets for Immune Responses to SARS-CoV-2. Cell Host Microbe 2020; 27(4): 671-680.e2.
[http://dx.doi.org/10.1016/j.chom.2020.03.002] [PMID: 32183941]

[39]   Tilocca B, Soggiu A, Sanguinetti M, *et al.* Comparative computational analysis of SARS-CoV-2 nucleocapsid protein epitopes in taxonomically related coronaviruses. Microbes Infect 2020; 22(4-5): 188-94.
[http://dx.doi.org/10.1016/j.micinf.2020.04.002] [PMID: 32302675]

[40]   Uddin MB, Hasan M, Harun-Al-Rashid A, Ahsan MI, Imran MAS, Ahmed SSU. Ancestral origin, antigenic resemblance and epidemiological insights of novel coronavirus (SARS-CoV-2): Global burden and Bangladesh perspective. Infect Genet Evol 2020; 84: 104440.
[http://dx.doi.org/10.1016/j.meegid.2020.104440] [PMID: 32622082]

[41]   Bai C, Warshel A. Critical Differences between the Binding Features of the Spike Proteins of SARS-CoV-2 and SARS-CoV. J Phys Chem B 2020; 124(28): 5907-12.
[http://dx.doi.org/10.1021/acs.jpcb.0c04317] [PMID: 32551652]

[42]   Wu C, Liu Y, Yang Y, *et al.* Analysis of therapeutic targets for SARS-CoV-2 and discovery of

potential drugs by computational methods. Acta Pharm Sin B 2020; 10(5): 766-88.
[http://dx.doi.org/10.1016/j.apsb.2020.02.008] [PMID: 32292689]

[43]   Hall DC Jr, Ji HF. A search for medications to treat COVID-19 *via in silico* molecular docking models of the SARS-CoV-2 spike glycoprotein and 3CL protease. Travel Med Infect Dis 2020; 35: 101646.
[http://dx.doi.org/10.1016/j.tmaid.2020.101646] [PMID: 32294562]

[44]   Feng S, Luan X, Wang Y, *et al.* Eltrombopag is a potential target for drug intervention in SARS-Co--2 spike protein. Infect Genet Evol 2020; 85: 104419.
[http://dx.doi.org/10.1016/j.meegid.2020.104419] [PMID: 32540428]

[45]   Qing X, Lee XY, De Raeymaeker J, *et al.* Pharmacophore Modeling: Advances, Limitations, And Current Utility in Drug Discovery. J Receptor Ligand Channel Res 2014; 7: 81-92.

[46]   Yang SY. Pharmacophore modeling and applications in drug discovery: challenges and recent advances. Drug Discov Today 2010; 15(11-12): 444-50.
[http://dx.doi.org/10.1016/j.drudis.2010.03.013] [PMID: 20362693]

[47]   Akram M, Waratchareeyakul W, Haupenthal J, Hartmann RW, Schuster D. Pharmacophore Modeling and *in Silico/in Vitro* Screening for Human Cytochrome P450 11B1 and Cytochrome P450 11B2 Inhibitors. Front Chem 2017; 5: 104.
[http://dx.doi.org/10.3389/fchem.2017.00104] [PMID: 29312923]

[48]   Schaller D, Šribar D, Noonan T, *et al.* Next Generation 3D Pharmacophore Modeling. Wiley Interdiscip Rev Comput Mol Sci 2020; 10(4): 1-20.
[http://dx.doi.org/10.1002/wcms.1468]

[49]   Khedkar SA, Malde AK, Coutinho EC, Srivastava S. Pharmacophore modeling in drug discovery and development: an overview. Med Chem 2007; 3(2): 187-97.
[http://dx.doi.org/10.2174/157340607780059521] [PMID: 17348856]

[50]   Sirois S, Wei DQ, Du Q, Chou KC. Virtual screening for SARS-CoV protease based on KZ7088 pharmacophore points. J Chem Inf Comput Sci 2004; 44(3): 1111-22.
[http://dx.doi.org/10.1021/ci034270n] [PMID: 15154780]

[51]   Radwan AA, Alanazi FK. *In Silico* Studies on Novel Inhibitors of MERS-CoV: Structure-Based Pharmacophore Modeling, Database Screening and Molecular Docking. Trop J Pharm Res 2018; 17(3): 513-7.
[http://dx.doi.org/10.4314/tjpr.v17i3.18]

[52]   Dhankhar P, Dalal V, Singh V, Tomar S, Kuma P. Computational Guided Identification of Novel Potent Inhibitors of NTD-N-Protein of SARS-CoV-2. ChemRxiv 2020.
[http://dx.doi.org/10.26434/chemrxiv.12280532.v1]

[53]   Idris MO, Yekeen AA, Alakanse OS, Durojaye OA. Computer-Aided Screening for Potential TMPRSS2 Inhibitors: A Combination of Pharmacophore Modeling, Molecular Docking and Molecular Dynamics Simulation Approaches. J Biomol Struct Dyn 2020; 1-19.
[PMID: 32672528]

[54]   Arun KG, Sharanya CS, Abhithaj J, Francis D, Sadasivan C. Drug Repurposing against SARS-CoV-2 Using E-Pharmacophore Based Virtual Screening, Molecular Docking and Molecular Dynamics with Main Protease as the Target. J Biomol Struct Dyn 2020; 0: 1-12.
[PMID: 32571168]

[55]   Yoshino R, Yasuo N, Sekijima M. Identification of key interactions between SARS-CoV-2 main protease and inhibitor drug candidates. Sci Rep 2020; 10(1): 12493.
[http://dx.doi.org/10.1038/s41598-020-69337-9] [PMID: 32719454]

[56]   Silva Andrade B, Ghosh P, Barh D, *et al.* Computational screening for potential drug candidates against the SARS-CoV-2 main protease. F1000 Res 2020; 9: 514.
[http://dx.doi.org/10.12688/f1000research.23829.2] [PMID: 33447372]

[57]   Jain P, Dorik R, Jain M, Campus I, Pradesh-india M. Identification of Pharmacophoric Features and

Novel Compounds for Inhibition of SARS-Cov-2 Main Protease. 2020.
[http://dx.doi.org/10.20944/preprints202004.0329.v1]

[58]   Gentile D, Patamia V, Scala A, Sciortino MT, Piperno A, Rescifina A. Putative Inhibitors of SARS-CoV-2 Main Protease from A Library of Marine Natural Products: A Virtual Screening and Molecular Modeling Study. Mar Drugs 2020; 18(4): 18.
[http://dx.doi.org/10.3390/md18040225] [PMID: 32340389]

[59]   Beura S, Chetti P. *In-Silico* Strategies for Probing Chloroquine Based Inhibitors against SARS-CoV-2. J Biomol Struct Dyn 2020.

[60]   Karaman M. Pharmacophore Analyses of SARS-CoV-2 Active Main Protease Inhibitors Using Pharmacophore Query and Docking Study. ChemRxiv. Cambridge: Cambridge Open Engage 2020.
[http://dx.doi.org/10.26434/chemrxiv.12443276.v1]

[61]   Haider Z, Muneeb Subhani M, Ansar Farooq M, *et al. In Silico* Discovery of Novel Inhibitors against Main Protease (Mpro) of SARS-CoV-2 Using Pharmacophore and Molecular Docking Based Virtual Screening from ZINC Database. Prepr. 2020.

[62]   J A, Francis D, C.S S, kumar Arun, C S, Variyar J. Repurposing Simeprevir, Calpain Inhibitor IV and a Cathepsin F Inhibitor Against SARS-CoV-2: A Study Using *in silico* Pharmacophore Modeling and Docking Methods. 2020.

[63]   Stefaniu A. Introductory Chapter: Molecular Docking and Molecular Dynamics Techniques to Achieve Rational Drug Design. In: Molecular Docking and Molecular Dynamics. IntechOpen 2019.

[64]   Pak Y, Wang S. Application of a Molecular Dynamics Simulation Method with a Generalized Effective Potential to the Flexible Molecular Docking Problems. J Phys Chem B 2000; 104(2): 354-9.
[http://dx.doi.org/10.1021/jp993073h]

[65]   Salmaso V, Moro S. Bridging Molecular Docking to Molecular Dynamics in Exploring Ligand-Protein Recognition Process: An Overview. Front Pharmacol 2018; 9: 923.
[http://dx.doi.org/10.3389/fphar.2018.00923] [PMID: 30186166]

[66]   Okimoto N, Futatsugi N, Fuji H, *et al.* High-performance drug discovery: computational screening by combining docking and molecular dynamics simulations. PLOS Comput Biol 2009; 5(10): e1000528.
[http://dx.doi.org/10.1371/journal.pcbi.1000528] [PMID: 19816553]

[67]   Kothandan G, Ganapathy J. A Short Review on the Application of Combining Molecular Docking and Molecular Dynamics Simulations in Field of Drug Discovery. J Chosun Nat Sci 2014; 7(2): 75-8.
[http://dx.doi.org/10.13160/ricns.2014.7.2.75]

[68]   Amin M, Sorour MK, Kasry A, Sorour MK, Kasry A. Comparing the Binding Interactions in the Receptor Binding Domains of SARS-CoV-2 and SARS-CoV. J Phys Chem Lett 2020; 11(12): 4897-900.
[http://dx.doi.org/10.1021/acs.jpclett.0c01064] [PMID: 32478523]

[69]   Ling R, Dai Y, Huang B, *et al. In silico* design of antiviral peptides targeting the spike protein of SARS-CoV-2. Peptides 2020; 130: 170328.
[http://dx.doi.org/10.1016/j.peptides.2020.170328] [PMID: 32380200]

[70]   Souza PFN, Lopes FES, Amaral JL, Freitas CDT, Oliveira JTA. A molecular docking study revealed that synthetic peptides induced conformational changes in the structure of SARS-CoV-2 spike glycoprotein, disrupting the interaction with human ACE2 receptor. Int J Biol Macromol 2020; 164: 66-76.
[http://dx.doi.org/10.1016/j.ijbiomac.2020.07.174] [PMID: 32693122]

[71]   Paasche A, Zipper A, Schäfer S, Ziebuhr J, Schirmeister T, Engels B. Evidence for substrate binding-induced zwitterion formation in the catalytic Cys-His dyad of the SARS-CoV main protease. Biochemistry 2014; 53(37): 5930-46.
[http://dx.doi.org/10.1021/bi400604t] [PMID: 25196915]

[72]   Suárez D, Díaz N. SARS-CoV-2 Main Protease: A Molecular Dynamics Study. J Chem Inf Model

2020; 60(12): 5815-31.
[http://dx.doi.org/10.1021/acs.jcim.0c00575] [PMID: 32678588]

[73] Thuy BTP, My TTA, Hai NTT, *et al.* Investigation into SARS-CoV-2 Resistance of Compounds in Garlic Essential Oil. ACS Omega 2020; 5(14): 8312-20.
[http://dx.doi.org/10.1021/acsomega.0c00772] [PMID: 32363255]

[74] Vardhan S, Sahoo SK. *In silico* ADMET and molecular docking study on searching potential inhibitors from limonoids and triterpenoids for COVID-19. Comput Biol Med 2020; 124: 103936.
[http://dx.doi.org/10.1016/j.compbiomed.2020.103936] [PMID: 32738628]

[75] Kiran G, Karthik L, Shree Devi MS, *et al.* *In Silico* computational screening of Kabasura Kudineer - Official Siddha Formulation and JACOM against SARS-CoV-2 spike protein. J Ayurveda Integr Med 2020; S0975-9476(20)30024-3.
[http://dx.doi.org/10.1016/j.jaim.2020.05.009] [PMID: 32527713]

[76] Mpiana PT, Ngbolua KT, Tshibangu DST, *et al.* Identification of potential inhibitors of SARS-CoV-2 main protease from *Aloe vera* compounds: A molecular docking study. Chem Phys Lett 2020; 754: 137751.
[http://dx.doi.org/10.1016/j.cplett.2020.137751] [PMID: 33518775]

[77] Rao P, Shukla A, Parmar P, *et al.* Reckoning a fungal metabolite, Pyranonigrin A as a potential Main protease (M^{pro}) inhibitor of novel SARS-CoV-2 virus identified using docking and molecular dynamics simulation. Biophys Chem 2020; 264: 106425.
[http://dx.doi.org/10.1016/j.bpc.2020.106425] [PMID: 32663708]

[78] Bharadwaj S, Lee KE, Dwivedi VD, Kang SG. Computational insights into tetracyclines as inhibitors against SARS-CoV-2 M^{pro} *via* combinatorial molecular simulation calculations. Life Sci 2020; 257: 118080.
[http://dx.doi.org/10.1016/j.lfs.2020.118080] [PMID: 32653520]

[79] Peele KA, Potla Durthi C, Srihansa T, *et al.* Molecular docking and dynamic simulations for antiviral compounds against SARS-CoV-2: A computational study. Informatics Med Unlocked 2020; 19: 100345.
[http://dx.doi.org/10.1016/j.imu.2020.100345] [PMID: 32395606]

[80] Barros RO, Junior FLCC, Pereira WS, Oliveira NMN, Ramos RM. Interaction of Drug Candidates with Various SARS-CoV-2 Receptors: An *in Silico* Study to Combat COVID-19. J Proteome Res 2020; 19(11): 4567-75.
[http://dx.doi.org/10.1021/acs.jproteome.0c00327] [PMID: 32786890]

[81] Kumar Y, Singh H, Patel CN. *In silico* prediction of potential inhibitors for the main protease of SARS-CoV-2 using molecular docking and dynamics simulation based drug-repurposing. J Infect Public Health 2020; 13(9): 1210-23.
[http://dx.doi.org/10.1016/j.jiph.2020.06.016] [PMID: 32561274]

[82] Marinho EM, Batista de Andrade Neto J, Silva J, *et al.* Virtual screening based on molecular docking of possible inhibitors of COVID-19 main protease. Microb Pathog 2020; 148: 104365.
[http://dx.doi.org/10.1016/j.micpath.2020.104365] [PMID: 32619669]

[83] Liang J, Pitsillou E, Karagiannis C, *et al.* Interaction of the prototypical α-ketoamide inhibitor with the SARS-CoV-2 main protease active site *in silico*: Molecular dynamic simulations highlight the stability of the ligand-protein complex. Comput Biol Chem 2020; 87: 107292.
[http://dx.doi.org/10.1016/j.compbiolchem.2020.107292] [PMID: 32485652]

[84] Bhowmik D, Nandi R, Jagadeesan R, Kumar N, Prakash A, Kumar D. Identification of potential inhibitors against SARS-CoV-2 by targeting proteins responsible for envelope formation and virion assembly using docking based virtual screening, and pharmacokinetics approaches. Infect Genet Evol 2020; 84: 104451.
[http://dx.doi.org/10.1016/j.meegid.2020.104451] [PMID: 32640381]

[85] Kumar S, Sharma PP, Shankar U, *et al.* Discovery of new hydroxyethylamine analogs against 3cl^{pro}

protein target of sars-cov-2: molecular docking, molecular dynamics simulation, and structure-activity relationship studies. J Chem Inf Model 2020; 60(12): 5754-70.
[http://dx.doi.org/10.1021/acs.jcim.0c00326] [PMID: 32551639]

[86]   Kumar A, Voet A, Zhang KYJ. Fragment based drug design: from experimental to computational approaches. Curr Med Chem 2012; 19(30): 5128-47.
[http://dx.doi.org/10.2174/092986712803530467] [PMID: 22934764]

[87]   Erlanson DA, Davis BJ, Jahnke W. Fragment-based drug discovery: advancing fragments in the absence of crystal structures. Cell Chem Biol 2019; 26(1): 9-15.
[http://dx.doi.org/10.1016/j.chembiol.2018.10.001] [PMID: 30482678]

[88]   Kirsch P, Hartman AM, Hirsch AKH, Empting M. Concepts and core principles of fragment-based drug design. Molecules 2019; 24(23): 4309.

[89]   Murray CW, Rees DC. The rise of fragment-based drug discovery. Nat Chem 2009; 1(3): 187-92.
[http://dx.doi.org/10.1038/nchem.217] [PMID: 21378847]

[90]   Tang B, He F, Liu D, Fang M, Wu Z, Xu D. AI-aided design of novel targeted covalent inhibitors against SARS-CoV-2. bioRxiv 2020.
[http://dx.doi.org/10.1101/2020.03.03.972133]

[91]   Gao J, Zhang L, Liu X, *et al.* Repurposing low-molecular-weight drugs against the main protease of severe acute respiratory syndrome coronavirus 2. J Phys Chem Lett 2020; 11(17): 7267-72.
[http://dx.doi.org/10.1021/acs.jpclett.0c01894] [PMID: 32787337]

[92]   Choudhury C. Fragment tailoring strategy to design novel chemical entities as potential binders of novel corona virus main protease. J Biomol Struct Dyn 2020; 0: 1-14.
[PMID: 32452282]

[93]   Verma M, Bansal D. Novel Potential Inhibitors Against SARS-CoV-2 Using Artificial Intelligence. ChemRxiv 2020.

[94]   Hartenfeller M, Schneider G. *De Novo* Drug Design. Chemoinformatics and Computational Chemical Biology. In: Bajorath J, Ed. Methods in Molecular Biology (Methods and Protocols). Totowa, NJ: Humana Press 2010; 672: pp. 299-323.
[http://dx.doi.org/10.1007/978-1-60761-839-3_12]

[95]   Kalyaanamoorthy S, Chen YPP. Structure-based drug design to augment hit discovery. Drug Discov Today 2011; 16(17-18): 831-9.
[http://dx.doi.org/10.1016/j.drudis.2011.07.006] [PMID: 21810482]

[96]   Loving K, Alberts I, Sherman W. Computational approaches for fragment-based and *de novo* design. Curr Top Med Chem 2010; 10(1): 14-32.
[http://dx.doi.org/10.2174/156802610790232305] [PMID: 19929832]

[97]   Yuan Y, Pei J, Lai L. LigBuilder V3: A Multi-Target *de novo* Drug Design Approach. Front Chem 2020; 8: 142.
[http://dx.doi.org/10.3389/fchem.2020.00142] [PMID: 32181242]

[98]   Bung N, Krishnan SR, Bulusu G, Roy A. *De Novo* Design of New Chemical Entities (NCEs) for SARS-CoV-2 Using. Artif Intell 2020.

[99]   Sousa SF, Cerqueira NM, Fernandes PA, Ramos MJ. Virtual screening in drug design and development. Comb Chem High Throughput Screen 2010; 13(5): 442-53.
[http://dx.doi.org/10.2174/138620710791293001] [PMID: 20236061]

[100] Subramaniam S, Mehrotra M, Gupta D. Virtual high throughput screening (vHTS)--a perspective. Bioinformation 2008; 3(1): 14-7.
[http://dx.doi.org/10.6026/97320630003014] [PMID: 19052660]

[101] Good AC, Krystek SR, Mason JS. High-throughput and virtual screening: core lead discovery technologies move towards integration. Drug Discov Today 2000; 5(12) (Suppl. 1): 61-9.

[http://dx.doi.org/10.1016/S1359-6446(00)00015-5] [PMID: 11564568]

[102] Bajorath J. Integration of virtual and high-throughput screening. Nat Rev Drug Discov 2002; 1(11): 882-94.
[http://dx.doi.org/10.1038/nrd941] [PMID: 12415248]

[103] Kontoyianni M. Docking and Virtual Screening in Drug Discovery. 2017; pp. 55-266.
[http://dx.doi.org/10.1007/978-1-4939-7201-2_18]

[104] Sharma K, Morla S, Goyal A, Kumar S. Computational guided drug repurposing for targeting 2'--ribose methyltransferase of SARS-CoV-2. Life Sci 2020; 259: 118169.
[http://dx.doi.org/10.1016/j.lfs.2020.118169] [PMID: 32738360]

[105] Wang J. Fast Identification of Possible Drug Treatment of Coronavirus Disease-19 (COVID-19) through Computational Drug Repurposing Study. J Chem Inf Model 2020; 60(6): 3277-86.
[http://dx.doi.org/10.1021/acs.jcim.0c00179] [PMID: 32315171]

[106] Iftikhar H, Ali HN, Farooq S, Naveed H, Shahzad-Ul-Hussan S. Identification of potential inhibitors of three key enzymes of SARS-CoV2 using computational approach. Comput Biol Med 2020; 122: 103848.
[http://dx.doi.org/10.1016/j.compbiomed.2020.103848] [PMID: 32658735]

[107] Cavasotto C, Di Filippo J. *In Silico* Drug Repurposing for COVID□19: Targeting SARS□CoV□2 Proteins through Docking and Consensus Ranking. Mol Inform 2020.
[PMID: 32722864]

[108] Gao K, Nguyen DD, Chen J, Wang R, Wei GW. Repositioning of 8565 Existing Drugs for COVID-19. J Phys Chem Lett 2020; 11(13): 5373-82.
[http://dx.doi.org/10.1021/acs.jpclett.0c01579] [PMID: 32543196]

[109] Gurung AB, Ali MA, Lee J, Farah MA, Al-Anazi KM. Unravelling lead antiviral phytochemicals for the inhibition of SARS-CoV-2 M^{pro} enzyme through *in silico* approach. Life Sci 2020; 255: 117831.
[http://dx.doi.org/10.1016/j.lfs.2020.117831] [PMID: 32450166]

[110] Bahadur Gurung A, Ajmal Ali M, Lee J, Abul Farah M, Mashay Al-Anazi K. Structure-based virtual screening of phytochemicals and repurposing of FDA approved antiviral drugs unravels lead molecules as potential inhibitors of coronavirus 3C-like protease enzyme. J King Saud Univ Sci 2020; 32(6): 2845-53.
[http://dx.doi.org/10.1016/j.jksus.2020.07.007] [PMID: 32837113]

[111] Gahlawat A, Kumar N, Kumar R, *et al.* Structure-Based Virtual Screening to Discover Potential Lead Molecules for the SARS-CoV-2 Main Protease. J Chem Inf Model 2020; 60(12): 5781-93.
[http://dx.doi.org/10.1021/acs.jcim.0c00546] [PMID: 32687345]

[112] Kandeel M, Al-Nazawi M. Virtual screening and repurposing of FDA approved drugs against COVID-19 main protease. Life Sci 2020; 251: 117627.
[http://dx.doi.org/10.1016/j.lfs.2020.117627] [PMID: 32251634]

[113] Jiménez-Alberto A, Ribas-Aparicio RM, Aparicio-Ozores G, Castelán-Vega JA. Virtual screening of approved drugs as potential SARS-CoV-2 main protease inhibitors. Comput Biol Chem 2020; 88: 107325.
[http://dx.doi.org/10.1016/j.compbiolchem.2020.107325] [PMID: 32623357]

[114] Ngo ST, Quynh Anh Pham N, Thi Le L, Pham D-H, Vu V V. Computational Determination of Potential Inhibitors of SARS-CoV-2 Main Protease. 2020.
[http://dx.doi.org/10.1021/acs.jcim.0c00491]

[115] Tsuji M. Potential anti-SARS-CoV-2 drug candidates identified through virtual screening of the ChEMBL database for compounds that target the main coronavirus protease. FEBS Open Bio 2020; 10(6): 995-1004.
[http://dx.doi.org/10.1002/2211-5463.12875] [PMID: 32374074]

[116] Mohammad T, Shamsi A, Anwar S, *et al.* Identification of high-affinity inhibitors of SARS-CoV-2

main protease: Towards the development of effective COVID-19 therapy. Virus Res 2020; 288: 198102.
[http://dx.doi.org/10.1016/j.virusres.2020.198102] [PMID: 32717346]

[117]   Santibáñez-Morán MG, López-López E, Prieto-Martínez FD, Sánchez-Cruz N, Medina-Franco JL. Consensus Virtual Screening of Dark Chemical Matter and Food Chemicals Uncover Potential Inhibitors of SARS-CoV-2 Main Protease. RSC Advances 2020; 10(42): 25089-99.
[http://dx.doi.org/10.1039/D0RA04922K]

[118]   Hage-Melim LIDS, Federico LB, de Oliveira NKS, *et al.* Virtual screening, ADME/Tox predictions and the drug repurposing concept for future use of old drugs against the COVID-19. Life Sci 2020; 256: 117963.
[http://dx.doi.org/10.1016/j.lfs.2020.117963] [PMID: 32535080]

[119]   Singh N, Decroly E, Khatib A-M, Villoutreix BO. Structure-based drug repositioning over the human TMPRSS2 protease domain: search for chemical probes able to repress SARS-CoV-2 Spike protein cleavages. Eur J Pharm Sci 2020; 153: 105495.
[http://dx.doi.org/10.1016/j.ejps.2020.105495] [PMID: 32730844]

[120]   Romeo A, Iacovelli F, Falconi M. Targeting the SARS-CoV-2 spike glycoprotein prefusion conformation: virtual screening and molecular dynamics simulations applied to the identification of potential fusion inhibitors. Virus Res 2020; 286: 198068.
[http://dx.doi.org/10.1016/j.virusres.2020.198068] [PMID: 32565126]

[121]   Naik B, Gupta N, Ojha R, Singh S, Prajapati VK, Prusty D. High throughput virtual screening reveals SARS-CoV-2 multi-target binding natural compounds to lead instant therapy for COVID-19 treatment. Int J Biol Macromol 2020; 160: 1-17.
[http://dx.doi.org/10.1016/j.ijbiomac.2020.05.184] [PMID: 32470577]

[122]   Ruan Z, Liu C, Guo Y, *et al.* SARS-CoV-2 and SARS-CoV: Virtual screening of potential inhibitors targeting RNA-dependent RNA polymerase activity (NSP12). J Med Virol 2021; 93(1): 389-400.
[http://dx.doi.org/10.1002/jmv.26222] [PMID: 32579254]

[123]   Mirza MU, Froeyen M. Structural elucidation of SARS-CoV-2 vital proteins: Computational methods reveal potential drug candidates against main protease, Nsp12 polymerase and Nsp13 helicase. J Pharm Anal 2020; 10(4): 320-8.
[http://dx.doi.org/10.1016/j.jpha.2020.04.008] [PMID: 32346490]

[124]   Wang X, Song K, Li L, Chen L. Structure-based drug design strategies and challenges. Curr Top Med Chem 2018; 18(12): 998-1006.
[http://dx.doi.org/10.2174/1568026618666180813152921] [PMID: 30101712]

[125]   Gelman R, Bayatra A, Kessler A, Schwartz A, Ilan Y. Targeting SARS-CoV-2 receptors as a means for reducing infectivity and improving antiviral and immune response: an algorithm-based method for overcoming resistance to antiviral agents. Emerg Microbes Infect 2020; 9(1): 1397-406.
[http://dx.doi.org/10.1080/22221751.2020.1776161] [PMID: 32490731]

CHAPTER 2

Potential Antiviral Medicinal Plants against Novel SARS-CoV-2 and COVID-19 Outbreak

Nazim Sekeroglu[1,2,*] and **Sevgi Gezici**[2,3]

[1] *Gaziantep University, Faculty of Science and Literature, Department of Biology, Gaziantep 27310, Turkey*

[2] *Gaziantep University, Faculty of Medicine, Department of Medical Biology, Gaziantep 27310, Turkey*

[3] *Department of Molecular Biology and Genetics, Faculty of Science and Literature, Kilis 7 Aralik University, 79000 Kilis, Turkey*

Abstract: Considering the significant worldwide threat of the Novel Corona Virus Disease 2019 (COVID-19), it is urgently needed to develop efficient prevention and treatment approaches in order to reduce the prevalence rate and mortality of the disease. Even though numerous experimental and clinical studies have been currently conducted for development of drug and vaccine througout the world, and some partially effective vaccines and chemical drugs have been developed against COVID-19. Herbal and dietary plants, including fruits, vegetables, herbs, spices, cereals, and edible tubers/roots, can play a significant role in enhancing the immune system and how to increase our defense barriers against virus-related diseases. Accordingly, medicinal plants with a wide range of bioactive compounds, which exhibit remarkable antiviral activities, can be used as a preventive treatment and cure for COVID-19. In order to combat SARS-CoV-2, rockrose (*Cistus* spp.), lemon balm (*Melissa officinalis* L.), rosemary (*Rosmarinus officinalis* L.), licorice root (*Glyrrhiza glabra* L.), olive leaf (*Olea europea* L.), peppermint (*Mentha piperita* L.), basil (*Ocimum bacilicum* L.), sumac (*Rhus coriaria* L.) and different species of thyme (*Origanum, Thymus* and *Thymbra*) are important medicinal plants that exhibit valuable antiviral activities. Since medicinal and aromatic plants are a worldwide hot topic, the aim of the current review was to provide an overview of the development of plant-based anti-coronavirus agents to the researchers based on an extensive literature survey.

Keywords: Antiviral, Bioactive compounds, *Cistus* spp., Coronavirus, COVID-19, Immune system, Lemon balm, Licorice root, Medicinal plants, *Melissa officinalis* L., *Ocimum bacilicum* L., Olive leaf, Outbreak, Peppermint, Pharmaceutical industry, Phytochemicals, *Rhus coriaria* L., Rockrose, Rosemary, Therapeutics.

* **Corresponding author Nazim Sekeroglu:** Department of Horticulture, Faculty of Agriculture, Kilis 7 Aralik University, Postal Code 79000 Kilis, Turkey; Fax: +90 (342) 360 1013; Tel: +90 (342) 360 1200 - 1922; E-mails: nazimsekeroglu@gantep.edu.tr, nsekeroglu@gmail.com

1. INTRODUCTION

Throughout history, pandemics of large-scale outbreaks of infectious diseases such as Cholera, Ebola, Bubonic Plague, AIDS (acquired immunodeficiency syndrome), Influenza, SARS (severe acute respiratory syndrome), MERS (Middle East Respiratory Syndrome), and currently COVID-19 (new type coronavirus, causative agent 2019-nCoV or SARS-CoV-2) have had a major impact worldwide. The Corona Virus Disease 2019 (COVID-19) has had similar outbreaks to other viral diseases because of its global spread, social and economic response, however, the recent coronavirus outbreak is different from other occurrences. It has different biological properties, cell surface proteins, and mechanisms of infection [1 - 4].

Coronaviruses (CoVs) belong to the family of Coronaviridae, Arteriviridae, Roniviridae and Mesoniviridae families. Of which, Coronaviridae is the largest family and includes the subfamily of Coronavirinae, which is now classified into four main genera including alpha (α)-coronavirus, beta (β)-coronavirus, gamma (γ)-coronavirus and delta (δ)-coronavirus, according to the 10th report on virus taxonomy from the International Committee on Taxonomy of Viruses (ICTV). α-coronaviruses and β-coronaviruses infect a variety of host cells and can cause life-threatening pneumonia in humans and some animals such as feline, porcine, canine, mice, bovine, bat and rodent, while γ-coronavirus and δ-coronavirus are specific of birds, but some of them can also infect other organisms [4 - 6].

CoV is an enveloped virus group that carries single-strand RNA (ribonucleic acid) genome, capable of infecting humans and a wide variety of animal species. This group of viruses, especially causing upper respiratory infections, lead symptoms that present with a sore throat, dry cough, runny nose, weakness, and fatigue. In coronavirus infections, the symptoms occur in the form of colds or flu; the virus infects the ciliated epithelial cells in the nasopharynx through the aminopeptidase N receptor or sialic acid receptors and leads to the development of damage to the epithelial cells as the virus multiplies. In addition, chemokines and interleukins released from the cells cause the development of local illnesses in the patients. In the following process, the virus can pass to pneumocytes, blood, urine (up to 2 months), and in some cases to feces [3, 7, 8].

Based on the ICTV, FECV (Feline Enteric Coronavirus) and FIPV (Feline Infectious Peritonitis Virus), the porcine TGEV (Transmissible Gastro- Enteritis Virus), Porcine PEDV (Epidemic Diarrhea Virus), PRCoV (Porcine Respiratory Coronavirus), CCoV (Canina Coronavirus), and human coronaviruses (HCoV-229E and HCoVNL63) are of α-coronaviruses. Betacoronaviruses also compromise Murine coronavirus (MHV) and Bovine Coronavirus (BCoV), and human coronaviruses (HCoV-OC43, HCoV-HKU1, SARS-CoV, MERS-CoV, and SARS-CoV-2 Interestingly, recent studies have shown that the new human CoV, namely SARS-CoV-2, shares high genome sequence similarity (almost 79.5%) with SARS-CoV, and similar to SARS-CoV, the new human CoV recognizes ACE2 (angiotensin-converting enzyme 2) cellular receptor to enter host cells. In addition to that, it has a similar genomic structure as SARS-CoV and MERS-CoV [2, 9 - 11].

Even though the history of CoVs began in the 1940's, the first human CoVs subsequently named as (i) human CoV 229E (HCoV-229E) and (ii) HCoV-OC43, were reported in the 1960's. After that, the virologist tried to identify the general structure of CoVs, as well as-replication and pathogenesis. The studies among the virologist provided to the discovery of other new human coronaviruses such as (iii) HCoV- Hong Kong University 1 (HKU1), (iv) HCoV-NL63, (v) severe acute respiratory syndrome (SARS)-CoV and (vi) the Middle East respiratory syndrome (MERS)-CoV [2, 9, 12]. Among these coronaviruses, SARS-CoV was identified as a global outbreak in 2003, and it had affected 8422 people in 32 countries, with a mortality rate of 10-15% [3, 13]. Then, almost after ten years, another highly pathogenic coronavirus MERS-CoV epidemic emerged in Middle Eastern countries in 2013. Although the major MERS-CoV pandemic has happened in the Republic of Korea, it was observed worldwide at any age of people with a fatality rate of 39% [12, 14]. Following this outbreak, the novel coronavirus outbreak, namely 2019-nCoV or COVID-19 emerged in Wuhan State, Hubei Province, China, in December 2019. It has spread to many countries and territories, United States (US), Spain, Italy, France, Germany, the United Kingdom, China, Iran, Turkey, Belgium and Netherlands are among the hardest hit countries. Since, it has infected many people and caused a high mortality rate in a short period, the World Health Organization (WHO) has declared the outbreak of the new coronavirus as a pandemic. As of 19 November 2021, more than 255,324,963 confirmed cases of COVID-19 have been reported in more than 180 countries and territories, resulting in approximately 5,127,696 deaths all around the world [15, 16]. Moreover, the number of infected patients with COVID-19 and death from this virus are alarmingly increasing day by day. Due to its rapid infection ability from person to person and high mortality rate, it has become vital to find efficient and accurate therapy strategies to urgently combat this disaster [17, 18]. Thus, scientists have been racing to understand the different coronavirus diseases in order to discover possible therapy strategies including drugs, therapeutic antibodies, cytokines, nucleic acid-based therapy, vaccines to treat and prevent coronavirus infections. Among the given strategies, researching effective antiviral drugs, which may be appropriate to cure the COVID-19, have apparently been the most certain option for immediate treatment. Nevertheless, no specific drug has been studied or made available for COVID-19 cases and clinical trials, as well as evaluations of potential antiviral drug candidates, are ongoing in various laboratories [3, 19].

Previous and current studies on developing drugs against many viral diseases reported that medicinal plants used in traditional folk medicine have significant importance for the ongoing development of therapeutic agents and broad-spectrum drugs for the treatment of coronavirus-related diseases because the medicinal plants are rich in bioactive and phytochemical compounds [20 - 23]. The information included in this review reveals that an extraordinary effort to develop efficient plant-based drugs against existing coronavirus outbreaks is urgently required to reduce the overwhelming impact the virus has on the worldwide healthcare systems. Some of the most important medicinal plants which could be used in the fight against various types of viruses are highlighted in the presented review (Fig. **1**). The emphasized plants not only prevent the replication of viral genome in virus infections, but they are also highly effective in strengthening the autoimmune system.

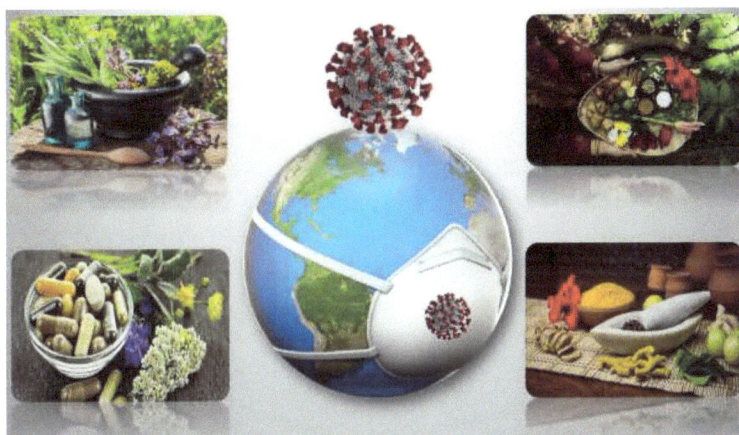

Fig. (1). Pictorial Abstract of the Chapter.

2. MEDICINAL PLANT-BASED ANTIVIRAL THERAPEUTICS

Even though almost all human coronaviruses had been threatened to human populations, SARS-CoVs and MERS-CoVs have been identified as the most harmful infections for humans until emerging the new coronaviruses infection in December 2019. So far, numerous antiviral agents have been discovered in order to block the virus entry to the host cells and inhibit viral replication and transcription in coronaviruses infections. Scientists have been putting huge effort into elucidating the structure and genomic organization of the virus, as well as discovering effective treatment regimens, and developing drugs and vaccines. Pfizer/BioNTech, Moderna, AstraZeneca, Sinovac, Sputnik V, and Johnson & Johnson (J&J) COVID-19 vaccines have been approved by the US Food and Drug

Administration (FDA) in clinically; however, there are over 200 vaccine candidates in clinical trials and preclinical studies being pursued around the worldwide. In addition to vaccines, antiviral drugs have been developed against COVID-19, and Remdesivir was the first drug approved by FDA [20 - 25].

Medicinal plants have offered many advantages in providing prevention and cure to a number of antiviral diseases as an alternative medicine throughout history. Bearing in mind the numerous benefits medicinal plants offer, they should be considered as an effective method of preventing and treating the COVID-19. Worldwide a large number of researches are focused on the utilization of plant-based antiviral therapeutics [26, 27]. Recent scientific reports related to potential medicinal plants on COVID-19, and commonly used other antiviral medicinal plants have been summarized below.

In a previous report, Praneem, a drug formulation obtained from neem tree (*Azadirachta indica*) extracts, was found as applicable herbal drugs for HIV therapy [28]. In another study, Geloy (*Tinospora cordifolia*) extract, was successfully used for controlling the severity of Dengue infections and has also been recommended for COVID-19 in India [24, 29].

Flavonoids compounds contained in mandarin (*Citrus reticulata*), pummelo (*Citrus maxima*) and sweet orange (*Citrus sinensis*) were tested in terms of antiviral activities. The results of *in vitro* and *in vivo* experiments indicated that they possess immune enhancer potentials in the host cells by inhibiting the expression of proinflammatory cytokines such as interleukin (IL), granulocyte colony-stimulating factor (GCSF), human interferon-inducible protein 10 (IP-10 or CXCL10), monocyte chemoattractant protein-1 (MCP-1/CCL2), macrophage inflammatory protein 1 alpha (MIP-1α), inducible nitric oxide synthase (iNOS), cyclooxygenase-2 (COX-2), and tumor necrosis factor-alpha (TNFα). In addition, molecular docking studies were revealed naringenin, naringin, hesperetin, hesperidin, neohesperidin and nobiletin showed binding affinity to the ACE-2 receptor of the coronavirus, of which especially naringin ($C_{27}H_{32}O_{14}$, Mw = 580 g/mol) and hesperetin ($C_{28}H_{34}O_{15}$, Mw = 302 g/mol), classified in to the flavonoids, had a stronger binding affinity to the ACE-2 [20].

Potential inhibitory effects of compounds obtained from *Citrus* sp., *Curcuma* sp., *Caesalpinia sappan*, and *Alpinia galanga* against SARS-CoV-2 infection were demonstrated based on the molecular docking studies by Utomo *et al.* (2020). In this study, *Citrus* sp. showed the best binding to ACE2, which resulted in inhibition on the development of the SARS-CoV-2, followed by *A. galanga, C. sappan*, and *Curcuma* sp., suggesting they could be used to overcome COVID-19 outbreak [30].

In Wuhan city of China, the researchers have tried a combination of western medicine and traditional medicine in treating a family case of COVID-19 with typical symptoms of the disease. Shuang Huang Lian oral liquid (SHL), containing extracts of three Chinese herbs, namely, *Lonicera japonica*, *Scutellaria baicalensis*, and *Forsythia suspensa*, is a Chinese traditional patent medicine. SHL has been used to treat cold, sore throat, cough, respiratory tract infection, bronchial asthma, acute bronchitis, and light pneumonia caused by bacteria/viruses clinically. Findings from these preliminary studies demonstrated that SHL is able to inhibit 2019-nCoV, and it might be an efficient treatment for COVID-19 patients after obtaining adequate clinical evidence [22].

Besides medicinal plants above suggested to combat COVID-19, commonly used and scientifically approved by their antiviral effects have been given in detail. Rockrose (*Cistus* spp.), lemon balm (*Melissa officinalis* L.), rosemary (*Rosmarinus officinalis* L.), licorice (*Glyrrhiza glabra* L.), olive leaf (*Olea europea* L.), peppermint (*Mentha piperita* L.), basil (*Ocimum bacilicum* L.), sumac (*Rhus coriaria* L.) and different species of thyme (*Origanum, Thymus* and *Thymbra*), which are grown naturally in Mediterranean countries and widely known in folk medicine, are presented in this section. The presented plants (Table **1**) have been known for their strong antioxidant capacities, broad antimicrobial activities and immune enhancer properties, along with powerful antiviral activities. Therefore, the use of these plants and natural products obtained from them may help to modulate the immune system in preventing viral diseases.

Table 1. Antiviral Medicinal Plants and Phytochemicals.

Medicinal Plant	Extract/Phytochemicals	Antiviral Activity	References
Melissa officinalis L.	Ethanol extract	Avian infectious bronchitis virus (IBV)	[100]
	EOs (lemon balm oil)	avian influenza virus (AIV) subtype H9N2	[47]
	EOs (lemon balm oil)	Herpes simplex virus (HSV-1 and HSV-2)	[51, 52]
	EOs (lemon balm oil)	Zika virus (ZIKV)	[57]
	leaves	Herpes simplex virus (HSV)	[48, 49]
	Extracts and EOs	herpes simplex virus (HSV), vaccinia virus, Semliki Forest and Newcastle virus	[50]
	Extracts	Herpes simplex virus type 1 (HSV-1), type 2 (HSV-2) and an acyclovir-resistant strain of HSV-1 (ACVres)	[58]
	Aqueous extracts	Herpes simplex virus (HSV-1)	[46, 53]
	Extracts and rosmarinic acid	Enterovirus 71 (EV71)	[54]

(Table 1) cont.....

Medicinal Plant	Extract/Phytochemicals	Antiviral Activity	References
Rosmarinus officinalis L.	oleanolic acid, rosmarinic acid and eucalyptol	Herpes simplex virus (HSV-1) and hepatitis B virus (HBV)	[55]
	Extracts	and an acyclovir-resistant strain of HSV-1 (ACVres)	[58]
	Extracts	Herpes simplex virus type 1 (HSV-1), type 2 (HSV-2) Newcastle disease virus (NDV), herpes simplex, vaccinia, Semliki Forest, and West Nile viruses	[59]
	Aqueous extracts	Measles, Mumps, Vesicular Stomatitis Virus (VSV), and Herpes simplex vius type-2 (HSV-2).	[60]
	EOs (rosemary) and 1.8 cineole	hepatitis A virus (HAV)	[56]
	EOs (rosemary) and rosemarinic acid	Zika virus (ZIKV)	[57]
	Extracts	Herpes simplex virus type 1 (HSV-1), type 2 (HSV-2)	[61]
	EOs (rosemary)	Herpes simplex virus type 1 (HSV-1)	[62]
	Extracts, cineol	Influenza A H1N1 and oral herpes simplex HSV-1	[63]
	EOs (rosemary)	avian infectious bronchitis (IBV),	[65]
Glycyrrhiza glabra L.	Extracts and kanzonol V	Zika virus (ZIKV)	[57]
	Extracts and glycyrrhizin	hepatitis A, B and C	[85]
	Extracts, glycyrrhizin and glycyrrhizic acid	Hepatitis (B and C), Human immmunodeficiency virus (HIV-1) and SARS coronavirus	[86, 87]
	Extracts and bioactive contituents (glycyrrhizin, glycocoumarin, lycopranocoumarin and lycocarbon A)	herpes simplex, Epstein-Barr, human cytomegalovirus, hepatitis A, B and C, influenza, HIV, varicella zoster virus (VZV) and SARS coronaviruses	[89]
	Aqueous extracts	herpes simplex virus (HSV-1)	[96]
	Extracts and glycyrrhizic acid	HIV, hepatitis B and C, SARS coronavirus and herpes simplex virus (HSV)	[97, 98]
	Extracts and glycyrrhizin	Swine epidemic diarrhea virus	[88]
	Extracts and glycyrrhizic acid	Kaposi's sarcoma herpes virus (KSHV)	[99]
	glycyrrhizic acid	hepatitis B virus	[93]

(Table 1) cont.....

Medicinal Plant	Extract/Phytochemicals	Antiviral Activity	References
Glycyrrhiza glabra L.	Extracts and glycyrrhizin	influenza A virus (FLUAV), Rift Valley fever virus (RVFV), Human metapneumotic virus (HMPV), echovirus 1 (EV1), chikungunya virus (CHIKV), Ross River virus (RRV), Zika virus (ZIKV), hepatitis C virus (HCV), Sindbis virus (SINV), HIV-1, cytomegalovirus (CMV), hepatitis B virus (HBV) and herpes simplex virus type 1 (HSV-1),	[90]
	Extracts and glycyrrhizin	influenza virus, SARS coronavirus and Human immmunodeficiency virus (HIV)	[85, 89]
	Extracts	influenza A virus	[95]
Cistus spp.	Extracts from *C. laurifolius*	Parainfluenza - 3 (PI - 3)	[42]
	Extracts from *C. incanus* subsp. *tauricus*	(H1N1, H5N1 and H7N7), Pathogenic avian influenza virus (HPAIV)	[43]
	Extracts from *C. incanus* subsp. *tauricus*	Influanza A and B virus and other viruses	[44]
Olea europea L.	Olea leaf aqueous extracts	Newcastle disease virus (NDV)	[67]
	Olea leaf and compounds (oleanolic acid and calcium elenolate)	Herpes simplex, polio viruses, rhinoviruses, mycoviruses, coxsackie virus, Varicella zoster, encephalo myocarditis	[66]
	Olea leaf	Herpes simplex virus (HSV-1) and infectious laryngotracheitis viruses	[68, 69]
	oleuropein glycosides and their enzyme hydrolysates [2- (4-hydroxyphenyl) ethyl and 2- (3,4-dihydroxyphenyl)]	rotavirus, rhinovirus, parvovirus, hepatitis, Epstein-Barr, herpes simplex, influenza, varicella zoster and cat leukemia viruses	[73]
	Olea leaf	Herpes simplex virus (HSV-1)	[70]
	Olea leaf and oleuropein	viral hemorrhagic septicemia virus (VHSV)	[71]
	Olea leaf aqueous extracts	rhesus rotavirus	[72]
Salvia officinalis L.	Ethanol extract	Avian infectious bronchitis virus (IBV)	[100]
	Aqueous extracts	Herpes simplex virus (HSV-1)	[46]
	Aqueous extracts	Measles, Mumps, Vesicular Stomatitis Virus (VSV), and Herpes simplex vius type-2 (HSV-2).	[60]
	EOs, 1,8-cineol and α-thujone	SARS☐CoV and HSV☐1	[102]
	Extracts and EOs	Zika virus (ZIKV)	[57]

(Table 1) cont.....

Medicinal Plant	Extract/Phytochemicals	Antiviral Activity	References
Mentha piperita L.	Ethanol extract	Avian infectious bronchitis virus (IBV)	[100]
	Aqueous extract, hydroalcoholic extract, essential oil	Herpes-simplex virus (HSV-1 and HSV-2)	[101]
	Aqueous extracts	Herpes simplex virus (HSV-1)	[46]
	Extracts	Herpes simplex virus type 1 (HSV-1), type 2 (HSV-2) and an acyclovir-resistant strain of HSV-1 (ACVres)	[58]
Origanum vulgare L.	Ethanol extract	Avian infectious bronchitis virus (IBV)	[100]
	Ethanol extracts and bioactive compounds	Respiratory syncytial virus (RSV), Coxsackievirus B3 (CVB3) and herpes simplex virus type 1 (HSV-1)	[79]
	Aqueous and ethanol extracts	equine arteritis virus (EAV), feline calicivirus (FCV), canine distemper virus (CDV), canine adenovirus (CAV), and canine cororavirus (CCoV)	[80]
	EOs and carvacrol	nonenveloped murine norovirus (NMN)	[81]
Thymus vulgaris L.	Ethanol extract	Avian infectious bronchitis virus (IBV)	[100]
	Aqueous extract, hydroalcoholic extract,	Herpes-simplex virus (HSV-1 and HSV-2)	[101]
	EOs	Herpes-simplex virus (HSV-1)	[51]
	Aqueous extracts	Measles, Mumps, Vesicular Stomatitis Virus (VSV), and Herpes simplex vius type-2 (HSV-2)	[60]
Thymus capitatus (L.) Hoffmans. & Link	EOs	Herpes simplex virüs (HSV-1), Echovirus 11 (ECV11) and Adenovirus (ADV)	[82]
	EOs	Herpes simplex virüs (HSV-2),	[84]
Ocimum bacilium L.	Aqueous extract	Herpes-simplex virus (HSV-1)	[101]
	Extracts and monoterpenes (camphor, thymol, linalool, and 1,8-cineole)	Bovine viral diarrhoea virus (BVDV)	[103]
	Extracts and purified compounds (apigenin, linalool and ursolic acid)	Herpes viruses (HSV), adenoviruses (ADV), hepatitis B virus), coxsackievirus B1 (CVB1) and enterovirus 71 (EV71)	[104]
Rhus coriaria L.	Fruit extracts	acyclovir resistant HSV-1	[105]
	Aqueous extract	hepatitis B virus (HBV)	[106]

2.1. Rockrose (*Cistus* spp.)

Cistus species, known as rockrose, are native to South Europe and North Africa, but they are naturally growing in Mediterranean climate. These plants are perennial, evergreen or semi-evergreen shrubs with hairy and stick left up to 30-100 cm height. Their attractive flowers, from white to dark pink, differ with species. Cistus genus contains about 20 different species and they spread in dry places, warm borders and coastal gardens. Cistus word comes from the Greek kiste "box" and refers to the shape of the capsules. "Laden", "Ladanum" or "Labdanum" with brown color, reminiscent, sticky, fragrant, easily crushed and softened between fingers, bitter taste and easily flammable oleoresin is a valuable natural product. This product is obtained especially from *Cistus albiflorus*, *Cistus creticus*, *Cistus ladanifer* and *Cistus maculatus* species [31, 32]. Labdanum is the best plant substitute for *ambergris* from sperm whales and is important for perfume manufacturing. This sticky substance is traditionally collected by whipping the bushes, so that the exudate adheres to the leather thongs or, in Crete by combing it from the hides of sheep and goats with a leather rake, or *ladanisterion*. Ladanum is now produced commercially in France and Spain [32]. According to scientific reports on different *Cistus* species, while the essential oils of *C. villosus* and *C. salviifolius* were rich in nonterpen compounds, *C. creticus* and *C. monspeliensis* had labdanum-type diterpenes [33]. *Cistus creticus* had tannins, heterosides, triterpenes, flavonoids and saponosides [34]. *C. salviifolius*, *C. creticus* and *C. laurifolius* species naturally grow in Turkey, first two species had mostly trans-tilirosid (mono-coumaroyl kaempferol glucoside), hyperin and myrsetin flavonoids compounds were the main compounds in *C. laurifolius* [35] Main used parts of the plant are oleoresin and essential oil. This medicinal plant has many properties like aromatic, stimulant, expectorant, astringent, antibiotic, mucus secretion enhancer and anti-diarrhea [31, 32]. The plant is economically used as a fumigant in Turkey and a fixative in lavender, fern and chypre perfumes, and as a commercial food flavoring for baked foods, soft drinks, ice cream and candies [32]. Five Cistus species (*C. creticus, C. parviflorus, C. salvifolius, C. monspeliensis* and *C. laurifolius*) naturally grow in coastal regions of Turkey. These plants are locally known as Pamucak, Karağan, Karahan and Tavşancıl. Plant leaves contain resin, essential oil, and tannins, and have been traditionally used as infusion (5%) as astringent, stimulant and expectorant in Anatolian Folk Medicine. Infusion (2%) of *C. laurifolius* is locally used for diabetes and wool dying in Konya district [30, 36, 37]. Scientific studies approved that different *Cistus* species, with rich phytochemical contents, have many pharmacological effects such as high antioxidant, strong antibacterial, antifungal, anti-inflammatory, antiviral, cytotoxic, and anticancer [38]. Having high phenolic and flavonoid content, *Cistus creticus* growing in Turkey was approved for its strong antibacterial, antioxidant and DNA protective effects [39]. Another scientific report indicated that Cistus is a higher antioxidant capacity than even green tea, which is known as the best antioxidant. In this study, Cistus and green tea were compared by their antioxidant capacities and the results showed that both plant extracts had a high content of polyphenols. Thus, they have strong antibacterial, antifungal and anti-inflammatory properties. In addition, a clinical study in 300 patients with upper respiratory tract infections demonstrated that patients treated with the Cistus product (Cistus incanus PANDALIS® (CYSTUS052®)) resulted in a more significant reduction in symptoms compared to treatment with the green tea product (Morgentau®) [40]. Different extracts (water, methanol, chloroform, ethyl acetate and bütanol) prepared from topsoil parts of five Cistus species (*C. creticus* L., *C. laurifolius* L., *C. monspeliensis* L., *C. parviflorus* Lam. and *C. salviifolius* L.) naturally growing in Turkey were studied for their antimicrobial activities against [*Staphylococcus aureus* (ATCC 29213 and ATCC 25923), *Streptococcus faecalis* (ATCC 29212), *Bacillus subtilis* (ATCC 6633), *Bacillus cereus* (RSKK 1122), *Pseudomonas aeruginosa* (ATCC 27853), *Escherichia coli* (ATCC 25922) and *Candida albicans* (ATCC 10231)], and the results showed that Cistus extracts had antimicrobial activity against all the investigated microbial except for *Pseudomonas aeruginosa* and *Candida albicans* [41]. The ethanolic extract and its fractions obtained using re-extraction by hexane, chloroform (CHCl3), butanol, and remaining-water (r-H2O) of *C. laurifolius* were investigated for their *in vitro* bioactivities. According to results, the *C. laurifolius* extracts had (minimum inhibitory concentration 32 µg/mL) exerted a strong antimicrobial activity against Gram-negative bacteria of *E. coli, P. mirabilis, K. pneumoniae*, and *A. baumannii*, and the Hexane extract of the plant (cytopathogenic effect of 32-8 µg/mL) had antiviral activity on PI-3 [42]. Various doses of *Cistus incanus* subsp. *tauricus* extracts had antiviral effects against different influenza viruses [A/Puerto-Rico/8/34 (H1N1), pathogenic avian influenza virus (HPAIV) A/FPV/Bratislava/79 (H7N7) and human isolate HPAIV (H5N1 sub-type (A/Thailand/1(KAN-1)/2004 (H5N1)] without any side effects [43]. Placebo-controlled clinical study was carried out to investigate the clinical effect of a *Cistus* extract (CYSTUS052) in 160 patients with infections of the upper respiratory tract caused by different microbial (*Staphylococcus aureus, Streptococcus pneumoniae, Mycoplasma pneumoniae, Chlamydia pneumonia, Haemophilus influenzae*, Influenza A Virus, Influenza B Virus and other viruses), and the results showed that a score of subjective symptoms decreased significantly over the course of treatment with Cistus, whereas treatment with placebo resulted in a less distinct decrease of symptoms [44].

2.2. Lemon Balm (*Melissa Officinalis* L.)

Lemon balm is an herbaceous perennial plant native to Europe, Eastern Mediterranean and Asia minor [32, 45]. Of three species in the *Melissa* genus,

Melissa officinalis L. is well-known and cultivated for over 2.000 years. Originally known as a honey plant, the name Melissa came from the Greek word "honey bee". Therapeutic properties of this ancient antiviral medicinal plant, with lemon scented essential oil, were discovered by Arab physicians around 10th century. In 1990s, its antiviral power was also clinically confirmed that topical applications of Melissa are effective in the treatment of Herpes Simplex infections if started in early stages. Lemon balm was called the "Elixir of life" by Paracelsus (1493-1541) and described it as "sovereign for the brain, strengthening the memory, and powerfully chasing away melancholy" by John Evelyn (1620-1706) [32]. Lemon balm has a valuable essential oil. The drug should contain at least 0.05% the oil having citronellal (30-40%) with small quantities as the main components of the oil together with citral (10-30%), which compromises two compounds as geranial (citral a) and neral (citral b), monoterpene glycosides, triterpenes, sesquiterpenes (germacrene D and ®-caryophyllene), phenolic acids (around 4% rosmarinic acid) and flavonoids. Lemon balm has many pharmacological properties such as cooling, sedative, carminative, digestive, antipyretic, spasmolytic, antiviral, antibacterial, and antifungal. The plant is used internally for nervous disorders, indigestion associated with nervous tension, hyperthyroidism, depression, and anxiety and popular as a calming and soothing herb, mainly for the treatment of minor sleeplessness and nervous stomach disorders in adults and children [32, 45]. Fresh leaves give a lemon flavor to salads, soups, sauces, herb vinegars, game and fish. Herbal tea can be prepared sole or combination with *Chamaemelum nobile* and *Filipendula ulmaria* and *Humulus lupulus* for nervous indigestion. Commercial volatile oil of the *Melissa* is commonly adulterated with lemon (*Citrus lemon*) or lemongrass (*Cymbopogon citratus*) [32].

Lemon balm (*Melissa officinalis* L.), peppermint (*Mentha × piperita* L.), and sage (*Salvia officinalis* L.) plant species, belonging to the family of Lamiaceae, exerted powerful activity for infection of HIV-1 in T-cell lines in a concentration dependently manner. It has been clearly concluded that the extracts from the tested plants may be used as candidate anti-HIV-1 agents at non-cytotoxic concentrations [46].

Essential oils of *M. officinalis* and synergistic effect with oseltamivir were evaluated against avian influenza virus (AIV) subtype H9N2 were evaluated *in vitro* in MDCK (Madin-Darby Canine Kidney) cells. The findings showed that lemon balm suppresses replication of AIV, also a synergetic activity was observed with oseltamivir and lemon balm [47].

In another work, a double-blind, placebo-controlled, randomized trial was carried out to treat HSV-infected patients who had a history of recurrent diseases using a standardized balm mint cream, Lomaherpan® (Natural Medicine Research, Emmenthal, Germany), prepared from *M. officinalis* leaves extract. The tested formulation of the cream was found to be efficient for the treatment of herpes simplex labilalis without any side toxic effects [48]. In a case study, involving 115 patients and another subsequent placebo-controlled double-blind 116 patients contributed significantly to the corroborative evidence of the antiviral activity of extract from *Melissa* leaves against herpes simplex infections. The finding of the study provided *M. officinalis* extracts were able to reduce the symptom scores of viral infections in the treated group [49].

The antiviral activity of water extracts from *M. officinalis* was established against herpes simplex virus, vaccinia virus, Semliki Forest virus and Newcastle virus. The EOs of the plant contains caffeic acid, rosmarinic, ferulic acid, linalool, oleanolic acid, ursolic acid, pomolic acid, protocatechuic acid, and luteolin--glucoside were also found to have anti-HSV-2 in the cell cultures [50].

The lemon balm oil was analyzed in regards to its antiviral capacities against herpes simplex virus type 1 (HSV-1) and herpes simplex virus type 2 (HSV-2) using *in vitro* plaque reduction assay on monkey kidney cells. Because of the lipophilic nature of the lemon balm, significant inhibition was observed in both herpesviruses. EO of *M. officinalis*, which is capable of suppressing virus penetration into the host cell, thus it might be useful for the treatment of herpetic infections [51]. The lemon oil was found to inhibit HSV-2 replication in the cell culture against human larynx epidermoid carcinoma cells (HEp-2) cells. The replication of HSV-2 was inhibited, indicating that the lemon oil contains anti-HSV-2 phytochemicals [52]. The virucidal and antiherpes effects of the extracts from *M. officinalis* were performed in cell culture, and a considerable anti-HIV effect was observed after treatment with a maximum tolerable concentration of 0.25% [53].

The results of the study conducted by Chen *et al*. (2017) indicate that *M. officinalis* and its constituent rosmarinic acid have anti-EV71 (Enterovirus 71) activities and could have to be potential therapeutic and prophylactic uses against EV71 infection [54].

2.3. Rosemary (*Rosmarinus Officinalis* L.)

Having two different species (*R. officinalis* L. and *R. eriocalix* syn. *lavandulaceus*, *R. officinalis* var. *prostrates*), *Rosmarinus* genus is native to Mediterranean climate and cultivated in Mediterranean countries. These aromatic, evergreen plants naturally grow on the dry, rock woodland and scrub in the coastal regions. Rosemary plants are a symbol for friendship, loyalty and remembrance throughout the world. The name Rosmarinus comes from the Latin word for dew of the sea, referring to dew-like appearance with its pale-blue flower far away. Rosemary is rich in secondary metabolites and is a well-known medicinal plant in history. Queen Elizabeth of Hungary, 72 years old, recovered from her serious illnesses after using the "Hungary Water" (rosemary tops macerated in alcohol) the King of Poland offered her. Greek scholars used rosemary garlands to improve their memory and concentration during their examinations [32]. Rosemary contains volatile oil (2.5%) with 1,8 cinole, α-pinene and camphor as main components; several flavonoids and their glycosides (diosmetin, luteolin and genkwainin), phenolic acids (rosmarinic acid), bitter diterpenes (carnosol, rosmanol), triterpenes (oleanic and ursolic acid), triterpen alcohols (α-amyrin, ®-amyrin and botulin), tannins, romaricine). The flavonoid diosmin is reputedly more effective than rutin (from *Ruta graveolens*). With these phytochemicals, rosemary has many useful pharmacological effects like strong antiseptic, antimicrobial, antibacterial, antifungal, antiviral, antioxidant, anti-inflammatory, astringent, antispasmodic, a stimulant, a painkiller and a tonic. This wonderful plant is used internally for depression, apathy, nervous exhaustion, headaches and migraines associated with nervous tension or feeling cold, poor circulation, carminative, stomachic and digestive problems associated with anxiety. Rosemary has useful externally for rheumatism, arthritis, neuralgia, muscular injuries, wounds, dandruff, scurf, and hair loss, as well. Besides its medicinal uses, fresh or dried rosemary leaves are important culinary herbs for flavoring meats, sausages, liqueurs, stuffings, soups and stews and also used as an ingredient in many cosmetics [32, 45].

Rosmarinus officinalis with bioactive compounds, namely oleanolic acid, rosmarinic acid and eucalyptol were found to possess strong antiviral and antimicrobial activities. Khwaza *et al.*, (2018) investigated the anti-HIV activity of carboxylic acid functional groups on oleanolic acid, which can inhibit HIV-1 replication in the host cell. These compounds also resulted in potent antiviral activity against influenza virus and hepatitis B virus by blocking the entry of the virus to the host cell, as well as inhibiting the virus compounds synthesis [55].

In a recent study, four essential oils, lemon (*Citrus limon*), sweet orange (*Citrus sinensis*), grapefruit (*Citrus paradisi*), and rosemary cineole (*Rosmarinus officinalis* chemotype 1.8 cineole) were analyzed for antiviral properties against hepatitis A virus (HAV). The findings demonstrated that cineole found in rosemary oil was found to be the most effective. Thus, it was capable of reducing viral infections in soft fruits [56].

An *in-silico* search for phytochemical anti-Zika virus (ZIKV) phytochemicals was carried out and generated ZIKV protease, methyltransferase, and RNA-dependent RNA polymerase using homology modeling techniques using molecular docking analyses. Overall, 2263 plant-derived secondary metabolites have been docked in the study. Some of the metabolites that have drug-like properties have exerted remarkable docking profiles to the ZIKV protein targets, and several of these are found in relatively common herbal medicines, including balsacone B is found in the buds of balsam poplar (*Populus balsamifera*), kanzonol V is found in licorice root (*Glycyrrhiza glabra*), cinnamoylechinaxanthol is found in *Echinacea* root; cimiphenol is found in black cohosh (*Actaea racemosa*, syn. *Cimicifuga racemosa*); and rosemarinic acid is found in several common herbs including rosemary (*Rosmarinus officinalis*), lemon balm (*Melissa officinalis*), and common sage (*Salvia officinalis*) [57].

The lemon balm (*Melissa officinalis*), peppermint (*Mentha x piperita*), prunella (*Prunella vulgaris*), rosemary (*Rosmarinus officinalis*), sage (*Salvia officinalis*) and thyme (*Thymus vulgaris*) extracts from species of the Lamiaceae family were screened for their antiviral inhibitory effects against Herpes simplex virus type 1 (HSV-1), type 2 (HSV-2) and an acyclovir-resistant strain of HSV-1 (ACVres). All the tested extracts exhibited anti-HSV activity; however; lemon balm, peppermint and thyme with high selectivity indices were found the most potent extracts. The results showed that the extracts inhibit HSV before adsorption, but have no effect on the intracellular virus replication. In this study, the researchers concluded that the extracts could be applied as supplementary topical treatment application against recurrent Herpes infections [58].

Several plants of the Labiaceae family were identified for antiviral activity on the Newcastle disease (NDV), herpes simplex, vaccinia, Semliki Forest, and West Nile viruses in cell culture. According to the findings of the study, aqueous extracts of sage (*Salvia cyprea*), marjoram (*Origanum maj*orana), wild thyme (*Thymus serpyllum*), American pennyroyal (*Hedeoma pulegioides*), Crea monda (*Satureia* sp.) and Spanish and French thymes (*Thymus* sp.) all had some antiviral effects against NDV and herpes simplex virus, while rosemary (*Rosmarinus officinalis*), horehound (*Marrubiutn vulgare*), and catnip (*Nepeta cataria*) extracts were not detectable as the most potent ones [59]. In another work performed with well-known plant species of Lamiacea family, aqueous extracts of the plants were assessed for their inhibitory potential against RNA and DNA viruses, namely Measles, Mumps, Vesicular Stomatitis Virus (VSV), and HSV-2. The work revealed that the rosemary (*Rosmarinus officinalis*) showed the highest antiviral potential followed by the thyme. On the other hand, Sage (*Salvia officinalis*) at a concentration of 1500 µg/ml, Rosemary (*Rosmarinus officinalis*) at a concentration of 500 µg/ml and Thyme (Thymus vulgaris) at a concentration of 2250 µg/ml exerted antiviral potentials [60].

Anti-biofilm and antiviral potential of leaf extracts from *Moringa oleifera* and *Rosmarinus officinalis* were aimed to evaluate by Nasr-Eldin *et al.* (2017). The antiviral results revealed that *M. oleifera* and rosemary extracts were not cytotoxic for Vero cells and showed inhibition on HSV-1and HSV-2 with inhibition percentages 43.2% and 21.4%, respectively [61].

In vitro antiviral activity of different concentrations of *Zataria multiflora*, *Eucalyptus caesia*, *Artemisia kermanensis*, *Satureja hotensis* and *Rosmarinus officinalis* essential oils against HSV-1 on Vero cells were analyzed in another study. The findings demonstrated that the oils studied in this research have a significant inhibitory effect on HSV-1. Additionally, anti- HSV activity of the tested EOs (concentration ≤ 0.02) did not show any cytotoxic effect on Vero cells viability [62].

Antiviral activity of the mixture plants was composed of equal parts (3.52% each) of *Eucalyptus globulus* CT cineol (leaf) and *Cinnamomum zeylanicum* CT cinnamaldehyde (bark), 3.00% of *Rosmarinus officinalis* CT cineol (leaf), 1.04% of *Daucus carota* CT carotol (seed), and 88.90% of *Camelina sativa* oil (seed) were tested on influenza A H1N1 and oral herpes simplex HSV-1. The mixture was found effective against H1N1 and HSV-1 viruses and may be valuable to treat influenza and post-influenza bacterial pneumonia infections. It can be concluded these plants could be very useful in clinical practice to combat common viral and bacterial infections [63].

In a research, effects of extracts from *R. officinalis* and some of the constituents isolated from ethyl acetate fraction of *R. officinalis* were evaluated using microneutralization assay and plaque assay against human respiratory syncytial virus (hRSV) replication. Among the tested bioactive constituents of *R. officinalis*, carnosic acid exhibited the most potent anti-hRSV activity [64].

In a recent study aimed to evaluate the capability of viral inhibition from the EOs obtained by hydrodistillation from *Lippia origanoides*, *Rosmarinus officinalis* and *Illicium verum* were tested against avian infectious bronchitis (IBV), belonging the genus of Coronavirus. It was observed that the three tested EOs in any concentration had statistically (p<0,05) significant antiviral effects, however the *R. officinalis* oil was found as the best [65].

2.4. Olive leaf (*Olea Europea* L.)

*Olea europe*a L. started to be mentioned since the existence of human beings. It has been considered as a symbol of peace and health since ancient times. All parts of this ancient plant, whose fruit and oil are used as food, can be found in every area of daily life. Olive seeds and olive leaves, which are considered as waste, are among the important elements of folk medicine. Olive leaf has traditionally been used against hypertension, urine enhancer, antipyretic, appetizing and constipation [31, 45]. In addition to the main active ingredient, oleuropein, which is thought to be effective on health, olive leaves contain numerous beneficial ingredients such as other seroiridoids (ligustrosite, oleasein), triterpenoids (oleanolic acid, uvaol), sterols, hydroxytyrosol, polyphenols (verbascosite, apigenin-7-glucoside, luteolin-7-glycoside), triterpenes (oleanolic acid), rutinoline (reolinolic acid) and diosmin), tannins, essential oils, organic acids, and resin [31, 45, 66].

Scientific studies indicate that olive fruit and oil contain a very high content of oleuropein; it even showed that the oleuropein substance found in the olive leaf are higher than the other parts, and it has proved to be an active phytochemical against many diseases. Oleuropein produces (-) elenolic acid compound, which is reported to have *in vitro* antiviral properties when hydrolyzed with acid. It has also been shown to have antiviral activity against many viruses such as parainfluenza, herpes simplex, pseudorabi, polio viruses (type-1, -2 and -3), rhinoviruses, mycoarditis, and two leukemia virus strains, thanks to rich oleanolic acid and calcium elenolate compounds of olive leaves [66]. Unlike the virus types studied by AMR, (2019), it was also revealed that water extracts obtained from olive leaves exhibit antiviral activity by decreasing the expression level of viral genes in chicken embryo fibroblast cells against the Newcastle disease virus (NDV), which is a highly contagious and economically important poultry virus [67]. In other studies, it has been demonstrated that olive leaves prevent HIV-1 and infectious laryngotracheitis viruses transition from cell to cell and acute infection of the viruses in the host. Moreover, most of the changes that occur in HIV-1 infected cells have been reported to reverse and regulate the expression of apoptosis inhibitor proteins (IAP1 and IAP2), calcium and protein kinase C pathway signal molecules (IL-2, IL-2Ra), and ornithine decarboxylase (ODC1) by olive leaves [68, 69]. In the study investigating *in vitro* antiviral activity of ethanol extracts from the olive leaf at different concentrations on Vero cells infected with herpes simplex virus-1 (HSV-1), olive leaf has been reported to significantly prevent HIV-1 development even at 1.25 mg/mL concentration, and decrease in virus proliferation depending on the concentration [70]. In another study conducted by Micol *et al.* (2005), the antiviral activity of olive extract and oleuropein, the main component of olive, were investigated against viral hemorrhagic septicemia virus (VHSV), which is a species of rapdovirus. It has been determined that both the extract and oleuropein can be used as natural antiviral agents against virus infection. Moreover, it has been suggested that oleuropein can be used to design antiviral agents [71]. In a study that tested the antiviral activity of about 150 plant species against rhesus rotavirus infections causing diarrhea, water extracts of olive leaf have been shown to be an agent that significantly inhibits rotavirus infections with $IC_{50}<300$ µg /mL inhibition concentration [72].

With drug development studies, William R. Fredrickson has created and patented orally available pharmaceutical forms of oleuropein glycosides in olive leaf and their enzyme hydrolysates [2- (4-hydroxyphenyl) ethyl and 2- (3,4-dihydroxyphenyl)] that can be used in the treatment of viral diseases in drug development studies. Oleuropein, the main active drug substance obtained by extracting olive leaves with different extraction techniques is used in this patent study, and different drug formulations have been developed to reduce viral symptoms caused by rotavirus, rhinovirus, parvovirus, hepatitis, Epstein-Barr, herpes simplex, influenza, varicella zoster and cat leukemia viruses [73].

Some mechanisms have been suggested regarding the mechanisms of olive leaf and oleuropein in preventing viral infections and their strong antiviral capacities. They are given as follows; (1) Reducing viral infection and / or spreading ability by preventing virus assembly to the host cell; (2) Inhibiting the production of amino acids that are crucial for viral development and protein synthesis; (3) Directly penetrating infected cells or reducing viral replication; (4) Neutralizing the production of reverse transcriptase and protease enzymes in the RNA viruses; (5) Increasing the release of the viral particle out of the host cell by stimulating phagocytosis [74].

2.5. Thyme Species (*Origanum, Thymus & Thymbra*)

Having distinguished phenolic compounds, like carvacrol and thymol that are isomers of each other, which give the thyme flavor, different plant species are commonly known as kekik in Turkey. These plant species (total 102 taxa) are native to the Mediterranean and belong to five different genera; *Thymus* (58 taxa), *Origanum* (26 taxa), *Satureja* (13 taxa), *Thymbra* (4 taxa) and *Coridothymus* (1 taxa) [37]. These kekik species are naturally grown throughout Turkey and are traditionally used by local people for many ethnobotanical purposes. Well-known and commercially traded kekik species are *Origanum onites* L. (Turkish Oregano), *Origanum vulgare* L. (Greek Oregano), *Origanum majorana* L. (Wild marjoram), *Thymbra spicata* L. (Zahter) and *Satureja hortensis* L. (Sater). Essential content and composition of these kekik species have already been investigated in many scientific studies. In previous scientific studies about *Origanum* species; essential oil contents varied between 1.3-7.7% in different species [75], and carvacrol contents as the main component of the essential oil, in commonly used *Origanum* taxa were highly variable that ranged from 47-89% (*O. onites*), 5-89% (*O. vulgare subsp. hirtum*), 53-80% (*O. majorana*). As an endemic kekik species, known as buckle kekik, *Origanum minutiflorum* had the highest carvacrol rate up to 98%. Other components of essential oils of *Origanum* species mentioned above were linalool, γ-terpinene, p-cymene, thymol and myrcene, and linalool type marjoram plants were also recorded [76]. As a natural element of Turkey flora, *Thymus* species had various essential oil contents (0.05-3.4%) by different taxa, and the main component of the essential oil of *Thymus* species, thymol content were determined from 17-70% in the *Thymus* species. Other determining components of the Thymus essential oil were carvacrol, linalyl acetate, linalool, γ-terpinene, p-cymene and geraniol, and some Thymus species apart from common Thymus had higher carvacrol (62%), geraniol (77%) and linalyl acetate (66) contents, as well [77]. Growing naturally in different parts of Turkey, zahter (*Thymbra spicata* var. *spicata* L.) plants were screened for their essential oil content and compositions. According to the results, it is found that essential contents were varied between 2.25% and 4.65%, and the main component of the zahter essential oil was found as carvacrol and thymol in the ranges of 14.34-91.77% and 0.27-40.68%, respectively. Another component of the zahter essential oil in the highest rates was γ-terpinene (0.40-21.83%) [78].

Six new phenolic compounds along with five known ones (2,5-dihydroxybenzoic acid, 3,4-dihydroxybenzoic acid, rosmarinic acid, origanoside, and maltol 60--(5-O-p-coumaroyl)-b-D-apiofuranosyl-b-Dglucopyranoside) were isolated from the ethanol extract of the whole plants of *Origanum vulgare*. The structures of the new compounds were identified with spectroscopic analyses and acid hydrolysis experiments. Moreover; the phenolic compounds combined with the previously isolated ones e-caffeic acid, amburoside A, oresbiusin A, (+)-(R)-butyl rosmarinate, apigenin, apigenin 7-O-b-D-glucoside, luteolin, 6,7,40-trihydroxyflavone, 5,7,30,40-tetrahydroxy-8-C-p-hydroxybenzylflavone and didymin). All these compounds were subjected to *in vitro* antioxidant evaluation with DPPH and FRAP assays. Additionally, their antiviral activities against the respiratory syncytial virus (RSV), Coxsackie virus B3 (CVB3) and herpes simplex virus type 1 (HSV-1) were determined by cytopathic effect (CPE) assay. In conclusion, all the examined compounds obtained from *Origanum vulgare* exerted high antioxidant capacity and antiviral [79].

In another study, antiviral activity of aqueous and ethanolic extracts of *Origanum vulgare* were determined against some viruses of veterinary importance (bovine viral diarrhea virus (BVDV), equine arteritis virus (EAV), equine influenza virus (EIV), feline calicivirus (FCV), canine distemper virus (CDV), canine adenovirus (CAV), and canine coronavirus (CCoV) by evaluating the possibility of inhibition of viral particles production. With respect to chemical analysis of the extracts of *O. vulgare*, identified in the water and ethanol extract phenolics were rosmarinic acid, caffeic acid, carnosol, p-coumaric acid, carnosic acid, luteolin, apigenin, kaempferol and quercetin. In conclusion, investigated compounds are responsible for the antiviral activity as well as which are the mechanisms involved. And, the results showed that the ethanolic extract of *O. vulgare* demonstrated lower cell viability than the aqueous extract and has significant antiviral activity against EAV and both aqueous and ethanolic extracts have antiviral action against CDV [80].

The antiviral activities of Oregano oil and its primary active component, carvacrol were studied against the non-enveloped murine norovirus (MNV), a human norovirus surrogate. The results demonstrated that carvacrol was effective in inactivating MNV within one hour of exposure by acting directly on the viral capsid and subsequently the RNA. It was also stated that the antiviral properties of oregano oil and carvacrol against MNV and demonstrate the potential of carvacrol as a natural food and surface (fomite) sanitizer to control human norovirus [81]. Essential oil samples distilled from *Thymus capitatus* (L.) Hoffmans. & Link was analyzed for their *in vitro* antiviral activity on Vero cells infected with Herpes simplex type 1 virus (HSV1), Echovirus 11 (ECV11) and Adenovirus (ADV). It was observed that thyme EOs significantly inhibited HSV1 and ECV11, while they affected ADV after penetration into the host cell. In this study, the EOs were also found to have strong antioxidant capacities, compared with synthetic Trolox antioxidants in this study [82].

Antioxidant and antimicrobial activities and chemical composition of essential oil and extracts of *Thymbra spicata* L. were investigated. In this study, eight different phenolic compounds (Protocatequic acid, p-OH benzoic acid, vanilic acid, syringic acid, ferulic acid, rutin, daizein and t-cinnamic acid) were determined in the plant extracts. The extracts were found to have strong antimicrobial activity and high antioxidant capacity [83]. Antiviral effect of the essential oils obtained from aerial parts of *T. spicata* L. was also investigated against HSV-2 (Herpes Simplex Virus type 2). It is found that *T. spicata* L., with a minimum concentration value of 40 µg/ml, significantly showed antiviral effect against HSV-2 compared to the control group and the essential oils had remarkable antiviral activity against HSV-2. This antiviral activity was attributed to the essential oil compounds of *T. spicata*, which were carvacrol, cymol, gama-terpinene and thymol [84]. In other work performed with essential oils of *T. vulgaris,* EOs were analyzed against Acyclovir-resistant clinical isolates of HSV-1, and it exhibited high levels of virucidal activity [51].

2.6. Licorice Root (*Glycyrrhiza Glabra* L.)

Glycyrrhiza genus, from the Leguminosae plant family, has 20 species found in a variety of habitats in the Mediterranean, tropical Asia, Australia and the Americas. This well-known ancient plant was processed in the liquorice extract in

Germany in the 11th century and cultivated in Italy in the 13th century [32]. Liquorice plant is native to Turkey and seven taxa (*Glycyrrhiza glabra* var. *glabra*, *Glycyrrhiza glabra* var. *glandulifera*, *Glycyrrhiza echinata*, *Glycyrrhiza aspera*, *Glycyrrhiza iconica*, *Glycyrrhiza flavescens* and *Glycyrrhiza asymmetrica*) are naturally growing in different part of the country [37]. Underground parts; roots and rhizomes, naturally or peeled from cortex, of *G. glabra* and other *Glycyrrhiza* species have been traditionally used in folk medicine for centuries throughout the world. *G. uralensis* is a key herb in Traditional Chinese Medicine (TCM) and other two species (*G. glabra* and *G. inflata*) known as *gan cao* (means as a sweet herb), and *Glycyrrhiza* plants have been used around 1250 different herbal formulations in TCM. The plant is called as "Yashtimadhu" in Ayurveda and is also an important medicinal herb in the Japanese Traditional Kampo Medicine system [32]. Fresh or dried roots of the plants are boiled in the water and then condensed with low pressure, thus liquorice extract, with bright black colored, distinguished sweet taste and water soluble, has been produced. This valuable natural product that is important for food and pharmaceutical industries called as "Meyanbalı" in Turkish language [31]. Liquorice root contains starch, sugars, gum, resin, flavone derivatives and glycyrrhizin (glycyrrhizic acid) [31], it also contains flavonoids, isoflavonoids and lactones that hydrolyzed when the fresh roots are dried [32]. Additionally, it contains triterpene saponins as glycyrrhizic acid (%2-15), and its aglicone glycyrrhetinic acid (24-hydroxy glycyrrhetinic) [45]. In southern part of Turkey, once dried and ponded into fiber, the liquorice is soaked with water and a special cold herbal infusion is prepared. This cold herbal drink has been abundantly consumed especially during hot summer months. A small amount of baking soda is added as a color enhancer; cinnamon and cloves are also added as a flavoring in the preparation of this dark colored sweet drink. Liquorice and its extract have been traditionally used as chest reliever, expectorant and cough suppressant in Turkey [31]. It is internally used for Addison's disease, asthma, bronchitis, coughs, peptic ulcer, arthritis, allergic complaints, and following steroid therapy. Not given to pregnant women or patients with anemia, high blood pressure, kidney diseases, or taking digoxin-based medication [32]. Liquorice and its extract have many pharmacological properties such as anti-inflammatory, antiviral, antimicrobial, cytotoxic (towards tumor cells), antihepatotoxic, antioxidant, anti-histaminic and immune stimulant [45].

Licorice and glycyrrhiza compounds have long been used as potential therapeutic agents for chronic hepatitis B and C, as well as human-induced immunodeficiency syndrome (AIDS) in folk medicine. Antiviral activity of glycyrrhizin and glycyrrhizic acid, which inhibit viral growth and cytopathology of hepatitis (A and C) and immunodeficiency virus (HIV) were clearly demonstrated in several studies [85]. Fiore *et al.* (2008) showed that glycyrrhizin and its derivatives from

G. glabra decrease hepatocellular damage in chronic hepatitis B and C, and antiviral activity against HIV-1, SARS-related coronavirus, respiratory syncytial virus, arboviruses, vaccinia virus, and vesicular stomatitis virus was also showed [86]. In a study conducted with glycyrrhizin, Crance *et al.* (2003) revealed antiviral effect of glycyrrhizin, through an inhibition of viral particles to host cell membrane binding, or *via* cellular signal transduction mechanisms. Thus, it was found to be a promising alternative treatment for viral diseases [87]. In swine epidemic diarrhea virus infection, glycyrrhizin has been reported to prevent viral proliferation by decreasing the virus entry into the cell and mRNA level of pro-inflammatory cytokines [88]. In another work, *in vitro* antiviral effects of *G. glabra* were observed against viruses leading respiratory tract infections such as influenza virus and the severe acute respiratory syndrome (SARS) corona virus, and human immunodeficiency virus (HIV) [85, 89].

Ianevski *et al.* (2019) were tested the broad spectrum antiviral activity of 108 active substances, including, acyclovir, famciclovir, phyllosiclovir, ganciclovir and valaciclovir; imatinib, erlotinib, gefitinib and dasatinib; telavancin, dalbavankin, oritavancin and teicoplanin; alisporivir and cyclo-sporin; minocycline and doxycycline; lovastatin and simvastatin, raloxifene and amiodarone; ritonavir and lopinavir; esomeprazole and omeprazole; camptothecin and topotecan; trifluridine and N-MCT; and quinine, brequinar, amodicuin, hydroxychloro-quinine, chloroquine, acetylsalicylic acid, azithromycin, pentosan polysulfate, thymmalfacin, camptothecin, topotecan, quinine and glycyrrhizin against 78 viruses with (-) single-stranded (ss)RNA, (+) ssRNA, double stranded (ds) RNA viruses like [influenza A virus (FLUAV), Rift Valley fever virus (RVFV), Human metapneumotic virus (HMPV), echovirus 1 (EV1), chikungunya virus (CHIKV), Ross River virus (RRV), Zika virus (ZIKV), hepatitis C virus (HCV), Sindbis virus (SINV), HIV-1, cytomegalovirus (CMV), hepatitis B virus (HBV) and herpes simplex virus type 1 (HSV-1), and others]. Among the tested active compounds, glycyrrhizin obtained from *G. glabra* root was determined as an effective immune booster against viral infections [90].

The pharmacological properties of the *G. glabra* extracts showed the presence of liquirtin, rhamnoliquirilin, glucoliquiritin apioside, liquiritigenin, prenyllicoflavone A, 1-metho-xyphaseolin, shinflavanone, semilicoisoflavone B, 1-methoxyficifolinol, shinpterocarpin, licopyranocoumarin, glisoflavone, licoarylcoumarin, isoangustone A, licoriphenone, and kanzonol R, glycyrrhizin, and several volatile components that possess anti-carcinogenic, antioxidant, antifungal, antibacterial and antiviral activities. Previous reports documented that the extracts of *G. glabra* were employed to assess potent antibacterial activities against *Bacillus subtilis, B. cereus, B. megaterium, Escherichia coli, Staphylococcus aureus, Enterococcus faecalis, Pseudomonas fluorescens, P.*

aeruginosa, Sarcina lutea, Salmonella paratyphi, S. dysenteriae, Vibrio parahaemolyticus and *V. mimicus* due to its rich phytochemical contents. Interestingly, it was revealed that chloroform, acetonic, ethyl acetate, and methanolic extracts of *G. glabra* inhibited bacterial growth of *S. typhimurium, E. coli* and *B. coagulans,* but no activity was observed towards *S. aureus, P. aeruginosa* and *E. faecalis* [91, 92]. In addition to antibacterial activities, Cinatl *et al.* (2003) demonstrated that the extracts of *G. glabra* and glycyrrhizic acid exerted strong antiviral effects against herpes simplex, Epstein-Barr, human cytomegalovirus, hepatitis (A, B and C), influenza, HIV, varicella zoster, and SARS coronaviruses and inhibited adsorption and penetration of the virus to the host cells. It was also reported that glycocoumarin, lycopranocoumarin, and lycocarbon A active substances found in licorice root inhibit the growth of giant cell structure in HIV-infected cell cultures by cellular signal transmissions such as protein kinase C, casein kinase II and transcription factors [89].

In recent research, licorice root and glycyrrhizic acid, a terpene isolated from the licorice roots, were found responsible for anti-viral, anti-inflammatory and hepatoprotective effects that causing a direct effect on hepatitis B virus through affecting the HBsAg (hepatitis B surface antigen) to extracellular secretion, evolving liver dysfunction in the patient, and finally enhancing the immune system in status of HBV [93].

In another study on the use of licorice root in traditional medicine, it was determined that licorice root and glycyrrhizinic acid have the effect of improving respiratory disorders, expectorant and enhancing immunity level. Furthermore, animal studies have revealed that licorice is able to prevent the replication and proliferation of influenza A virus and hepatitis B and C virus. Besides these viruses, licorice root has been shown to have *in vitro* antiviral activity against HIV-1 and SARS coronavirus-related infections [94]. In another study, licorice root has been reported to protect cells against influenza A virus infection and significantly reduce the number of infected cells [95].

Ghannad *et al.* (2014) investigated antiviral effects of liquorice root extracts on Vero cells infected with herpes simplex virüs-1 (HSV-1). It has been reported that licorice root at different concentrations had been found to be effective on the attachment of the virus to the host cell surface and it may be used as a potential anti-HIV-1 agent [96].

Clinical studies revealed that glycyrrhizic acid and its derivatives, triterpene glycosides, obtained from licorice root (*G. glabra* L. and *G. uralensis* Fisher) are a promising way of designing new and efficient drugs for the treatment of HIV, hepatitis B and C, SARS coronavirus and herpes simplex virus infections [97]. In a pilot study, it has also been concluded that licorice root extract has a synergistic effect with interferons and shows the capacity of inhibiting the expression of the hepatitis C virus particle at both RNA and protein levels and therefore can be an antiviral agent [98]. In a later study, glycyrrhizic acid has been shown to regulate the expression of latent-related nuclear antigen B lymphocytes in cells infected with the caposisarcoma-associated herpes virus (KSHV), thereby demonstrating that it significantly reduces viral infection [99].

2.7. Other Antiviral Medicinal Plants

Fifteen selected medicinal plants (*Satureja montana, Chamaemelum nobile, Perilla frutescens, Agastashe foeniculum, Origanum vulgare, Mentha piperita, Geranium macrorrhizum, Melissa officinalis, Angelica archangelica, Thymus vulgaris, Hssopus officinalis, Nepeta cataria, Echinacea purpurea, Salvia officinalis*, and *Desmodium canadence*) were extracted to evaluate their antiviral activities on avian infectious bronchitis virus (IBV), a coronavirus that belongs to the Coronaviridae family. Extracts of *S. montana, O. vulgare, M. piperita, M. officinalis, T. vulgaris, H. officinalis, S. officinalis* and *D. canadense* demonstrated antiviral activity prior to and during IBV-infection, whereas *S. montana* displayed anti-IBV activity prior to and after infection. Among the tested extracts *M. piperita, T. vulgaris* and *D. canadense* were found the most effective in the study [100]. Yamasaki *et al.*, (1998) reported that aqueous extract of *M. piperita* exerted antiviral effect on Herpes-simplex virus type-1 (HSV-1), further its hydroalcoholic extracts and peppermint oil was found to have significantly anti-HIV-1 and anti-HIV-2 activities by blocking virus penetration into the host cell [101].

In another study conducted with essential oils distilled from *Laurus nobilis, Juniperus oxycedrus* ssp. *oxycedrus, Thuja orientalis, Cupressus sempervirens* ssp. *pyramidalis, Pistacia palaestina, Salvia officinalis*, and *Satureja thymbra* were evaluated in terms of their *in vitro* antiviral activities. Among the tested medicinal plants, *S. officinalis* and bioactive compounds of EOs such as 1,8-cineol and α-thujone demonstrated strong activity against SARS-CoV and HSV-1 infections [102].

In vitro inhibition of the bovine viral diarrhoea virus (BVDV) using essential oil of *Ocimum basilicum* and monoterpenes, namely camphor, thymol, linalool, and 1,8-cineole, were studied in cell culture on Madin-Darby bovine kidney cells (MDBK). They were found as antiviral agents against BVDV depending on the concentration [103]. In other work, *O. bacilium* extracts and selected purified components, including apigenin, linalool and ursolic acid, were identified antiviral effects on herpes viruses (HSV), adenoviruses (ADV), hepatitis B virus, coxsackievirus B1 (CVB1) and enterovirus 71 (EV71). Among these compounds, ursolic acid demonstrated the strongest activity against tested viruses, while linalool showed the highest activity against AVD [104].

The antiviral effects of fruit extracts from *Rhus coriaria* L. against acyclovir resistant HSV-1 were shown both before viral infection and after viral replication in the host cell. The highest inhibition on acyclovir resistant HSV-1 infectivity was obtained 2 and 4 hours after the infection. In other words, the anti-HSV-1 effects of the extracts on acyclovir resistant HSV-1 after virus infection were more remarkable than before virus adsorption [105]. In another research, the aqueous extract of *R. coriaria* L. was observed on the release of HBsAg as a consequence of HBV replication in the human hepatoma cell line (HuH-7). It can be concluded that aqueous sumac extract has a significant inhibition effect on the multiplication and antigen secretion of HBV [106].

CONCLUSION AND FUTURE DIRECTIONS

Coronaviruses (CoVs) are one of the largest families of viruses that interact with components of host cells at many levels, suggesting this causes pathogenesis. After two highly pathogenic human CoVs, namely SARS and MERS, many genetic and molecular mechanisms of CoVs have been identified, but there are some challenges about the new coronavirus and COVID-19. One of the main reasons for that is that RNA viruses can quickly modify their genomes therefore the identified agents, drugs, or vaccines cannot properly be evaluated in *in vitro* and *in vivo* studies. Scientists have been putting huge effort into elucidating the structure and genomic organization of the virus, as well as discovering effective treatment regimens and developing drugs and vaccines. As a matter of fact, medicinal plants are proven to be effective in strengthening the host's immune system against viral pathogens because they contain a wide range of bioactive components. Therefore, medicinal plants can be considered as alternative treatment options to combat the virus, specifically, medicinal plants with active phytochemicals, which are sustainable natural sources that the pharmaceutical industry could use in order to develop new drugs. On account of its broad-spectrum of medicinal properties, its biologically active ingredients and its lower negative side effects on human health, medicinal plants should be closely investigated whilst avoiding the loss of the ethnobotanical heritage.

LIST OF ABBREVIATIONS

ACE2	Angiotensin-converting enzyme 2;
AIV	Avian influenza virus;
CMV	Cytomegalovirus;
COVID-19	Corona Virus Disease 2019;

DPP4: FPV	Favipiravir;
HBV	Hepatitis B virus;
HIV	Human immunodeficiency virus;
HKU1	HCoV- Hong Kong University 1;
HMPV	Human metapneumotic virus;
HSV	Herpes simplex virus;
IBV	Avian infectious bronchitis virus;
KSHV	Kaposi's sarcoma herpes virus;
LASV	Arenavirus Lassa virus;
MERS	Middle East Respiratory Syndrome;
NDV	Newcastle disease virus;
NMN	Non-enveloped murine norovirus;
PI-3	Parainfluenza - 3;
POLIO	Poliomyelitis-1 virus;
RSV	Respiratory syncytial virus;
RVFV	Rift Valley fever virus;
SARS	Severe Acute Respiratory Syndrome;
SARS-CoV-2 (2019-nCoV)	The Severe Acute Respiratory Syndrome Coronavirus 2;
SINV	Sindbis virus;
VSV	Vesicular stomatitis virus;
VZV	Varicella zoster virus;
WHO	World Health Organization;
ZIKV	Zika virus.

CONSENT FOR PUBLICATION

Not applicable.

CONFLICT OF INTEREST

The authors declare no conflict of interest, financial or otherwise.

ACKNOWLEDGEMENTS

Declared none.

REFERENCES

[1]   Cheever FS, Daniels JB, Pappenheimer AM, Bailey OT. A murine virus (JHM) causing disseminated encephalomyelitis with extensive destruction of myelin. J Exp Med 1949; 90(3): 181-210.

[http://dx.doi.org/10.1084/jem.90.3.181] [PMID: 18137294]

[2]   Walsh EE, Shin JH, Falsey AR. Clinical impact of human coronaviruses 229E and OC43 infection in diverse adult populations. J Infect Dis 2013; 208(10): 1634-42.
[http://dx.doi.org/10.1093/infdis/jit393] [PMID: 23922367]

[3]   Pillaiyar T, Meenakshisundaram S, Manickam M. Recent discovery and development of inhibitors targeting coronaviruses. Drug Discov Today 2020; 25(4): 668-88.
[http://dx.doi.org/10.1016/j.drudis.2020.01.015] [PMID: 32006468]

[4]   Geller C, Varbanov M, Duval RE. Human coronaviruses: insights into environmental resistance and its influence on the development of new antiseptic strategies. Viruses 2012; 4(11): 3044-68.
[http://dx.doi.org/10.3390/v4113044] [PMID: 23202515]

[5]   King AM, Lefkowitz E, Adams MJ, Carstens EB, Eds. Virus taxonomy: ninth report of the International Committee on Taxonomy of Viruses Elsevier 2011; 9.

[6]   Kanwar A, Selvaraju S, Esper F. Human coronavirus (hcov) infection among adults in cleveland, ohio: an increasingly recognized respiratory pathogen. Open Forum Infect Dis. Oxford University Press 2017; 4: pp. (2)1-6.
[http://dx.doi.org/10.1093/ofid/ofx052]

[7]   Li G, Fan Y, Lai Y, *et al.* Coronavirus infections and immune responses. J Med Virol 2020; 92(4): 424-32.
[http://dx.doi.org/10.1002/jmv.25685] [PMID: 31981224]

[8]   Phan T. Novel coronavirus: From discovery to clinical diagnostics. Infect Genet Evol 2020; 79: 104211.
[http://dx.doi.org/10.1016/j.meegid.2020.104211] [PMID: 32007627]

[9]   Lau SK, Woo PC, Yip CC, *et al.* Coronavirus HKU1 and other coronavirus infections in Hong Kong. J Clin Microbiol 2006; 44(6): 2063-71.
[http://dx.doi.org/10.1128/JCM.02614-05] [PMID: 16757599]

[10] Chan JF, Lau SK, To KK, Cheng VC, Woo PC, Yuen KY. Middle East respiratory syndrome coronavirus: another zoonotic betacoronavirus causing SARS-like disease. Clin Microbiol Rev 2015; 28(2): 465-522.
[http://dx.doi.org/10.1128/CMR.00102-14] [PMID: 25810418]

[11] Zhou F, Yu T, Du R, *et al.* Clinical course and risk factors for mortality of adult inpatients with COVID-19 in Wuhan, China: a retrospective cohort study. Lancet 2020; 395(10229): 1054-62.
[http://dx.doi.org/10.1016/S0140-6736(20)30566-3] [PMID: 32171076]

[12] Park SY, Lee JS, Son JS, *et al.* Post-exposure prophylaxis for Middle East respiratory syndrome in healthcare workers. J Hosp Infect 2019; 101(1): 42-6.
[http://dx.doi.org/10.1016/j.jhin.2018.09.005] [PMID: 30240813]

[13] World Health Organization. Middle East respiratory syndrome coronavirus (MERS-CoV) summary and literature update-as of 20 January. Switzerland: Geneva 2014.

[14] World Health Organization. Clinical mamagment of severe acute respiratory infection when MERS-CoV infection is suspected: interim guidance. 2019. Available at: https://www.who.int/emergencies/diseases/novel-coronavirus-2019/situation-reports/

[15] World Health Organization. Novel Coronavirus (2019-nCoV) situation report 2021. [published online ahead of print November 19, 2021]. https://covid19.who.int

[16] GISAID. (Global Initiative on Sharing All Influenza Data) Accessed https://www.gisaid.org/

[17] Paraskevis D, Kostaki EG, Magiorkinis G, Panayiotakopoulos G, Sourvinos G, Tsiodras S. Full-genome evolutionary analysis of the novel corona virus (2019-nCoV) rejects the hypothesis of emergence as a result of a recent recombination event. Infect Genet Evol 2020; 79: 104212.
[http://dx.doi.org/10.1016/j.meegid.2020.104212] [PMID: 32004758]

[18]   Xu Z, Shi L, Wang Y, *et al.* Pathological findings of COVID-19 associated with acute respiratory distress syndrome. Lancet Respir Med 2020; 8(4): 420-2.
       [http://dx.doi.org/10.1016/S2213-2600(20)30076-X] [PMID: 32085846]

[19]   Xu J, Shi PY, Li H, Zhou J. Broad spectrum antiviral agent niclosamide and its therapeutic potential. ACS Infect Dis 2020; 6(5): 909-15.
       [http://dx.doi.org/10.1021/acsinfecdis.0c00052] [PMID: 32125140]

[20]   Cheng L, Zheng W, Li M, *et al.* Citrus fruits are rich in flavonoids for immunoregulation and potential targeting ACE2. Preprints 2020.https://www.preprints.org/manuscript/202002.0313/v1

[21]   Luo H, Tang QL, Shang YX, *et al.* Can Chinese medicine be used for prevention of corona virus disease 2019 (COVID-19)? A review of historical classics, research evidence and current prevention programs. Chin J Integr Med 2020; 26(4): 243-50.
       [http://dx.doi.org/10.1007/s11655-020-3192-6] [PMID: 32065348]

[22]   Ni L, Zhou L, Zhou M, Zhao J, Wang DW. Combination of western medicine and Chinese traditional patent medicine in treating a family case of COVID-19. Front Med 2020; 14(2): 210-4.
       [http://dx.doi.org/10.1007/s11684-020-0757-x] [PMID: 32170559]

[23]   Khalifa I, Zhu W, Nafie MS, Dutta K, Li C. Anti-COVID-19 effects of ten structurally different hydrolysable tannins through binding with the catalytic-closed sites of COVID-19 main protease: an *in-silico* approach. Preprints 2020.
       [http://dx.doi.org/10.20944/preprints202003.0277.v1]

[24]   Chhikara BS, Rathi B, Singh J, Poonam FNU. Corona virus SARS-CoV-2 disease COVID-19: Infection, prevention and clinical advances of the prospective chemical drug therapeutics. Chem Biol Lett 2020; 7(1): 63-72.

[25]   Stebbing J, Phelan A, Griffin I, *et al.* COVID-19: combining antiviral and anti-inflammatory treatments. Lancet Infect Dis 2020; 20(4): 400-2.
       [http://dx.doi.org/10.1016/S1473-3099(20)30132-8] [PMID: 32113509]

[26]   Ben-Shabat S, Yarmolinsky L, Porat D, Dahan A. Antiviral effect of phytochemicals from medicinal plants: Applications and drug delivery strategies. Drug Deliv Transl Res 2019; 1-14.
       [PMID: 31788762]

[27]   Manivannan R, Punniyamoorthy A, Tamilselvan C. Plant secondary metabolites of antiviral properties a rich medicinal source for drug discovery: a mini review. J Drug Deliv Ther 2019; 9(5): 161-7.
       [http://dx.doi.org/10.22270/jddt.v9i5.3471]

[28]   D'Cruz OJ, Uckun FM. Clinical development of microbicides for the prevention of HIV infection. Curr Pharm Des 2004; 10(3): 315-36.
       [http://dx.doi.org/10.2174/1381612043386374] [PMID: 14754390]

[29]   Dhama K, Sachan S, Khandia R, *et al.* Medicinal and beneficial health applications of *Tinospora cordifolia* (Guduchi): a miraculous herb countering various diseases/disorders and its Immunomodulatory effects. Recent Pat Endocr Metab Immune Drug Discov 2017; 10(2): 96-111.
       [http://dx.doi.org/10.2174/1872214811666170301105101] [PMID: 28260522]

[30]   Utomo RY, *et al.* Revealing the . Preprints 2020.
       [http://dx.doi.org/10.20944/preprints202003.0214.v1]

[31]   Baytop T. Türkiye'de Bitkilerle Tedavi – Geçmişte ve Bugün. Nobel Tıp Kitabevleri. İstanbul: İlaveli II. Baskı 1999.

[32]   Bown D. Encyclopedia of Herbs and Their Uses, The Herb Society of America. Darling. London: Kindersley 2004; 167: pp. 16-8.

[33]   Politeo O, Burčul AMF, Carev I, Kamenjarin J. Phytochemical Composition and Antimicrobial Activity of Essential Oils of Wild Growing Cistus species in Croatia. Nat Prod Commun 2018; 13(6): 771-4.

[http://dx.doi.org/10.1177/1934578X1801300631]

[34] Sahraoui R, Djellali S, Chakera AN. Morphological, anatomical, secondary metabolites investigation and physicochemical analysis of Cistus creticus. Pharmacol Commun 2013; 3(4): 58-63.

[35] Gürbüz P, Koşar M, Güvenalp Z, Kuruüzüm UZ. A, Demirezer EÖ. Simultaneous determination of selected flavonoids from different Cistus species by HPLC-PDA. Marmara Pharm J 2018; 22(3): 405-10.

[36] Coode MJE, Cistaceae. P Davis, Mill R, Tan K. Flora of Turkey and the East Aegean Islands. Edinburgh, UK.: Edinburgh University Press. 1988; 10: p. 61.

[37] TUBIVES. Turkish Plants Data Service 2020. Last Accessed Date: 30 June http://www.tubives.com/

[38] Stępień A, Aebisher D, Bartusik-Aebisher D. Biological properties of "Cistus species". Eur J Clin Exp Med 2018; 16(2): 127-32.
[http://dx.doi.org/10.15584/ejcem.2018.2.8]

[39] Kilic DD, Siriken B, Erturk O, Tanrikulu G, Gül M, Başkan C. Antibacterial, Antioxidant and DNA Interaction Properties of Cistus creticus L. Extracts. J Int Environ Appl Sci 2019; 14(3): 110-5.

[40] Kalus U, Kiesewetter H, Radtke H. Effect of CYSTUS052 and green tea on subjective symptoms in patients with infection of the upper respiratory tract. Phytother Res 2010; 24(1): 96-100.
[http://dx.doi.org/10.1002/ptr.2876] [PMID: 19444821]

[41] Guvenc A, Yıldız S, Özkan AM, *et al.* Antimicrobiological Studies on Turkish Cistus Species. Pharm Biol 2005; 43(2): 178-83.
[http://dx.doi.org/10.1080/13880200590919537]

[42] Ustun U, Ozcelik B, Baykal T. Bioactivities of Ethanolic Extract and its Fractions of Cistus laurifolius L. (Cistaceae) and Salvia wiedemannii Boiss. (Lamiaceae) Species. Pharmacogn Mag 2016; 12: pp. (45)82-5.

[43] Ehrhardt C, Hrincius ER, Korte V, *et al.* A polyphenol rich plant extract, CYSTUS052, exerts anti influenza virus activity in cell culture without toxic side effects or the tendency to induce viral resistance. Antiviral Res 2007; 76(1): 38-47.
[http://dx.doi.org/10.1016/j.antiviral.2007.05.002] [PMID: 17572513]

[44] Kalus U, Grigorov A, Kadecki O, Jansen JP, Kiesewetter H, Radtke H. Cistus incanus (CYSTUS052) for treating patients with infection of the upper respiratory tract. A prospective, randomised, placebo-controlled clinical study. Antiviral Res 2009; 84(3): 267-71.
[http://dx.doi.org/10.1016/j.antiviral.2009.10.001] [PMID: 19828122]

[45] Wyk BE, Wink M. Medicinal Plants of the World. Portland, Oregon, USA: Timber Press 2004.

[46] Geuenich S, Goffinet C, Venzke S, *et al.* Aqueous extracts from peppermint, sage and lemon balm leaves display potent anti-HIV-1 activity by increasing the virion density. Retrovirology 2008; 5(1): 27.
[http://dx.doi.org/10.1186/1742-4690-5-27] [PMID: 18355409]

[47] Pourghanbari G, Nili H, Moattari A, Mohammadi A, Iraji A. Antiviral activity of the oseltamivir and Melissa officinalis L. essential oil against avian influenza A virus (H9N2). Virusdisease 2016; 27(2): 170-8.
[http://dx.doi.org/10.1007/s13337-016-0321-0] [PMID: 27366768]

[48] Koytchev R, Alken RG, Dundarov S. Balm mint extract (Lo-701) for topical treatment of recurring herpes labialis. Phytomedicine 1999; 6(4): 225-30.
[http://dx.doi.org/10.1016/S0944-7113(99)80013-0] [PMID: 10589440]

[49] Wölbling RH, Leonhardt K. Local therapy of herpes simplex with dried extract from Melissa officinalis. Phytomedicine 1994; 1(1): 25-31.
[http://dx.doi.org/10.1016/S0944-7113(11)80019-X] [PMID: 23195812]

[50] Todorov D, Hinkov A, Shishkova K, Shishkov S. Antiviral potential of Bulgarian medicinal plants.

Phytochem Rev 2014; 13(2): 525-38.
[http://dx.doi.org/10.1007/s11101-014-9357-1]

[51]   Schnitzler P, Schuhmacher A, Astani A, Reichling J. Melissa officinalis oil affects infectivity of enveloped herpesviruses. Phytomedicine 2008; 15(9): 734-40.
       [http://dx.doi.org/10.1016/j.phymed.2008.04.018] [PMID: 18693101]

[52]   Allahverdiyev A, Duran N, Ozguven M, Koltas S. Antiviral activity of the volatile oils of Melissa officinalis L. against Herpes simplex virus type-2. Phytomedicine 2004; 11(7-8): 657-61.
       [http://dx.doi.org/10.1016/j.phymed.2003.07.014] [PMID: 15636181]

[53]   Dimitrova Z, Dimov B, Manolova N, Pancheva S, Ilieva D, Shishkov S. Antiherpes effect of Melissa officinalis L. extracts. Acta Microbiol Bulg 1993; 29: 65-72.
       [PMID: 8390134]

[54]   Chen SG, Leu YL, Cheng ML, *et al.* Anti-enterovirus 71 activities of Melissa officinalis extract and its biologically active constituent rosmarinic acid. Sci Rep 2017; 7(1): 12264.
       [http://dx.doi.org/10.1038/s41598-017-12388-2] [PMID: 28947773]

[55]   Khwaza V, Oyedeji OO, Aderibigbe BA. Antiviral activities of oleanolic acid and its analogues. Molecules 2018; 23(9): 2300.
       [http://dx.doi.org/10.3390/molecules23092300] [PMID: 30205592]

[56]   Battistini R, Rossini I, Ercolini C, *et al.* Antiviral activity of essential oils against hepatitis a virus in soft fruits. Food Environ Virol 2019; 11(1): 90-5.
       [http://dx.doi.org/10.1007/s12560-019-09367-3] [PMID: 30684236]

[57]   Byler KG, Ogungbe IV, Setzer WN. *In-silico* screening for anti-Zika virus phytochemicals. J Mol Graph Model 2016; 69: 78-91.
       [http://dx.doi.org/10.1016/j.jmgm.2016.08.011] [PMID: 27588363]

[58]   Nolkemper S, Reichling J, Stintzing FC, Carle R, Schnitzler P. Antiviral effect of aqueous extracts from species of the Lamiaceae family against Herpes simplex virus type 1 and type 2 *in vitro.* Planta Med 2006; 72(15): 1378-82.
       [http://dx.doi.org/10.1055/s-2006-951719] [PMID: 17091431]

[59]   Herrmann EC Jr, Kucera LS. Antiviral substances in plants of the mint family (labiatae). 3. Peppermint (Mentha piperita) and other mint plants. Proc Soc Exp Biol Med 1967; 124(3): 874-8.
       [http://dx.doi.org/10.3181/00379727-124-31874] [PMID: 4290278]

[60]   El-Awady SI, Essam T, Hashem A, Boseila AA, Mohmmed AF. Assessment of antiviral activity for Lamiaceae family members against RNA and DNA virus models using cell-culture: *in vitro* study. World J Med Sci 2014; 11(1): 111-9.

[61]   Nasr-Eldin MA, Abdelhamid A, Baraka D. Antibiofilm and Antiviral Potential of Leaf Extracts from *Moringa oleifera* and Rosemary (*Rosmarinus officinalis Lam.*). Egypt J Microbiol 2017; 52(1): 129-39.

[62]   Gavanji S, Sayedipour SS, Larki B, Bakhtari A. Antiviral activity of some plant oils against herpes simplex virus type 1 in Vero cell culture. J Acute Med 2015; 5(3): 62-8.
       [http://dx.doi.org/10.1016/j.jacme.2015.07.001]

[63]   Brochot A, Guilbot A, Haddioui L, Roques C. Antibacterial, antifungal, and antiviral effects of three essential oil blends. MicrobiologyOpen 2017; 6(4): e00459.
       [http://dx.doi.org/10.1002/mbo3.459] [PMID: 28296357]

[64]   Shin HB, Choi MS, Ryu B, *et al.* Antiviral activity of carnosic acid against respiratory syncytial virus. Virol J 2013; 10(1): 303.
       [http://dx.doi.org/10.1186/1743-422X-10-303] [PMID: 24103432]

[65]   Giraldo HJA, Salazar DFS, Diaz SU, Isaza JA. Inhibición del virus de Bronquitis Infecciosa Aviar mediante el uso de aceites esenciales. REDVET. Rev Electrón Vet 2017; 18(10): 1-9.

[66]   AMR. Alternative Medicine Review. Olive Leaf Monograph - Foundational Med Rev 2009; 14(1)http://www.altmedrev.com/archive/publications/14/1/62.pdf

[67]   Salih RH, Odisho SM, Al-Shammari AM, Ibrahim OMS. Antiviral effects of olea europaea leaves extract and interferon-beta on gene expression of newcastle disease virus. Adv Anim Vet Sci 2017; 5(11): 436-45.
[http://dx.doi.org/10.17582/journal.aavs/2017/5.11.436.445]

[68]   Lee-Huang S, Zhang L, Huang PL, Chang YT, Huang PL. Anti-HIV activity of olive leaf extract (OLE) and modulation of host cell gene expression by HIV-1 infection and OLE treatment. Biochem Biophys Res Commun 2003; 307(4): 1029-37.
[http://dx.doi.org/10.1016/S0006-291X(03)01292-0] [PMID: 12878215]

[69]   Zaher KS. *In vitro* studies on the antiviral effect of olive leaf against infectious laryngotracheitis virus. Glob Vet 2007; 1(1): 24-30.

[70]   Motamedifar M, Nekoueian AA, Moatari A. The effect of hydroalcoholic extract of olive leaves against herpes simplex virus type 1. Iran J Med Sci 2007; 32(4): 222-6.

[71]   Micol V, Caturla N, Pérez-Fons L, Más V, Pérez L, Estepa A. The olive leaf extract exhibits antiviral activity against viral haemorrhagic septicaemia rhabdovirus (VHSV). Antiviral Res 2005; 66(2-3): 129-36.
[http://dx.doi.org/10.1016/j.antiviral.2005.02.005] [PMID: 15869811]

[72]   Knipping K, Garssen J, van't Land B. An evaluation of the inhibitory effects against rotavirus infection of edible plant extracts. Virol J 2012; 9(1): 137-44.
[http://dx.doi.org/10.1186/1743-422X-9-137] [PMID: 22834653]

[73]   Fredrickson WR. U.S. Patent No. 6,117,844. Washington, DC: U.S: Patent and Trademark Office 2000.

[74]   Khan Y, Panchal S, Vyas N, Butani A, Kumar V. Olea europaea: a phyto-pharmacological review. Pharmacogn Rev 2007; 1(1): 114-8.http://www.phcogrev.com

[75]   Baser KHC, Ozek T, Tümen G, Sezik E. Composition of the Essential Oil of Turkish Origanum Species with Commercial Importance. J Essent Oil Res 1993; 5(6): 619-23.
[http://dx.doi.org/10.1080/10412905.1993.9698294]

[76]   Baser KHC, Kırımer N. Essential Oils of Anatolian Lamiaceae – An Update Nat Vol Essent Oils (NVEO). 2018; 5(4): 1-28.

[77]   Tumen G, Kırımer N, Başer KHC. Composition of the Essential Oils of Thymus Species Growing in Turkey. Khim Prir Soedin 1995; 1: 55-60.

[78]   Kizil S, Toncer O, Dıraz E, Karaman S. Variation of agronomical characteristics and essential oil components of zahter (*Thymbra spicata* L. var. spicata) populations in semi-arid climatic conditions. Turk J Field Crops 2015; 20(2): 242-51.
[http://dx.doi.org/10.17557/tjfc.46517]

[79]   Zhang XL, Guo YS, Wang CH, *et al.* Phenolic compounds from *Origanum vulgare* and their antioxidant and antiviral activities. Food Chem 2014; 152: 300-6.
[http://dx.doi.org/10.1016/j.foodchem.2013.11.153] [PMID: 24444941]

[80]   Blank DE, de Oliveira Hübner S, Alves GH, Cardoso CAL, Freitag RA, Cleff MB. Chemical Composition and Antiviral Effect of Extracts of Origanum vulgare. Adv Biosci Biotechnol 2019; 10(07): 188-96.
[http://dx.doi.org/10.4236/abb.2019.107014]

[81]   Gilling DH, Kitajima M, Torrey JR, Bright KR. Antiviral efficacy and mechanisms of action of oregano essential oil and its primary component carvacrol against murine norovirus. J Appl Microbiol 2014; 116(5): 1149-63.
[http://dx.doi.org/10.1111/jam.12453] [PMID: 24779581]

[82]   Salah-Fatnassi KBH, Slim-Bannour A, Harzallah-Skhiri F, *et al.* Activités antivirale et antioxydante *in vitro* d'huiles essentielles de *Thymus capitatus* (L.) Hoffmans. & Link de Tunisie. Acta Bot Gallica 2010; 157(3): 433-44.
[http://dx.doi.org/10.1080/12538078.2010.10516220]

[83]   Erturk O, Tanrıkulu GI, Yavuz C, Can Z, Çakır HE. Chemical compositions, antioxidant and antimicrobial activities of the essential oil and extracts of Lamiaceae family (*Ocimum basilicum* and *Thymbra spicata*) from Turkey. Int J Secon Metab 2017; 4(3, Special Issue 2): 340-8.

[84]   Duran N, Kaya A, Gulbol Duran G, Eryilmaz N. *In vitro* antiviral effect of the essential oils of *Thymbra spicata* L. on Herpes simplex virus type 2. ICAMS – 4th International Conference on Advanced Materials and Systems.

[85]   Mamedov NA, Egamberdieva D. Phytochemical constituents and pharmacological effects of licorice: a review. Plant and Human Health. Cham: Springer 2019; Vol. 3: pp. 1-21.
[http://dx.doi.org/10.1007/978-3-030-04408-4_1]

[86]   Fiore C, Eisenhut M, Krausse R, *et al.* Antiviral effects of Glycyrrhiza species. Phytother Res 2008; 22(2): 141-8.
[http://dx.doi.org/10.1002/ptr.2295] [PMID: 17886224]

[87]   Crance JM, Scaramozzino N, Jouan A, Garin D. Interferon, ribavirin, 6-azauridine and glycyrrhizin: antiviral compounds active against pathogenic flaviviruses. Antiviral Res 2003; 58(1): 73-9.
[http://dx.doi.org/10.1016/S0166-3542(02)00185-7] [PMID: 12719009]

[88]   Huan CC, Wang HX, Sheng XX, Wang R, Wang X, Mao X. Glycyrrhizin inhibits porcine epidemic diarrhea virus infection and attenuates the proinflammatory responses by inhibition of high mobility group box-1 protein. Arch Virol 2017; 162(6): 1467-76.
[http://dx.doi.org/10.1007/s00705-017-3259-7] [PMID: 28175983]

[89]   Cinatl J, Morgenstern B, Bauer G, Chandra P, Rabenau H, Doerr HW. Glycyrrhizin, an active component of liquorice roots, and replication of SARS-associated coronavirus. Lancet 2003; 361(9374): 2045-6.
[http://dx.doi.org/10.1016/S0140-6736(03)13615-X] [PMID: 12814717]

[90]   Ianevski A, Andersen PI, Merits A, Bjørås M, Kainov D. Expanding the activity spectrum of antiviral agents. Drug Discov Today 2019; 24(5): 1224-8.
[http://dx.doi.org/10.1016/j.drudis.2019.04.006] [PMID: 30980905]

[91]   Nirmala P, Selvaraj T. Anti-inflammatory and anti-bacterial activities of *Glycyrrhiza glabra* L. J Agr Tech 2011; 7(3): 815-23.

[92]   El-Saber Batiha G, Magdy Beshbishy A, El-Mleeh A, Abdel-Daim MM, Prasad Devkota H. Traditional uses, bioactive chemical constituents, and pharmacological and toxicological activities of *Glycyrrhiza glabra* L. Fabaceae). Biomolecules 2020; 10(3): 1-21.
[http://dx.doi.org/10.3390/biom10030352] [PMID: 32106571]

[93]   Sun ZG, Zhao TT, Lu N, Yang YA, Zhu HL. Research progress of glycyrrhizic acid on antiviral activity. Mini Rev Med Chem 2019; 19(10): 826-32.
[http://dx.doi.org/10.2174/1389557519666190119111125] [PMID: 30659537]

[94]   Fiore C, Eisenhut M, Ragazzi E, Zanchin G, Armanini D. A history of the therapeutic use of liquorice in Europe. J Ethnopharmacol 2005; 99(3): 317-24.
[http://dx.doi.org/10.1016/j.jep.2005.04.015] [PMID: 15978760]

[95]   Yasmin AR, Chia SL, Looi QH, Omar AR, Noordin MM, Ideris A. Herbal extracts as antiviral agents. Feed Additives. Academic Press 2020; pp. 115-32.
[http://dx.doi.org/10.1016/B978-0-12-814700-9.00007-8]

[96]   Sabouri Ghannad M, Mohammadi A, Safiallahy S, Faradmal J, Azizi M, Ahmadvand Z. The effect of aqueous extract of Glycyrrhiza glabra on herpes simplex virus 1. Jundishapur J Microbiol 2014; 7(7): e11616.

[http://dx.doi.org/10.5812/jjm.11616] [PMID: 25368801]

[97]   Baltina LA, Kondratenko RM, Baltina LA Jr, Plyasunova OA, Pokrovskii AG, Tolstikov GA. Prospects for the creation of new antiviral drugs based on glycyrrhizic acid and its derivatives (a review). Pharm Chem J 2009; 43(10): 539-48.
[http://dx.doi.org/10.1007/s11094-010-0348-2] [PMID: 32214533]

[98]   Ashfaq UA, Masoud MS, Nawaz Z, Riazuddin S. Glycyrrhizin as antiviral agent against Hepatitis C Virus. J Transl Med 2011; 9(1): 112.
[http://dx.doi.org/10.1186/1479-5876-9-112] [PMID: 21762538]

[99]   Pastorino G, Cornara L, Soares S, Rodrigues F, Oliveira MBPP. Liquorice (Glycyrrhiza glabra): A phytochemical and pharmacological review. Phytother Res 2018; 32(12): 2323-39.
[http://dx.doi.org/10.1002/ptr.6178] [PMID: 30117204]

[100]   Lelešius R, Karpovaitė A, Mickienė R, *et al.* *In vitro* antiviral activity of fifteen plant extracts against avian infectious bronchitis virus. BMC Vet Res 2019; 15(1): 178.
[http://dx.doi.org/10.1186/s12917-019-1925-6] [PMID: 31142304]

[101]   Yamasaki K, Nakano M, Kawahata T, *et al.* Anti-HIV-1 activity of herbs in Labiatae. Biol Pharm Bull 1998; 21(8): 829-33.
[http://dx.doi.org/10.1248/bpb.21.829] [PMID: 9743251]

[102]   Loizzo MR, Saab AM, Tundis R, *et al.* Phytochemical analysis and *in vitro* antiviral activities of the essential oils of seven Lebanon species. Chem Biodivers 2008; 5(3): 461-70.
[http://dx.doi.org/10.1002/cbdv.200890045] [PMID: 18357554]

[103]   Kubiça TF, Alves SH, Weiblen R, Lovato LT. *In vitro* inhibition of the bovine viral diarrhoea virus by the essential oil of *Ocimum basilicum* (basil) and monoterpenes. Braz J Microbiol 2014; 45(1): 209-14.
[http://dx.doi.org/10.1590/S1517-83822014005000030] [PMID: 24948933]

[104]   Chiang LC, Ng LT, Cheng PW, Chiang W, Lin CC. Antiviral activities of extracts and selected pure constituents of *Ocimum basilicum*. Clin Exp Pharmacol Physiol 2005; 32(10): 811-6.
[http://dx.doi.org/10.1111/j.1440-1681.2005.04270.x] [PMID: 16173941]

[105]   Parsania M, Rezaee MB, Monavari SH, Jaimand K. Mousavi Jazayeri SM, Razazian M, Nadjarha MH. Evaluation of antiviral effects of sumac (*Rhus coriaria* L.) fruit extract on acyclovir resistant Herpes simplex virus type 1. Med Sci J Islamic Azad Univesity-Tehran Medical Branch 2017; 27(1): 1-8.

[106]   Gharabolagha AF, Sabahia F, Karimib M, *et al.* Effects of *Rhus coriaria* L.(sumac) extract on hepatitis B virus replication and Hbs Ag secretion. J Rep Pharm Sci 2018; 7(1): 100-7.

CHAPTER 3

Infections Caused by SARS: Main Characteristics, Targets and Inhibitors

Herbert Igor Rodrigues de Medeiros[1], Gabriela Cristina Soares Rodrigues[1], Mayara dos Santos Maia[1], Marcus Tullius Scotti[1] and Luciana Scotti[1,*]

[1] *Laboratory of Cheminformatics, Program of Natural and Synthetic Bioactive Products (PgPNSB), Health Sciences Center, Federal University of Paraíba, João Pessoa-PB, Brazil*

Abstract: SARS-coronavirus (SARS-CoV) originated in China from 2002 to 2003 and caused a global outbreak with 8098 cases and 774 confirmed deaths. More than 15 years later, in less than a year, the new coronavirus (2019-nCoV) has infected more than 44 million people and killed more than 1 million. The COVID-19 pandemic has brought serious consequences for several countries and a worldwide alert about coronaviruses. Severe acute respiratory syndrome (SARS) is an emerging infectious viral disease characterized by severe clinical manifestations of the lower respiratory tract that lead to severe lung damage and the spread of the virus to several other organs. Phylogenetic analyzes demonstrate that SARS-CoV-2 shares a 79% identity with SARS-CoV, and just as there was no effective treatment against SARS-CoV, it does not yet exist against SARS-CoV-2. However, researchers from all over the world are dedicating themselves to several studies in an attempt to find the best treatment and prevention against the coronavirus. Thus, this book chapter addresses the main characteristics of SARS, the main targets and drugs that have achieved excellent results in clinical trials.

Keywords: Drugs, SARS, SARS-CoV, Sar-CoV-2, Target.

1. INTRODUCTION

Coronaviruses (CoVs) are RNA viruses that cause respiratory and enteric diseases with variable pathogenicity in humans and animals. All CoVs are known to infect humans are zoonotic, or of animal origin, and many believe they originate from host bats [1, 2]. Due to the large size of the genome (the largest non-segmented RNA viral genome), single-stranded and positive sense of about 26–32 kb in size, frequent recombination and high genomic plasticity, CoVs are prone to transmission between species and are able to adapt quickly to new hosts [2, 3].

---

* **Corresponding author Luciana Scotti:** Laboratory of Cheminformatics, Program of Natural and Synthetic Bioactive Products (PgPNSB), Health Sciences Center, Federal University of Paraíba, João Pessoa-PB, Brazil; Tel: +5583996245075; E-mail: luciana.scotti@gmail.com

Luciana Scotti and Marcus T. Scotti (Eds.)

Severe acute respiratory syndrome (SARS), which emerged as a pandemic in 2002 and 2003, was caused by Severe acute respiratory syndrome coronavirus (SARS-CoV), a virus previously unknown [4, 5]. This virus was first isolated in 2003 from samples from three SARS patients. According to the World Health Organization (WHO), SARS has infected more than 8,000 people and caused at least 813 deaths [6, 7].

SARS-CoV has been identified as a clinical entity in which patients have a fever, dry cough, dyspnoea, headache and hypoxemia. Typical laboratory findings are lymphopenia and slightly elevated aminotransferase levels. Death can result from progressive respiratory failure due to alveolar damage caused by an infectious agent transmitted from human to human [8].

The pathological features available for SARS-CoV infections were mainly obtained at autopsies. The predominant visceral macroscopic were changes in fatal cases of SARS - CoV mainly in edematous lungs with increased gross weight and multiple areas of congestion, increased lymph nodes in the pulmonary hiluses and in the abdominal cavity, as well as decreased spleen size and reduced spleen weight [9, 10].

A large number of SARS-CoV particles and genomic sequences have been detected in circulating lymphocytes, monocytes and lymphoid tissues, as well as in epithelial cells of the respiratory tract, intestinal mucosa, epithelium of renal distal tubules, neurons in the brain and macrophages residing in tissues that reside in different organs [11]. The therapeutic agent effective against SARS was unavailable at the time of the initial outbreak. Fortunately, SARS has been successfully contained, and no SARS outbreaks have been reported since 2004 [4].

An outbreak of pneumonia with unknown cause was reported in Wuhan, Hubei province, China, in December 2019, associated with the Huanan Seafood Wholesale Market [12]. The causative agent of the outbreak was identified by the WHO as the severe acute respiratory syndrome coronavirus-2 (SARS-CoV-2), producing the disease called coronavirus disease-2019 (COVID-19) (13). SARS-CoV-2 shares 96.3%, 89% and 82% of nucleotide similarity with the bat CoV RaTG13, SARS-like CoV ZXC21 and SARS-CoV, respectively, which confirms its zoonotic origin, based on the analysis phylogenetics [13 - 15]. Human-t--human transmission has been confirmed even in asymptomatic carriers.

The virus has spread to at least 219 countries and territories and in October 2020, the global epidemiological situation is over 42 million cases and 1.1 million deaths reported globally, with massive global increases in the number of daily cases with more 2.8 million new cases and nearly 40,000 new deaths reported in the past few days [16].

2. ORIGIN AND EPIDEMIOLOGY

At the beginning of the SARS epidemic, most patients had animal exposure rates before developing the disease. Subsequently, the causative agent of SARS was identified, SARS-CoV and / or anti-SARS-CoV antibodies were found in palm civets (Paguma larvata) and animals handled in a market [17 - 20]. However, research using breeding and wild civets revealed that the SARS-CoV strains found in market civets were passed on to them by other animals [21, 22].

Research has also identified the coronavirus in zoonotic reservoirs, including horseshoe bats (genus Rhinolophus), Himalayan palm civets (*Paguma larvata*) and raccoon dogs (*Nyctereutes procyonoides*), and determined that the virus that infected human hosts is from southern China, in Guangdong province [2, 7 - 9].

Subsequent studies have shown that wild horseshoe bats (Family Rhinolophidae), which can also be found in LAM in China and served in some Chinese restaurants in Guangdong, China, have detectable levels of antibodies against SARS-CoV, suggesting a bat origin for the SARS-CoV [22].

The evolutionary relationship between coronavirus and bats was proposed, in which the ancestor for SARS-CoV first spread to bats of the Hipposideridae family, then to Rhinolophidae and then to palm civets and, eventually, to humans [23].

In 2013, two new SARS-like CoVs were isolated from Rhinolophus bats in China, and these viruses showed a high relationship with SARS-CoV of all bat coronaviruses [24]. ORF8 analysis of SARS-identical CoVs in bats suggests that Chinese horseshoe bats are the natural reservoirs of SARS-CoV, these viruses are identified by a set of unique accessory open reading structures (Open Read Frame - ORFs) that are located between the M genes and N [25].

According to their antigenic and genetic characteristics, CoVs are classified into three groups. The main group of CoVs comprises Porcine Transmissible Gastroenteritis Virus (TGEV), Feline Coronavirus (FCoV), Canine Coronavirus (CCoV), HCoV-229E and Porcine Epidemic Diarrhea Virus (PEDV). The second group consists of murine hepatitis Virus (MHV), Bovine Coronavirus (BCoV), HCoV-OC43, Swine Hemagglutinating Encephalomyelitis Virus (HEV), Rat Coronavirus (RtCoV) and Equine Coronavirus (ECoV). The third group is formed by Avian Infectious Bronchitis Virus (IBV), Turkey Coronavirus (TCoV) and Coronavirus Pheasant [26]. This subfamily is formed by four genera,

Alphacoronavirus, Betacoronavirus, Gammacoronavirus and Deltacoronavirus, based on their phylogenetic relationships and genomic structures, the first two genera include only mammalian CoVs, with human CoVs found in each of these groups, while the other two genera are confined to birds CoVs [17].

In late December 2019, several viral pneumonia patients were identified and associated with the Huanan seafood market in Wuhan, Hubei Province, China, where several non-aquatic animals like birds and rabbits were also on sale before the outbreak [27, 28]. Subsequently, China confirmed the WHO on the outbreak and Huanan's seafood stores were closed. In early January 2020, the virus was recognized as a coronavirus with about 95% symmetry with the coronary bat virus and about 70% similarity to SARS-CoV [27 - 29].

In January 2020, China confirmed more than 5,900 confirmed and more than 9,000 suspected 2019-nCoV infection cases in 33 Chinese provinces or municipalities, with 106 deaths, with reports in Thailand, Japan, South Korea, Malaysia, Singapore and the USA. Infections in medical workers and family groups have also been reported and transmission from person to person has been confirmed, with the majority of infected patients having a high fever and some having dyspnoea, with chest X-rays revealing invasive lesions in both lungs [27].

In April 2020, 210 countries and territories reported more than 1,998,111 confirmed cases and 126,604 deaths caused by the SARS-CoV-2 virus and show the presence on six continents, with a mortality rate of about 3.4% of cases reported, however, it depends on the number of factors, such as general health, age, sex and the local health system [30].

Initially, the new virus was named 2019-nCoV. Subsequently, the task of the specialists of the International Committee on Virus Taxonomy (ICTV) called it the SARS-CoV-2 virus because it is very similar to what caused the SARS outbreak (SARS-CoVs). In research with international gene banks, such as GenBank, the researchers published several sequences of SARS-CoV-2 genes. This gene mapping is of fundamental relevance because it allows researchers to track the phylogenetic tree of the virus and, especially, the recognition of strains that differ according to mutations. According to recent studies, a peak mutation, which possibly occurred in late November 2019, triggered the jump for humans [31]. Thus, Angeletti *et al.* checked the sequence of the SARS-CoV-2 gene with that of SARS-CoV. They analyzed the transmembrane helical segments in coded ORF1ab 2 (nsp2) and nsp3 and found that position 723 has a serine instead of a glycine residue, while position 1010 is occupied by proline instead of isoleucine [32].

This data provides us with important information about the potential source of the virus. Interestingly, the pangolin's Covs (Manis javanica) have a receptor-binding domain (RBD) domain identical to that of the human spike SARS-CoV2 protein. However, neither the CoVs of bats nor those present in pangolins have the sequence of the polybasic site for furin, suggesting that natural selection must also have favored the acquisition of that site for the transition to human-human transmission, being the viral mutations a key to elucidating the potential relapses of the disease [31].

The research developed by Lu and collaborators (2020) [27], shows 2019-nCoV is sufficiently divergent from SARS-CoV to be considered a new human infective betacoronavirus. Although our phylogenetic analysis suggests that bats may be the original host of this virus, an animal sold in the seafood market in Wuhan may represent an intermediate host that facilitates the emergence of the virus in humans. It is important to note that structural analysis suggests that 2019-nCoV may be able to bind to the angiotensin-converting enzyme 2 receptors in humans.

3. SARS PATHOGENESIS

SARS is an emerging infectious viral disease characterized by severe clinical manifestations of the lower respiratory tract. The pathogenesis of SARS is highly complex, with several factors leading to serious lung damage and the spread of the virus to several other organs [33]. The SARS coronavirus targets the epithelial cells of the respiratory tract, resulting in diffuse alveolar damage, just as various organs and cell types can be contaminated in the course of the disease, including mucosal cells from the intestines, tubular epithelial cells from the kidneys, brain neurons and various types of immune cells, and certain organs can suffer indirect damage [34].

Patients infected with (SARS-CoV) often have fever and evidence of respiratory disease, general malaise and respiratory tract symptoms, including coughing and shortness of breath, and a mortality rate of approximately 10% [35, 36].

A SARS disease model has been suggested based on three stages: viral replication, immune hyperactivity, and lung destruction [37]. SARS pathology of the lung has been related to diffuse alveolar damage, epithelial cell proliferation and macrophage increase, and is generally considered to be viral pneumonia [18, 38]. In addition, SARS patients may still exhibit gastrointestinal symptoms [39], splenic atrophy and lymphadenopathy [10], as well, diarrhea is very common in patients with SARS (30 to 40% of patients).

Pro-inflammatory cytokines released by macrophages stimulated in the alveoli may play a role in the pathogenesis of SARS [5, 7, 38, 39]. The underlying mechanisms caused by the most serious SARS-CoV infection remain not fully understood [40]. Extensive lung lesions in patients infected with SARS-CoV appear to be associated with high virus titers, 13 increased infiltration of monocytes, macrophages and neutrophils into the lungs [41], and high levels of pro-inflammatory cytokines and serum chemokines [42]. Thus, the clinical deterioration of SARS-CoV infection may result from a combination of direct virus-induced cytopathic effects and immunopathology induced by hypercytokinaemia. Research on changes in cytokine / chemokine profiles during SARS - CoV infection showed high levels of circulating cytokines, such as tumor necrosis factor α (TNF - α), CXCL □ 10, interleukin - 6 (IL - 6) and IL - 8, possibly contributed to the poor prognosis in SARS-CoV infections [40].

High serum levels of proinflammatory cytokines (IL - 1, IL - 6, IL - 12, Interferon γ [IFN - γ] and transforming growth factor - β) and chemokines (CCL2, CXCL9, CXCL10 and IL - 8) were identified in SARS patients with severe disease compared to individuals with uncomplicated SARS [40, 43]. In addition, high mutation rates of RNA viruses allow them to adapt quickly to changes in their environment, resulting in a complex virus system and restriction of factor evolution [36, 44].

SARS-CoV has been detected in respiratory secretions, feces, urine and tears in infected individuals [45]. Nosocomial transmission of SARS was facilitated by the use of nebulizers, suction, intubation, bronchoscopy or cardiopulmonary resuscitation in patients with SARS, when a large number of infectious droplets were generated [46, 47].

With symptomatic similarities to its predecessor, (SARS-CoV), (SARS-CoV-2) symptoms cause flu-like symptoms in infected people. Although symptoms appear in infected people, they can vary from person to person; this virus is affecting different people in different ways. Most infected people may experience mild to moderate symptoms. The clinical symptoms of patients infected with SARSCoV-2 are mainly fever (> 38 ° C), fatigue and dry cough [13, 28, 30, 48]. Infected people may experience pain, nasal congestion, cold, sore throat, dyspnea and diarrhea. Currently, the disease control center (CDC) has added symptoms that can be felt by infected people, such as chills, muscle aches, tremors, headaches and loss of smell and taste. It can take an average of 5 to 6 days for the infected person to show symptoms, but in some cases, it can take up to 14 days [49, 50].

Studies by Lu *et al.* (2020) state that the pathogenic mechanism of SARS-CoV-2 is similar to that of SARS-CoV. Both viruses bind to the surface receptor cell by angiotensin-converting enzyme 2 (ACE2) into the epithelium of human airway cells *via* protein S in the envelope and entering the host cell [51 - 53]. ACE2 is highly expressed in type 2 alveolar cells as well as in the esophagus, ileum, colon, heart, kidney, bladder and testicles [54].

The incubation period is indicated from the moment that the causative agent invades the cell or produces action commonly to the cell when the cell comes to demonstrate the reaction or clinical symptom. The incubation period for different infectious diseases is different, depending on the number of pathogens, pathogenicity and the autoimmunity of the infected person [55].

The pathogenic mechanism that produces SARS-CoV-2-induced pneumonia appears to be particularly complex. Some patients infected with SARSCoV-2 in severe cases may progress to acute respiratory distress syndrome or even to multiple organ failure (ECMO). In addition to respiratory symptoms, some infected people also experience digestive symptoms, such as loss of appetite, nausea and vomiting, diarrhea which are common symptoms of SARS-CoV-2 infection [55 - 57].

While several cytokines, such as tumor necrosis factor α (TNF-α), IL-1β, IL-8, IL-12, interferon-gamma-inducible protein (IP10), inflammatory macrophage protein 1A (MIP1A) and monocyte a chemoattractive protein 1 (MCP1) is implicated in the pathogenic cascade of the disease, the protagonist of this storm is interleukin 6 (IL-6) [58, 59]. IL-6 is produced mainly by activated leukocytes and acts on a large number of cells and tissues, being able to promote the differentiation of B lymphocytes, promote the growth of some sets of cells and block the growth of others [31, 60]. It is also implicated in the pathogenesis of cytokine release syndrome (CRS), which is an acute systemic inflammatory syndrome characterized by fever and multiple organ dysfunction. IL-6 is not the only protagonist in the scene. It has been proven, for example, that the binding of SARS-CoV-2 to the Toll-Like Receptor (TLR) induces the release of pro-IL-1β that is cleaved in lung inflammation mediating active mature IL-1β, up to fibrosis [60].

4. TAXONOMY

The designation coronavirus was assigned based on the morphology similar to the crown or corona in Latin observed for these viruses in the electron microscope [20, 38, 61]. CoVs arc onc of the largest groups of viruses that belong to the order Nidovirales, suborder Cornidovirineae and family Coronaviridae [38]. Coronaviridae is classified into two subfamilies, namely, Letovirinae and Orthocoronavirinae. Letovirinae includes the genus Alphaletovirus, while Orthocoronaviridae is further classified based on phylogenetic analysis and genome structure into four genera: Alphacoronavirus (α-CoV), Betacoronavirus (β-CoV), Gammacoronavirus (γ-CoV) and Deltacoronavirus (δ-CoV), which contain 17, 12, 2 and 7 unique species, respectively (ICTV 2018) [3, 12]. In addition, the genus (β-CoV) is divided into five subgenera or strains [62]. Genomic characterization showed that probably bats and rodents are the genetic sources of alpha-CoVs and beta-CoVs. In contrast, avian species appear to represent the genetic sources of delta-CoVs and gamma-CoVs [31].

The Coronaviridae family was established by the International Committee on the taxonomy of viruses and just like the families, Arteviridae and Roniviridae belong to the order Nidovirales [63]. The Coronaviridae family consists of viruses enveloped with a single-stranded positive sense RNA genome approximately 26-32 kilobases in size, which is the largest known genome of an RNA virus [20]. Depending on their host targets, coronaviruses can be divided into animal and human coronaviruses. Many diseases in domestic animals are related to animal coronaviruses, such as canine respiratory coronavirus [64].

Schwartz and Graham (2020), state that the determinant virus, SARS-CoV-2, is a newly described coronavirus belonging to the Coronaviridae family and to the genus Betacoronavirus [51] and subgenus Sarbecovirus [65, 66], the same genus of two previously described harmful human coronaviruses that have caused previous epidemics disease - SARS-CoV, causing SARS and Middle East coronavirus respiratory syndrome (MERS-CoV), causing MERS [67, 68]. Studies show estimates suggest that generally 2% of the population are healthy carriers of a CoV and that these viruses are responsible for approximately 5% to 10% of acute respiratory infections [69].

Thus, encompassing the newly discovered SARS-CoV-2, there are seven coronaviruses that infect humans [70]. Human coronavirus (HCoV) -229E, HCoV-NL63, HCoV-OC43 or HCoV-HKU1 cause only the common cold, while severe acute respiratory syndrome coronavirus (SARS-CoV) or Middle Eastern respiratory syndrome (MERS-CoV) coronavirus caused relatively high mortality and appeared in 2002 6 and 2012,7 respectively [40, 70]. SARS-CoV and MERS-CoV belong to subgroups 2b and 2c of betacoronaviruses, respectively, while SARS-CoV-2 is a new member of betacoronaviruses distinct from SARS-CoV and MERS-CoV [51]. In Fig. (**1**), we can see the phylogenetic tree of RNA viruses [3].

Fig. (1). Coronavirus phylogenetic tree based on complete genome sequences. The seven known coronaviruses that infect humans are indicated with a red star [3].

5. MAIN TARGETS OF SARS-COV AND SARS-COV-2

The most important structural proteins in CoV are Spike protein (S), membrane protein (M), an envelope protein (E) and nucleocapsid protein (N) [71] (Fig. **2**). Protein S mediates the binding of the virus to receptors on the host cell surface, resulting in fusion and subsequent viral entry. Protein M is the most abundant protein and plays a central role in directing the assembly and sprouting of the virus through interaction with E, S and N. Protein E participates in viral assembly. The N protein is the only one that binds to the RNA genome and is also involved in viral formation [72]. In addition to these proteins, a part of the CoV RNA genome is covered by ORF1a/b, which produces the two viral replicase proteins that are polyproteins (PP1a and PP1ab). Sixteen other mature non-structural proteins (NSPs) arise from the additional processing of these two PPs, which participate in different viral functions, such as the formation of the replicase transcriptase complex [71]. Non-structural proteins produced by the coronavirus include M^{pro} (main protease), also known as 3-chymotrypsin cysteine protease (3CL^{pro}), papain-like protease and RNA-dependent RNA polymerase (RdRp), helicase, structural proteins (glycoprotein from peak) and accessory proteins. Non-structural proteins play a key role during the virus's life cycle, and the peak glycoprotein is necessary for virus interactions with host cell receptors during viral entry, so they are considered promising targets for the design and development of antiviral agents against SARS [73].

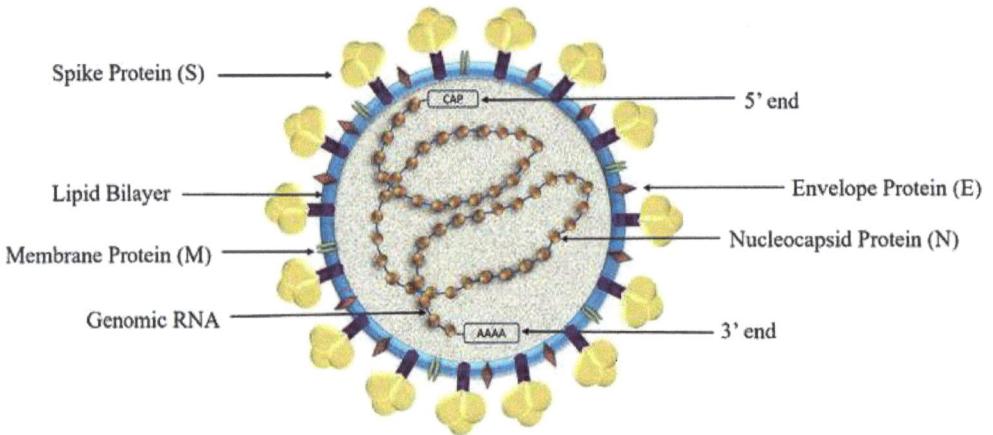

Fig. (2). Structural proteins and genetic material of CoV [74].

5.1. Glycoprotein Spike (S)

The transmembrane peak glycoprotein (S) is synthesized as a single polypeptide chain precursor of -1 300 amino acids and then cleaved by host furin-like proteases in an amino terminal S1 (N) subunit and an S2 terminal subunit carboxyl (C) [75]. Spike forms homotrimers that protrude from the viral surface and enter host cells. The glycoprotein comprises two functional subunits responsible for binding to the host cell receptor and fusing the viral and cell membranes [76]. The distal S1 subunit comprises the receptor binding domain (s) and contributes to stabilizing the pre-fusion state of the S2 subunit anchored in the membrane containing the fusion machinery. The S1 subunit contains a receptor binding domain (RBD), while the S2 subunit contains a hydrophobic fusion peptide and two heptal repeat regions [77]. Within S the receptor binding domain (RBD) mediates the interaction with angiotensin-converting enzyme 2 (ACE2)

[78] (Fig. **3**). The SARS-CoV S1 pre-fusion subunit is organized into four distinct domains: NTD, CTD1, CTD2 and CTD3 [79]. Among these, CTD1 is the receptor-binding domain, and a CTD1 in the trimer adopts an "upward" conformation as a prerequisite for the binding of SARS-CoV to the ACE2 enzyme cell receptor [77]. The glycoprotein in SARS-CoV-2 is cleaved by host proteases in the so-called S2′ to activate the protein for membrane fusion through conformational changes. Thus, entry of the coronavirus into susceptible cells is a process that requires the combined action of receptor binding and proteolytic processing of protein S to promote virus-cell fusion [76].

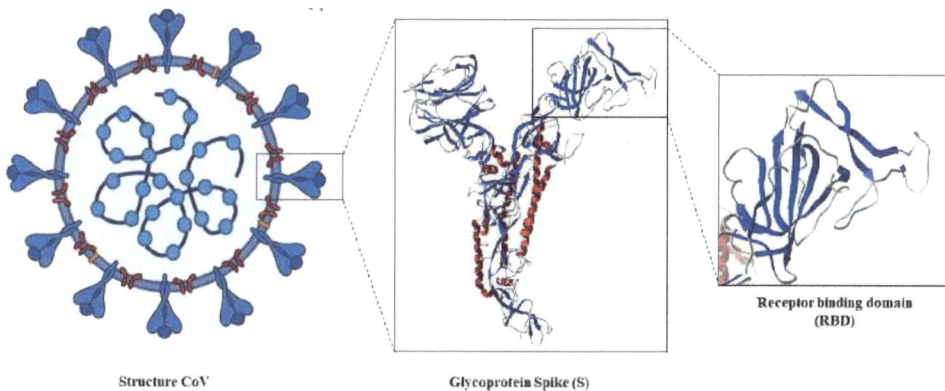

Structure CoV   Glycoprotein Spike (S)   Receptor binding domain (RBD)

Fig. (3). Structure of the Spike glycoprotein and the RBD binding domain.

Spike is the primary target for neutralizing antibodies, to bind to its receptor and mediate membrane fusion and virus entry. SARS-CoV-2 S proteins share about 76% of amino acid identity with SARS-CoV and the potential RBD amino acid sequence of SARS-CoV-2 is only about 74% homologous to that of SARS-CoV [80].

A study by Lan *et al.* [81], showed critical residues of interaction of the RBD portion of the peak and compared the residues that interact with ACE2 in the SARS-CoV-2 and SARS-CoV RBDs (Fig. **4**). The study revealed that among the 14 shared amino acid positions used by both RBMs for interacting with ACE2, eight have identical residues between the two RBDs, including Tyr449 / Tyr436, Tyr453 / Tyr440, Asn487 / Asn473, Tyr489 / Tyr475, Gly496 SARS-CoV-2 / SARS-CoV / Gly482, Thr500 / Thr486, Gly502 / Gly488 and Tyr491, respectively. In addition, five positions have residues that have similar biochemical properties, despite having different side chains, including Leu455 / Tyr442, Phe456 / Leu443, Phe486 / Leu472, Gln493 / Asn479 and Asn501 / Thr487 of SARS-CoV-2 / SARS-CoV, respectively. Another study by Liu *et al.* [82], showed that the SARS-CoV-2 protein S can bind to ACE2 through Leu455,

Phe486, Gln493, Asn501 and Tyr505, only the fourth is equal to SARS-CoV. In the external subdomain of SARS-CoV, residues L472, N479 and T487 are the main interface positions; mutations at these sites support the S adaptation for binding to human ACE2.

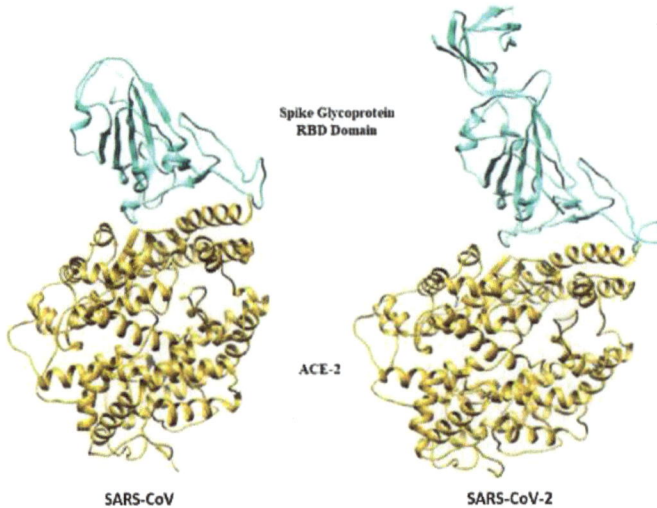

Fig. (4). Structure of the RBD domain of the Spike protein (blue) of SARS-CoV and SARS-CoV-2 complexed with the human ACE-2 receptor (yellow).

A study by Ou *et al.* [80], showed that SARS-CoV-2 enters 293 / hACE2 cells mainly by endocytosis, that PIKfyve, TPC2 and cathepsin L are critical for entry, and that the SARS-CoV-2 S protein is less stable than SARS-CoV S In addition, they observed that polyclonal anti-SARS S1 T62 antibodies inhibit the entry of SARS-CoV S, but not SARS-CoV -2 S pseudovirions. Thus, they suggest that recovering from one infection may not protect against the other.

To understand why SARS-CoV-2 Spike leads to a stronger infection than SARS-CoV, Shang *et al.* [83], gathered a series of evidence from biochemical assays and pseudovirus entry and SARS-CoV as a comparison. Thus, it was possible to identify the main mechanisms of entry into the SARS-CoV-2 cell that potentially contribute to immune evasion, cellular infectivity and wide spread of the virus. The study showed that SARS-CoV-2 RBD has a higher affinity for hACE2 binding than SARS-CoV RBD because at the peak of SARS-CoV, RBD is mainly in the standing state; however, at the peak of SARS-CoV-2, RBD is mainly in the lying state, even as less accessible RBD. To maintain its high infectivity, SARS-CoV-2 Spike is pre-activated by furin, increasing the entry of pseudovirus into different types of cell lines that express hACE2, including pulmonary epithelial and pulmonary fibroblast cell lines. In addition, TMPRSS2 cell surface protease and lysosomal cathepsins also activate the entry of the SARS-CoV-2 pseudovirus. However, compared to the entry of the SARS-CoV pseudovirus, the activation occurs only by TMPRSS2 and cathepsins, but not by furin.

Several peptides have been developed in recent months to neutralize one of the main targets of SARS-CoV and SARS-CoV-2. Xia *et al*. [84], generated a series of EK1-derived lipopeptides and found that EK1C4 was the most potent fusion inhibitor against SARS-CoV-2 mediated membrane fusion with IC^{50} of 1.3 and 15.8 nM, about 241 and 149 times more potent than the original EK1 peptide, respectively. EK1C4 was also highly effective against membrane fusion and infection of other tested human coronavirus pseudoviruses, including SARS-CoV. Pinto *et al*. [85], identified an antibody (called S309) that was able to potently neutralize the SARS-CoV-2 and SARS-CoV pseudoviruses by involving the glycoprotein S receptor binding domain. S309 recognizes an epitope containing a glycan that is conserved within the subgenus Sarbecovirus, without competing with the recipient. Tian *et al*. [86], reported for the first time that a SARS-Co--specific human monoclonal antibody, CR3022, could potently bind to 2019-nCoV RBD (6.3 nM KD). The CR3022 epitope does not overlap the ACE2 binding site in 2019-nCoV RBD and the results suggest that CR3022 may have the potential to be developed as a candidate therapy, alone or in combination with other neutralizing antibodies.

5.2. Membrane Protein (M)

The SARS-CoV membrane proteins (M) are responsible for assembling the release of vesicles wrapped in the membrane and for forming virus-like particles (VLPs) when co-expressed with the N protein [87]. The M-membrane glycoprotein is co-translationally inserted into the endoplasmic reticulum (ER) and transported to Golgi complexes [74].

Hu *et al*. [88], based on comparative analysis of sequence characteristics, phylogenetic investigation and experimental results, were able to characterize the structure of protein M. According to the study, protein M is characterized by a typical TM (transmembrane) region composed of three putative TM domains of 80 residues that represent about a third of all protein. The first TM domain (TMI) consists of 19 residues with 83% formed by neutral amino acids, making it highly hydrophobic. The second domain (TMII) is between codons 50-72 (23 residues), with 81% of neutral, non-polar residues and with physical and chemical characteristics similar to TMI. The TMIII domain is located between codons 76-98 (23 residues), with 68.2% of non-polar neutral residues and, therefore, is not as hydrophobic as the other two. The segment between TMII and TMIII is possibly located abroad.

The self-assembly process of the M protein is complex, involving signaling and interactions with other proteins. Data suggest that SARS-CoV M contains a plasma membrane localization signal involving the third transmembrane domain and that glycosylation is not necessary for the localization, self-assembly and release of the plasma membrane M [89]. Codons 50 of the amino terminal carrying the first transmembrane domain are apparently sufficient for Golgi retention, efficient membrane binding and multimerization of the M SARS-CoV protein. Second Tseng *et al.* [87], a leucine motif on the endodomain tail (218LL219) is necessary for efficient packaging of N in VLPs. In addition, they observed that cysteine residues 63, 85 and 158 are not in close proximity to the M dimer interface and a significant reduction in M secretion due to the substitution of serine for C158, but not for C63 or C85. Further analysis suggests that C158 is involved in the MN interaction. Mutations of the highly conserved 107-SWWSFNPE-114 motif, leading to substitutions at codons W19, W57, P58, W91, Y94 or F95 resulted in significantly reduced VLP yields, largely due to defective M secretion. An additional functional analysis of truncated M proteins showed that the 134 N-terminal amino acids comprising the three transmembrane domains are sufficient to mediate the accumulation of M in the Golgi complex and to reinforce the recruitment of the viral peak S protein to the assembly sites and budding of the virus in the ERGIC [74].

In the host, the NF-κB and TBK1-IRF3 signaling cascades are activated by-products of the M gene. The M protein, instead of the mRNA M, is responsible for the induction of M-mediated IFN-β that is preferentially associated with the activation of MyD88, TIRAP and TICAM2 TLR adapter proteins, but not the RIG-I signaling cascade [90]. Another study indicates that SARS - CoV M suppresses NF-κB activity probably through direct interaction with IKKβ, resulting in less expression of Cyclooxygenase 2 (COX-2), contributing to the pathogenesis of SARS [91].

5.3. Envelope Protein (E)

CoV E protein is a short, integral, 76–109 amino acid protein, ranging from 8.4 to 12 kDa in size. The primary and secondary structure reveals a short hydrophilic amino terminal region consisting of 7-12 amino acids, followed by a large hydrophobic transmembrane domain (TMD) of 25 amino acids and ends with a long hydrophilic carboxyl terminal [92]. Protein E is located in secretory pathways in the space between the endoplasmic reticulum and the Golgi apparatus [93].

CoV (E) envelope protein is a small protein that participates in aspects of the virus life cycle, such as assembly, budding, envelope formation and pathogenesis [94].

Regarding the general sequence similarity, the E SARS-CoV-2 protein has the greatest similarity with SARS-CoV (94.74%) with only minor differences [94]. The SARS-CoV-2 protein E differs from that of SARS by only three substitutions and one deletion. Substitutions and insertions are positioned in flexible cytoplasmic regions, where they are not expected to affect the protein structure [95] (Fig. **5**).

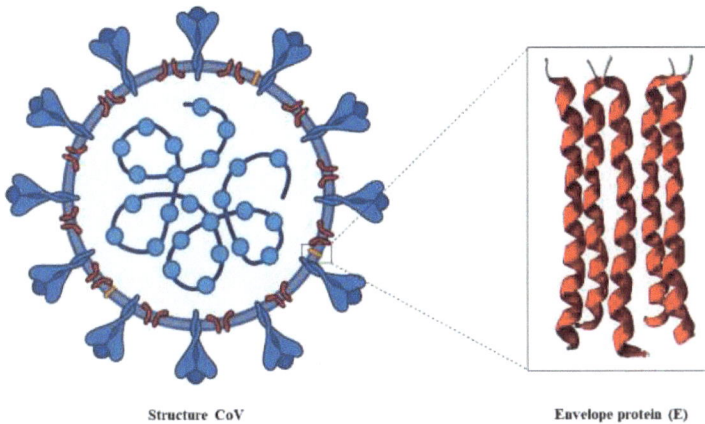

Structure CoV   Envelope protein (E)

Fig. (5). Structure of the CoV envelope protein.

Protein E of all SARS viruses preserves its critical motives used for pathogenesis and should be considered as an alternative target to be tested for therapies against COVID-2019 [95, 96]. Gupta *et al.* [97], used several computational approaches to study the structure and function of the human protein SARS-CoV-2 E, as well as its interaction with various phytochemicals. The result revealed that the α helix and the loops present in this protein experience random movement under ideal conditions, modulating the activity of the ion channel and contributing to pathogenesis. The compounds Belachinal, Macaflavanone E and Vibsanol B, managed to inhibit the function of protein E, through interactions with the amino acids Val25 and Phe26.

5.4. Nucleocapsid Protein (N)

CoV N protein is a multifunctional protein that plays essential roles in the formation of helical ribonucleoproteins during the packaging of the viral RNA genome, regulating viral RNA synthesis in replication / transcription and modulating the metabolism of infected cells [98, 99].

Protein N is expressed in host samples during the early stages of infection and is known to bind to viral RNA to form a nucleus of a ribonucleoprotein that helps it enter the host cell and interact with cellular processes after fusion of the virus [74]. Thus, its main function is to package the RNA molecule of the viral genome in a ribonucleoprotein complex (RNP) called a capsid. Therefore, ribonucleocapsid packaging is essential in viral self-assembly and the RNP complex is the essential model for replication by the RNA-dependent RNA polymerase complex [100].

The N SARS-CoV protein is a 46 kDa phosphoprotein containing 422 amino acids. It forms a dimer, which constitutes the basic building block of the nucleocapsid through its C-terminal. The structure of the N-terminal domain solution called RBD (residues 45-181) is capable of binding to RNA with micromolar affinity [100]. The structure of the dimerization domain (residues 248-365) also binds to nucleic acid. The complete SARS-CoV-2 genome is 29.9 kb in length and 419 amino acids. The structural base of the SARS-CoV-2 nucleocapsid has several residues in the ribonucleotide binding domain to distinctly recognize CoV RNA substrates. The tail residues N-terminal (Asn48, Asn49, Thr50 and Ala51) are considered more flexible and extended [98]. The SARS-CoV N protein contains two distinct RNA binding domains (the N-terminal [NTD] domain and the C-terminal [CTD] domain) linked by a poorly structured binding region (LKR) containing a serine / arginine (SR -rich) domain (SRD) [101]. The two folded domains do not interact significantly with each other, so the full-length N protein is a flexible, multivalent RNA binding protein [102].

The SARS-CoV-2 protein N sequence shows almost 90% similarity to the SARS-CoV N protein [103]. The high level of the sequence alignment between the SARS-CoV-2 and SARS-CoV N proteins suggests that these proteins exhibit substantial overlap in the organization, structure and general function of the domain [99].

According Cascarina e Ross [99], the SARS-CoV-2 N protein can take advantage of the ability to form or join biomolecular condensates to deregulate stress granules, increase viral replication or translation of viral proteins and package the viral RNA genome into new virions. Therefore, recognizing the role of protein N at various stages of the viral life cycle, the authors conclude that modulation of protein N regulation by treatments targeting host cell or organelle kinases may be viable strategies to fight infections caused by SARS- CoV-2.

Ye *et al.* [104], studied the strong and early antibody responses to the nucleocapsid exhibited by patients infected with SARS-CoV-2. They observed more than 10,000 occurrences of amino acid substitutions in the N protein, verifying the variability in the N2a domain, especially in residues 203 and 204, which mutate in large part of infections. However, they found that these substitutions within the N1b and N2b domains are grouped away from their functional RNA binding and dimerization interfaces, which can contribute to drug design and antibody-based testing.

5.5. 3-chymotrypsin-like Cysteine Protease (3CL^pro)

3CL[pro] or M[pro] is a dimer consisting of two highly conserved cysteine protease monomers [105]. Each monomer is formed by three domains and has a catalytic dyad (His41 and Cys145) located in a gap between domains I and II (residues 10-99 and 100-182, respectively). The catalytic residues are located in the double fold β of the chymotrypsin type in domains I and II. The catalytic domains are connected by a long loop region to the C-terminal III domain (residues 198-303) composed of five antiparallel α helices [106]. Dimerization is necessary for enzymatic activity since the N finger of each of the two monomers interacts with Glu166 of the other monomer, which helps in the correct orientation of the S1 pocket of the substrate binding site [107]. It was also observed that only 12 of the 306 residues are different in SARS-CoV-2 M[pro] compared to SARS-CoV M[pro] (96% sequence identity). In addition, none of the 12 variant residues are involved in any major roles in the enzymatic activity of SARS-CoV-2 M[pro] [106] (Fig. **6**).

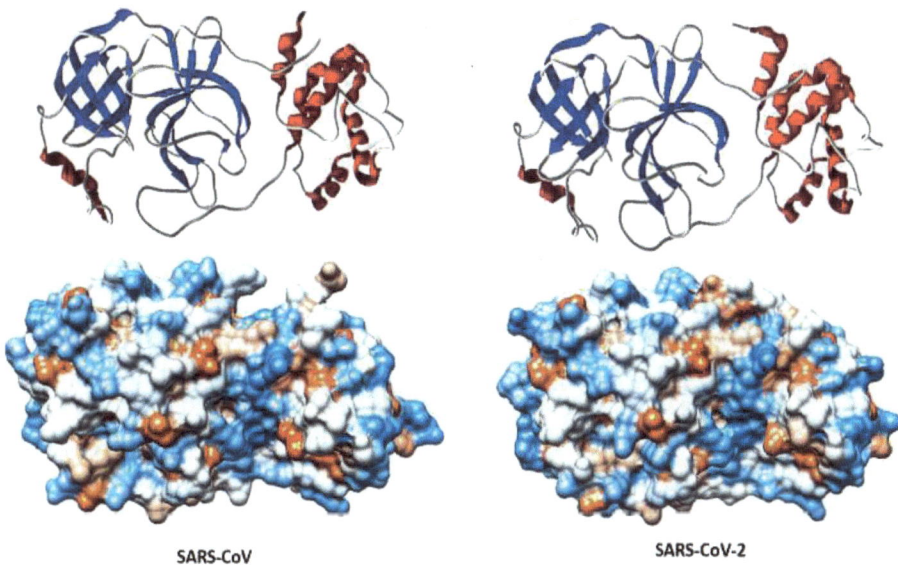

SARS-CoV　　　　　　　　　　　　　SARS-CoV-2

Fig. (6). Structures of 3CL[pro] proteins and hydrophobicity of SARS-CoV and SARS-CoV-2. In proteins with blue hydrophobicity, they are represented by positive amino acids and in orange, the negative amino acids.

SARS-CoV-2 M[pro] plays a key role in the processing of polyproteins and is therefore considered a promising target for the development of anti-coronavirus therapeutic agents [73]. Provides a critical role in the replication of virus particles and, unlike genes encoding structural/accessory proteins, is located at the 3' and, which exhibits excessive variability [108]. Inhibiting the activity of this enzyme would block viral replication. As human proteases with similar cleavage specificity are not known, such inhibitors are unlikely to be toxic [109]. In addition, due to high mutation rates, proteins that are conserved have a great advantage for drug development. Thus, drugs that target M[pro] are generally able to prevent virus replication and proliferation and exhibit broad-spectrum antiviral activity, also decreasing the risk of mutation-mediated drug resistance in future deadly viral strains [73].

In order to design potent inhibitors against this enzyme, it is important to know the molecular structure and the catalytic site well. A study by Wang *et al.*, allowed to identify a pair of residues (Glu-His) and His164 conserved as critical for the binding; a GSCGS motif conserved as important for the beginning of the catalysis, a partial negative charge cluster (PNCC) formed by Arg-Tyr-Asp as essential for the catalysis and a conserved water molecule mediating the remote interaction between PNCC and catalytic dyad [105]. M[pro] has a catalytic Cys-His dyad instead of a Ser8 (Cys) -His-Asp (Glu) triad. The catalytic residues Cys145 and His41 in 3CL Mpro are within an active site cavity located on the surface of the protein and can accommodate four substrate residues at positions P1 'to P4, flanked by residues from both domains I and II [110]. M[pro] has a unique substrate preference for glutamine at the P1 site (Leu-Gln ↓ (Ser, Ala, Gly), a feature that is absent in closely related host proteases, suggesting that it is feasible to achieve high selectivity targeting viral M[pro] [111].

Several studies have shown potent, selective inhibitors and drug candidates against SARS-CoV and SARS-CoV-2 Mpro. Sacco *et al*. Reported that inhibitors of calpain II and XII and boceprevir have low IC^{50} values in μM against SARS-CoV-2 M[pro] [112]. The boceprevir compounds showed an IC^{50} inhibitory activity of 4.13 μMm, while Calpain II and Calpain XII showed values of 0.907 and 0.45, respectively [111]. This is because these compounds have a hydrophobic side chain in the P1 position, challenging the notion that a necessary hydrophilic fraction in this position [112].

To facilitate the rapid discovery of antiviral compounds with clinical potential, several researchers have developed strategies that combine virtual drug screening and high-throughput screening to reuse existing drugs to achieve SARS-CoV-2 M[pro] [113]. Excellent results were obtained by Jin, Du, Yang; from a library of 10,000 FDA approved drugs and natural products, selected the best *in silico* results for assays of enzymatic activity against M^{pro} from SARS-CoV-2. Experimental tests showed that Ebselen, disulfiram, Tideglusib and Carmofur, presented IC^{50} values of 0.76, 9.35, 1.55 and 1.82, respectively [113]. Narkhede *et al.*, also used computer resources to track potent natural products against SARS-CoV-2 M^{pro}. With the aid of *in silico* techniques, such as molecular docking and druggability studies, it was possible to select natural active compounds, including glycyrrhizin, bicylogermecrene, triptantrin, β-sitosterol, indirubine, indigo, indigo, hesperetin, chrysophanic acid, reine, berberine and β -cariophylene [114]. Fisher *et al.*; in order to find new inhibitors, did a computational search from a library of more than 606 million compounds for binding to the newly resolved crystal structure of the SARS-CoV-2 main protease (M^{pro}). After the screening of shapes, two docking protocols were applied, followed by the determination of molecular descriptors relevant to pharmacokinetics and simulations of molecular dynamics. After evaluating the potential link, a list of 12 acquirable compounds was obtained, among them, the compound Rhamnetin, is now commercially available in pharmacies [115]. Several other studies have contributed to the investigation and selection of potential compounds against M^{pro} [72, 116 - 121].

5.6. Angiotensin Converting Enzyme (ACE)-2

ACE-2 is a monocarboxypeptidase and its gene is located on chromosome 17 in humans, encoding a 180 kDa protein with 805 amino acids [122]. Each domain has an active zinc binding motif, His-Glu-XX-His (HEXXH motif). The HEXXH histidine motif identified as an important component in a wide variety of zinc-dependent metalloproteases consists of five residues, the first histidine followed by glutamic acid being conserved, then the two variable amino acids and a final histidine [123]. ACE is a type I transmembrane glycoprotein, which is anchored to the plasma membrane through a single carboxy-terminal transmembrane domain, that is, with a single extracellular catalytic domain. ACE-2 has been reported in a subset of human monocytes CD14 + CD16, also expressed by enterocytes of the small intestine and is present in arterial and venous endothelial cells and arterial smooth muscle, in alveolar epithelial cells of lungs type I and II and epithelial cells of the oral mucosa [123].

ACE-2 is responsible for the conversion of angiotensin II, showing protection in the cardiovascular system and in many organs [122]. In addition, it is considered one of the main receptors for the entry of coronavirus in humans. Although ACE-2 is an important receptor for coronavirus infection, the type of coronavirus can cause different effects in the body, between mild and severe. One explanation is that the binding site for both viruses is distinct from the active enzyme site, which gives SARS-CoV-2 greater binding efficiency in ACE-2 than in other types of coronaviruses [124].

According Samavati and Uhal [123], the binding of the coronavirus peak protein to ACE2 leads to the release of ACE2 receptors by various proteases, which in turn leads to the loss of the protective function of the ACE2 / MAS axis in the lungs and other organs. In addition, the activation of the classical pathway (ACE / RAS / Ang II) and alternative pathways through tissue-specific proteases, including cathepsins chymase-type proteases, leads to excessive production of Ang II at the tissue level. The excess of AngII leads to an imbalance of Ang (1-7) / MAS and ACE2 protection, contributing to epithelial and endovascular lesions. Therefore, induction of the ACE2 downstream pathway, activating ACE2 / Ang1-Axis 7 / MAS can be a useful strategy in preventing pulmonary and cardiovascular damage associated with SARS-CoV2 infections.

6. DRUGS AND INHIBITORS AGAINST SARS

The new coronavirus 2019 (COVID-19) is the seventh coronavirus capable of infecting humans, called SARS-CoV-2 by the International Committee on Virus Taxonomy [125]. Some drugs already on the market, such as Remdesivir, Favipiravir and Chloroquine / Hydroxychloroquine have shown potential inhibitors against SARS-CoV-2, however, to date, no specific clinically approved medication or vaccines are available to treat the disease [125]. In this sense, it is vital to develop specific drugs against SARS-CoV-2, given that researchers are rushing to develop antiviral compounds for use in therapy and a range of natural and synthetic compounds are being analyzed to achieve this goal.

Choy *et al.*, 2020 [126] in their analysis, reported the *in vitro* antiviral effect of drugs cited in the literature as inhibitors of SARS-CoV-2 replication and those currently under evaluation in clinical trials for patients with SARS-CoV-2. Among the 16 drugs analyzed against cells of the *Vero E6* lineage previously infected by SARS-CoV-2, only remdesivir and lopinavir (Fig. **7**), as well as homoringtonine and emetin (Fig. **8**) presented an EC_{50} below 100 µM. In this sense, the compounds mentioned above had an EC_{50} of 23.15 µM, 26.63 µM, 2.55 µM and 0.46 µM, respectively. In addition, ribavirin and favipiravir, currently evaluated in clinical trials, showed no inhibition at 100 µM. In addition, a synergy was observed between remdesivir and emetina, since remdesivir at 6.25 µM in combination with emetine at 0.195 µM reached 64.9% inhibition in viral yield.

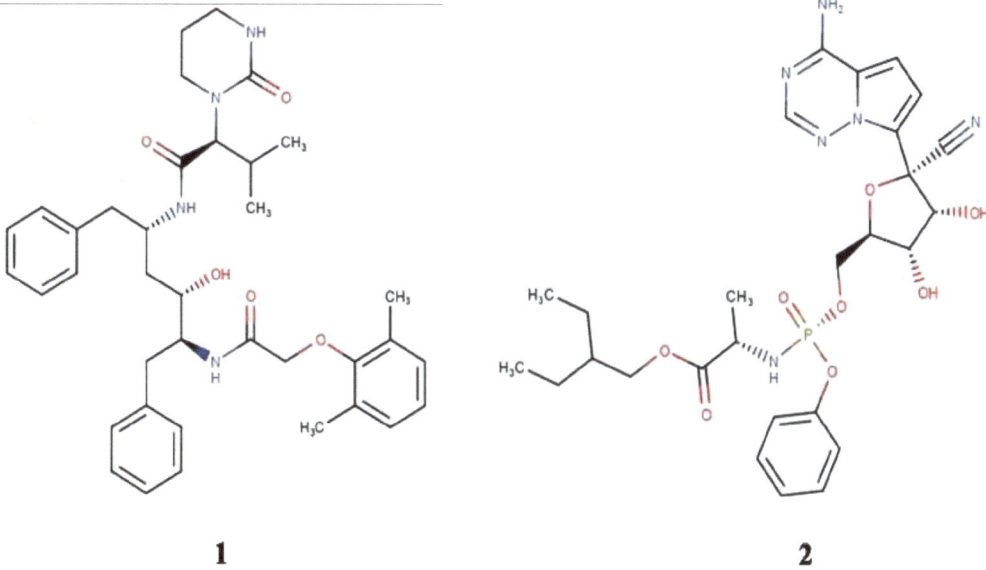

1   **2**

Fig. (7). 2d structures of remdesivir (**1**) and lopinavir (**2**).

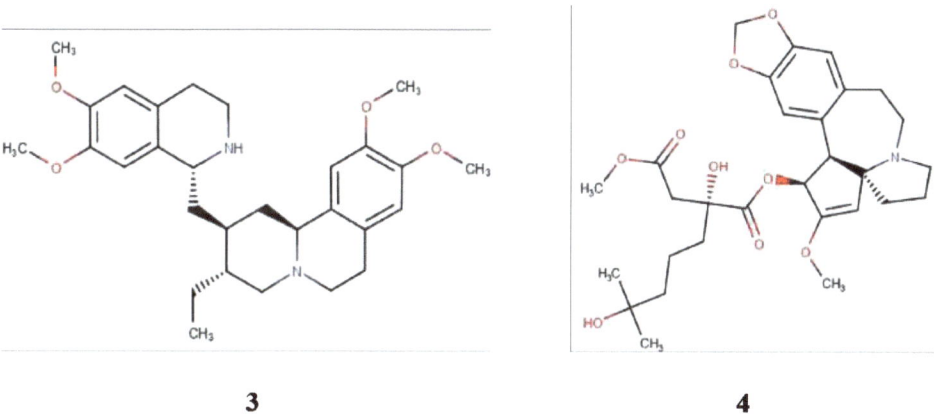

3   **4**

Fig. (8). 2d structures of homoringtonine (**3**) and emetine (**4**).

Zhang *et al.*, 2020 [109] evaluated the inhibitory profile of 4 compounds derived from α-ketoamides (Fig. **9**) by *in silico*, *in vitro* and *in vivo* methods. After using *Molecular Docking*, several interactions of the compounds in question were seen with the amino acids present in SARS-CoV-2, however, compounds 13a and 13b were the ones that showed the most expressive results against the virus. Compound 13b showed an IC_{50} of 0.67 μM and an EC_{50} of 4-5 μM against lung cells of the *Calu-3* strain infected with SARS-CoV-2. In pharmacokinetic studies in CD1 lineage mice using the subcutaneous route, the half-life of compound 13b was 1.8 hrs, in addition, the inhalation route with this compound was used, which proved to be quite promising. In addition, compounds 13a and 13b did not show adverse effects in the assays against mice. As a result, studies with α-ketoamide inhibitors showed that compound 13a inhibited SARS-CoV-2 replication *in vitro*, while compound 13b remained in lung tissue for more than 24h. The authors conclude that compounds 13a and 13b are safe and effective, making them excellent candidates for treatment against SARS-CoV-2.

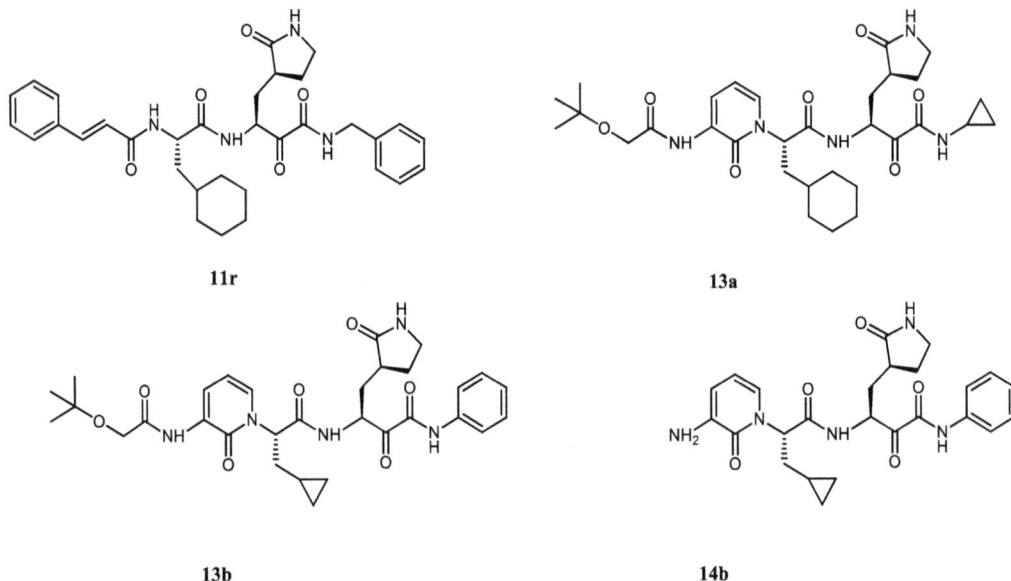

11r

13a

13b

14b

Fig. (9). 2d structures of the α-ketoamide derivatives analyzed.

Jin *et al.* (2020) [4] analyzed *in silico* and *in vitro* compounds that inhibit the main protease (M^{pro}) of SARS-CoV-2, a fundamental enzyme for viral replication and transcription. For this purpose, more than 10,000 compounds, including approved drugs, drug candidates in clinical trials and other pharmacologically active M^{pro} inhibitor compounds, were analyzed by virtual screening. Of the analyzed compounds, only 6 demonstrated potential inhibitors, to mention: ebselen, disulfiram, tideglusib, carmofur, shikonin and PX-12, as shown in Fig. **(10)**. In *in vitro* assays using Vero E6 cells previously infected, the compounds showed significant IC$_{50}$, citing: 0.67 μM (ebselen), 9.35 μM (disulfiram), 1.55 μM (tideglusib), 1.82 μM (carmofur), 15.75 μM (shikonin) and 21.39 μM (PX-12). In addition, the EC$_{50}$ of ebselen (4.67 μM) was compared and compared to that of a promising inhibitor of the protease Mpro called N3 (EC$_{50}$ of 16.77 μM).

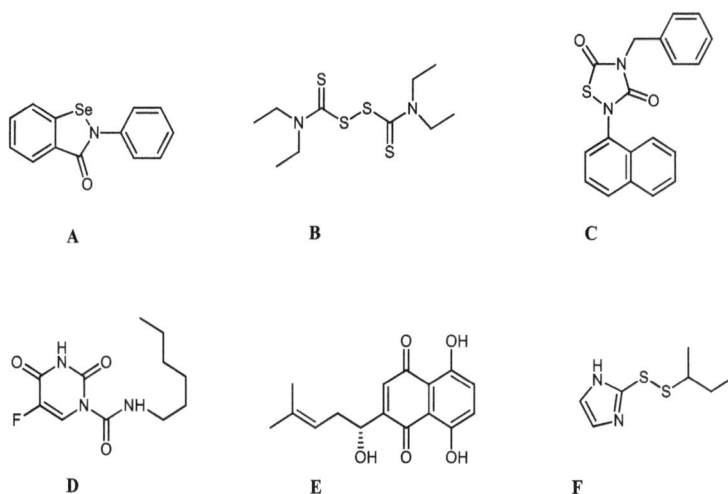

Fig. (10). 2d structures of the compounds: A - ebselen; B - disulfiram; C -tideglusib; D - Carmofur; E - shikonin; F- PX-12.

Dai *et al.* (2020) [116] designed two synthetic inhibitors, 11a and 11b (Fig. **11**), based on the analysis of the structure of the SARS-CoV-2 M^{pro} protease active site and evaluated their inhibitory profile, using *in silico*, *in vitro* and *in vivo* methods. In view of the *in silico* analyzes, both compounds showed several interactions with the amino acid residues of SARS-CoV-2, showing promising potential inhibitors. Motivated by such results, the authors analyzed the inhibitory profile of these compounds against the recombinant SARS-CoV-2 M^{pro} from *Escherichia coli* and against such method, excellent inhibitory potentials were found, with an IC$_{50}$ of 0.053 μM for compound 11a and 0.040 μM for compound 11b. In addition, compounds 11a and 11b showed an EC$_{50}$ 0.53 and 0.72 μM, respectively, compared to *Vero E6* cells.

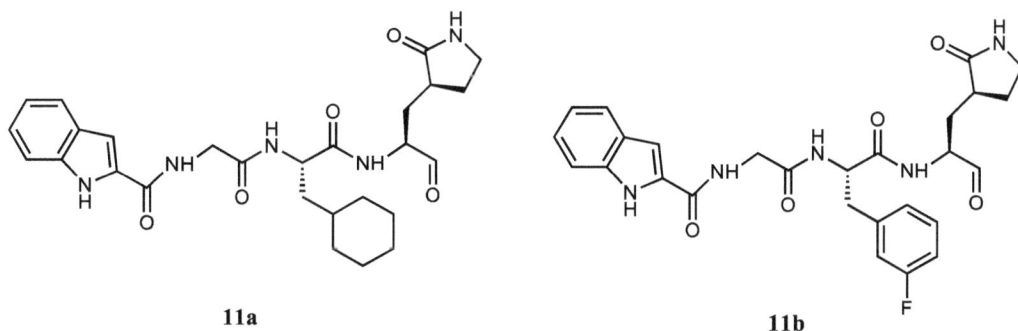

Fig. (11). Two-dimensional structure of compounds 11a and 11b.

Additionally, the compounds were evaluated against mice using the intraperitoneal and intravenous routes. Compound 11a showed, through the intraperitoneal route, a bioavailability of 87.8% and a half-life of 4.27 hrs, while by the intravenous route, it also showed bioavailability above 80% and a half-life of 4.41 hrs. Compound 11b, on the other hand, had an intraperitoneal route, bioavailability above 80% and a half-life of 5.21 hrs, while intravenously, it also had good bioavailability and a half-life of 1.65 hrs. In view of the results, compound 11a had better potential and thus, it was subjected to *in vivo* tests using now, intravenous drip in beagle rats and dogs. The results showed that compound 11a exhibited long half-life values for rats (7.6 hrs) and beagle dogs (5.5 hrs), in addition, no significant toxicity was observed in the animals. Thus, compound 11a showed better pharmacokinetic properties and low toxicity when tested in mice, rats and dogs, suggesting that this compound is a promising drug candidate.

Caly *et al.* (2020) [127] evaluated the drug ivermectin against SARS-CoV-2 using *in vitro* methods. Ivermectin has been approved by the Food and Drug Administration (FDA) for the treatment of parasitic infections, however, several studies report its inhibitory potential against SARS-CoV-2. The researchers used cells from the Vero strain infected by the virus and analyzed the inhibitory profile of ivermectin at a concentration of 5 μM. After 48 hrs, ivermectin inhibited about 99.98% of the virus in cell culture, presenting an IC_{50} of 2 μM. These results demonstrate that ivermectin has a potent antiviral action *in vitro* against SARS-CoV-2, with a single concentration capable of controlling viral replication in 24–48 h.

Ngo *et al.*, (2020) [128] investigated *in silico* methods compounds that inhibit the main SARS-CoV-2 protease, M^{pro}. The authors used rigorous computational methodologies to determine the probable natural inhibitors, to mention: *molecular docking* (Autodock Vina *software*) to determine the ligand binding posture and affinity for SARS-CoV-2 M^{pro}, the molecular dynamics simulation (GROMACS *software*), to simulate the structural change of the solvated SARS-CoV-2 M^{pro} + inhibitor complex. In addition, the calculation of free energy by the FPL (Fast Pulling of Ligand) approach and the simulation of disturbance of free energy by the FEP (Free Energy Perturbation) approach, as shown in Scheme (**1**). In view of the methodologies used, certain filtering was done, through the analysis of a database containing approximately 4,600 compounds. In view of these hundreds of compounds analyzed, the authors concluded that two natural compounds, cannabisin A and isoactoside, as well as an HIV-1 PR inhibitor, darunavir, showed promising results, with great SARS-free energy -CoV-2 M^{pro}.

```
┌─────────────────────┐   ┌─────────────────────┐   ┌─────────────────────┐   ┌─────────────────────┐
│ Molecular Docking   │   │   FPL Simulation    │   │   FEP Calculation   │   │ Potential Inhibitors│
│                     │ → │                     │ → │                     │ → │                     │
│ ~ 4600 compounds    │   │   35 compounds      │   │   3 compounds       │   │   2 compounds       │
└─────────────────────┘   └─────────────────────┘   └─────────────────────┘   └─────────────────────┘
```

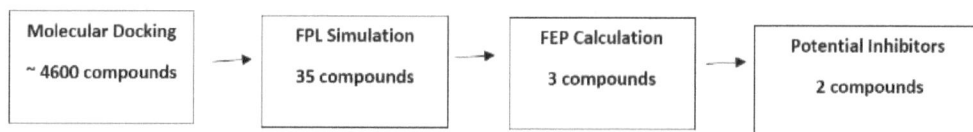

Scheme (1). Computational strategy to determine the likely natural inhibitors of the SARS-CoV-2 M^{pro} protease

Based on the premise that natural compounds can add value to the development of specific therapies against SARS-CoV-2, Neto *et al.* (2021) [129] conducted a survey of the literature on the antiviral activity of Indian Neem (*Azadirachta indica A. Juss.*) against SARS-CoV-2. This medicinal plant has been widely studied for having several therapeutic properties, such as anti-inflammatory, antiviral, antitumor, antibiotic, antifungal, among others. Motivated by such properties, these researchers analyzed in the literature the main studies involving this plant in relation to SARS-CoV-2 and in view of the analyzes, it was possible to identify some potential inhibitors of the SARS-CoV-2 membrane (M) and Envelope (E) proteins using *molecular docking*, MD simulation and bond-free energy calculations. The compounds derived from Indian Neem, showed stable binding and interactions with crucial regions of E and M necessary for the assembly and were expected to have good pharmacokinetic properties. One of the constituents, nimbolin A showed the strongest binding free energy with proteins E and M. In addition, other compounds such as Nimocin and Cycloartanols (24-Methylenocycloartanol and 24-Methylenocycloartan-3-one) were also strongly bound to both proteins.

In addition, studies involving molecular coupling tools have evaluated the binding efficacy of natural compounds from Neem against three main targets of SARS-CoV-2, namely: 1) surface glycoprotein (6VSB) responsible for viral binding, 2) dependent RNA polymerase of RNA (6M71) responsible for viral replication and 3) main protease (6Y84) responsible for viral replication. Phytochemicals methyl eugenol, oleanolic acid and ursolic acid had high binding efficiency against the peak glycoprotein surface and SARS-CoV-2 RNA polymerase. Epoxy-azadiradione, gedunine, methyl eugenol, oleanolic acid and ursolic acid showed high binding efficacy against the main SARS-CoV-2 protease.

In view of the results found, the binding efficacy of the natural compounds of Neem was superior to that of the standard drugs Lopinavir / Ritonavir and Remdesivir (used against SARS-CoV-2), showing that these natural compounds have a high binding efficiency against SARS- CoV-2, on targets involved in viral binding and replication, therefore, can be useful in managing infection caused by

SARS-CoV-2. From the data analysis, it was found that Indian Neem contains an antiviral potential, evidencing both through its extract and isolated phytochemicals, among the mechanisms of antiviral action, the action on viral protease stands out.

Lopes *et al.* (2020) [130] investigated in the literature the main findings on the antiviral activity of ivermectin (Fig. **12**) against SARS-CoV-2. Through the analysis of the works contained in the literature, it was demonstrated in initial studies, *in vitro*, that there is a significant reduction in the viral load of SARS-CoV-2 in approximately 5000 times, equivalent to 99.98% of the viral RNA, after 48 hours of starting this medication. It was also found that there was no additional benefit reported after increasing the medication administration time by up to 72 hours. In addition, studies claim that Ivermectin acts by inhibiting the nuclear import of host and viral proteins mediated by IMPα/β1, thus interrupting the evasion mechanism of the virus, considering that RNA viruses depend on the integrase protein and the heterodimer α/β1 of the importin (IMPα/β1) during infection.

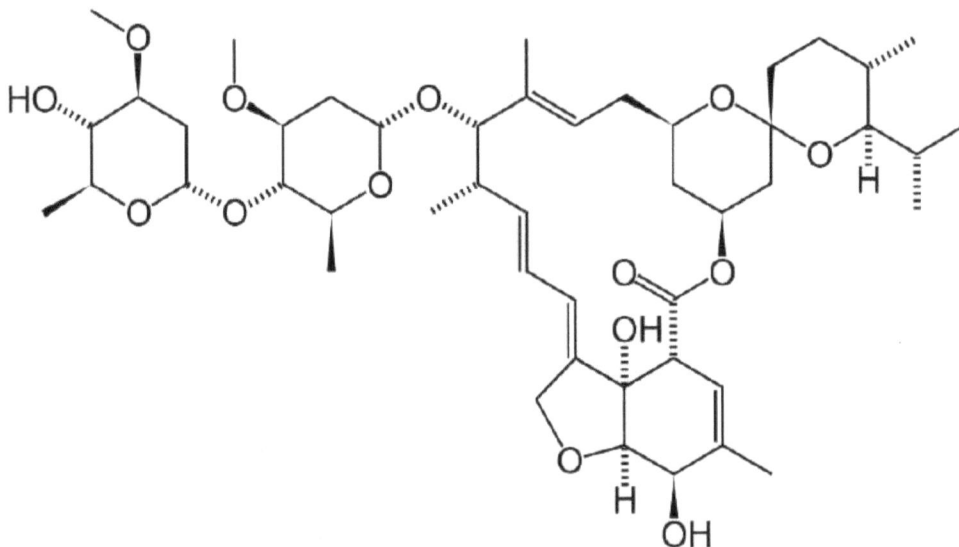

Fig. (12). Two-dimensional structure of ivermectin.

Regarding toxicity, no toxicity was observed in relation to the studies analyzed, however, some studies suggest that there may be adverse effects, however, the conventional dose of a maximum of 200 μg/kg is considered safe in therapy in humans. In view of this, the results revealed that interventions using ivermectin *in vitro* are statistically significant, with the main effect of decreasing viral replication.

Fu *et al.* (2020) [125] selected a group of 18 drugs (Table **1**) already on the market to assess their inhibitory potentials against SARS-CoV-2 using *in silico* and *in vitro* methods. After a virtual screening of the 18 drugs used to target different viral proteases, only boceprevir (Fig. **13**) and GC376 demonstrated significant inhibitory potentials, with an IC_{50} of 8.0 μM and 0.15 μM, respectively. For this, *molecular docking* and enzymatic assays of fluorescence resonance energy transfer (FRET) in a single concentration (100 μM) were performed. Additionally, in the *in vitro* method using previously infected *Vero* cells and remdesivir as a positive control (currently approved for emergency use for severe infections by COVID-19), both boceprevir and GC376 showed potential inhibitors against protease M pro SARS-CoV-2, with EC_{50} values of 15.57 μM and 0.70 μM, respectively. In addition, remdesivir inhibited SARS-CoV-2 replication with an EC_{50} value of 0.58 μM and it has been shown that the combination of 1 μM GC376 and 1 μM remdesivir can completely inhibit viral replication.

Table 1. Drugs selected for virtual screening as potential inhibitors of SARS-CoV-2 M^{pro} protease.

ID	Target	Drug
1	HIV Protease	Saquinavir
2	HIV Protease	Ritonavir
3	HIV Protease	Indinavir
4	HIV Protease	Nelfinavir mesylate
5	HIV Protease	Amprenavir
6	HIV Protease	Lopinavir
7	HIV Protease	Atazanavir Sulfate
8	HIV Protease	Fosamprenavir
9	HIV Protease	Tipranavir
10	HIV Protease	Darunavir
11	HCV NS3 protease	Boceprevir
12	HCV NS3 protease	Telaprevir
13	HCV NS3 protease	Simeprevir
14	HCV NS3 protease	Asunaprevir
15	HCV NS3 protease	Grazoprevir
16	Proteasome	Carfilzomib
17	Proteasome	Bortezomib
18	3C-like protease	GC376 sodium

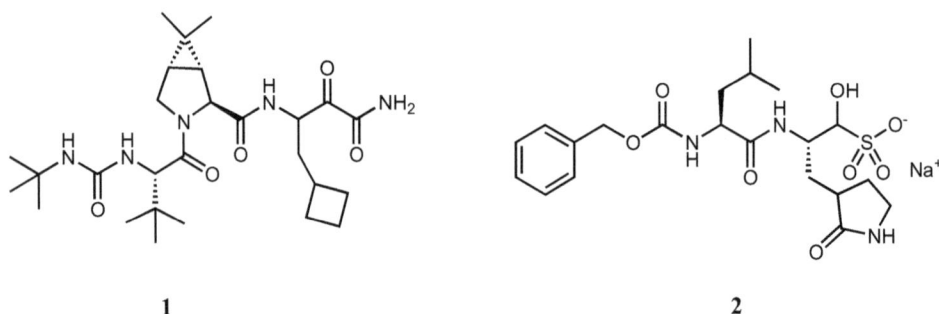

Fig. (13). Two-dimensional structure of boceprevir (1) and GC376 (2).

Kwon *et al.* (2020) [131] evaluated the inhibitory potential *in vitro* and *in silico* of sulfated polysaccharides using cells of the *Vero* strain infected with SARS-CoV-2 and *molecular docking*. Among the polysaccharides that showed potential, were NACH (derived from non-anticoagulant heparin), TriS-heparin (trisulfated heparin), heparin, RPI-28 and RPI-27 (polysaccharides extracted from Japanese saccharine algae). Using cells of the *Vero* strain previously infected by the virus, the polysaccharide that showed the greatest inhibitory potential was RPI-27, with an EC_{50} of 8.3 ± 4.6 µg/mL, which corresponds to 83 nM, more potent than the remdesivir (used in emergencies against COVID-19) with an EC_{50} value reported *in vitro* of 770 nM in *Vero* cells. The RPI-28 showed an EC_{50} of 1.2 µM, while heparin and TriS-heparin also showed potent antiviral activity, with an EC_{50} 2.1 and 5.0 µM, respectively, while NACH presented an EC_{50} of 55 µM .

The marked activity of RPI-27 and RPI-28 in relation to the other tested polysaccharides may be a result of multivalent interactions between the polysaccharide and the SARS-CoV-2 viral particle, considering that heparin, TriS-heparin and NACH are linear polysaccharides, whereas RPI-27 and RPI-28 are highly branched, which justifies the difference in antiviral activity. Additionally, in order to try to understand the mechanism for such inhibition of these compounds, *molecular docking* studies were carried out. The results demonstrated that these sulfated polysaccharides bind strongly to the SARS-Co--2 protein S, suggesting that they can act as baits to interfere in the binding of protein S to the heparan sulfate co-receptor in host tissues, inhibiting viral infection.

Xia *et al.* (2019) [132] demonstrated in their studies the probable mechanism for the fusion and viral entry of SARS-CoV-2 in the host cells, as well as the inhibitory potential of a promising peptide called EK1. The group of researchers reported that glycoprotein S plays an important role in mediating viral infection by SARS-CoV-2. For a better understanding, the glycoprotein S consists of two subunits, S1 and S2. The S1 subunit binds to the cell receptor through its RBD, followed by conformational changes in the S2 subunit, which allows the fusion peptide to enter the membrane of the host's target cell. The heptal repeat region 1 (HR1) in the S2 subunit forms a homotrimeric set, which exposes three highly conserved hydrophobic grooves on the surface that connect heptal repeat 2 (HR2). This central six-helix beam structure (6-HB) is formed during the fusion process and helps to bring viral and cell membranes in close proximity for fusion and viral entry.

In this sense, it is justifiable that protein S is one of the target proteins for the development of specific drugs. In particular, Xia *et al.* (2019) [132] stresses that S1 RBD is a significant target site, and both RBD-specific antibodies and RBD-based vaccines in the test phase, exhibited effective antiviral activity or protective effect in blocking the virus from binding to host receptors. In addition, the HR region in the S2 subunit also plays a central role in SARS-CoV-2 infections, forming 6-HB that mediates viral fusion. In view of this, peptides derived from the HR2 regions of the SARS-CoV and MERS-CoVS proteins can competitively inhibit the formation of viral 6-HB, thus preventing viral fusion and entry into host cells. Thus, these researchers performed a virtual screening of a peptide called OC43-HR2P by *in silico* methods, which showed broad spectrum fusion inhibitory activity, while another peptide derived from it, EK1, showed promising potency and amplitude in inhibiting infection. Still, *in vivo* studies have demonstrated that the administration of EK1 through the nasal route has highly protective effects and safety profiles, highlighting its clinical potential.

Continuing the research, the group of researchers Xia *et al.* (2020) [84] found that SARS-CoV-2 showed superior plasma membrane fusion capacity compared to SARS-CoV and based on this, as they had previously developed a pan-coronavirus fusion inhibitor, EK1, which targeted the HR1 domain and could inhibit infection with divergent human coronaviruses tested, including SARS-CoV and MERS-CoV, now, in the present study, a series of EK1-derived lipopeptides has been generated, which has been shown that EK1C4 was the most potent fusion inhibitor against the SARS-CoV-2 S protein-mediated membrane fusion and pseudovirus infection with an IC_{50} of 1.3 and 15.8 nM, respectively, about 241 and 149 times more potent than the previously developed EK1 peptide. EK1C4 was also highly effective against membrane fusion and infection of other tested human coronavirus pseudoviruses, including SARS-CoV and MERS-CoV, as well as SARSr-CoVs, and potently inhibited the replication of 5 examined live human coronaviruses, including SARS-CoV-2. Furthermore, the intranasal application of EK1C4 before or after the challenge with HCoV-OC43 protected mice from infection, which raises high expectations for being a drug candidate.

Chien *et al.* (2020) [13] based on their analysis of the activities of 3 viral inhibitors that they had previously demonstrated for themselves, that is, three nucleotide analogs, sofosbuvir triphosphates, allovudine and zidovudine (AZT), which inhibited the dependent RNA polymerase of the SARS-CoV RNA (RdRp). Given the similarity of 98% of the SARS-CoV amino acids to the SARS-CoV-2 RdRp, it was concluded that these 3 nucleotide analogs should also inhibit the SARS-CoV-2 RdRP. In view of this and based on the promising results of these three drug forms of active triphosphates, the present study was selected by *in silico* methods, specifically molecular docking, the active triphosphate forms of six antiviral agents, alovudine, tenofovir alafenamide, AZT, abacavir, lamivudine and emtricitabine, for evaluation as inhibitors of SARS-CoV-2 viral RNA polymerase (RdRp). Additionally, based on promising results published in the sofosbuvir literature, it was evaluated together. In this sense, Chien *et al.* (2020) [133], after *in silico* analysis, demonstrated by *in vitro* methods (Rosetta cells 2 pLysS *E. coli*) the inhibitory capacity of these analogs against the SARS-CoV-2 viral polymerase, however, only sofosbuvir, alovudine, tenofovir alafenamide and abacavir showed results significantly and thus can be considered as potential candidates in clinical trials for the treatment and prevention of COVID-19.

Mahmud *et al.* (2020) [134] used combinatorial bioinformatics approaches to analyze promising natural plant-derived compounds against SARS-CoV-2. For this, we used a database (taken from PubChem) containing 1480 natural compounds derived from plants, in order to find molecules active against the main protease (M^{Pro}) of SARS-CoV-2. In this sense, virtual screening was used, simulations of ADMET properties (absorption, distribution, metabolism, excretion and toxicity) with analysis of the five-rule by Lipinski, simulation of molecular dynamics and *molecular docking* to reach potential compounds. Among all, a total of 14 compounds showed significant results, and of these, 3 were separated, based on those that showed the best results.

In this sense, the 3 best natural compounds that proved to be strong drug candidates, were carinol, albanine A and myricetin (Fig. **14**), since they had a better binding profile than the rest of the compounds with energy binding –8.476, –8.036, –8.439 kcal/mol, respectively. In addition, as this study represents a perfect model for inhibiting the SARS-CoV-2 M^{Pro} protease through the study of bioinformatics, these potential drug candidates can help researchers find a superior and effective solution against COVID-19 after future experiments.

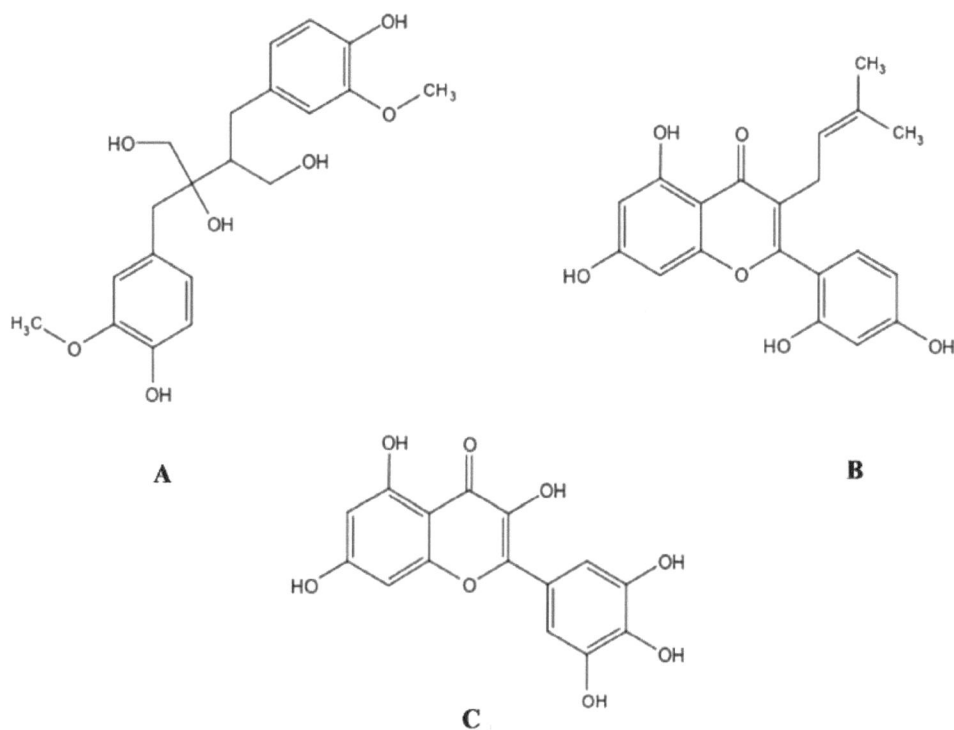

Fig. (14). Structures 2d of carinol (A), albanina A (B) and miricetina (C).

Gentile *et al.* (2020) [135] used computational techniques based on a screening of compounds taken from the Natural Marine Product (MNP) library, in order to identify natural marine inhibitors of the SARS-CoV-2 M^{pro} protease. At first, a virtual screening of 14,064 molecules was carried out in the MNP library and of these, only 180 molecules were separated for further studies. In this sense and using *molecular docking* and molecular dynamics simulation, only 17 molecules showed potentials against the M^{pro} protease, most of which are represented by mainly a class of molecules called florotanins, floroglucinol oligomers (1,3,5-trihydroxybenzene) and isolated from the brown seaweed *Sargassum spinuligerum*. Among them, it was found that the most active inhibitors were molecules 7 (8,8'-Bieckol), 10 (6,6'-Bieckol) and 11 (Dieckol), belonging to the family of florotanins and isolated from the brown alga *Ecklonia cava*, as shown in Fig. (**15**).

7

10

11

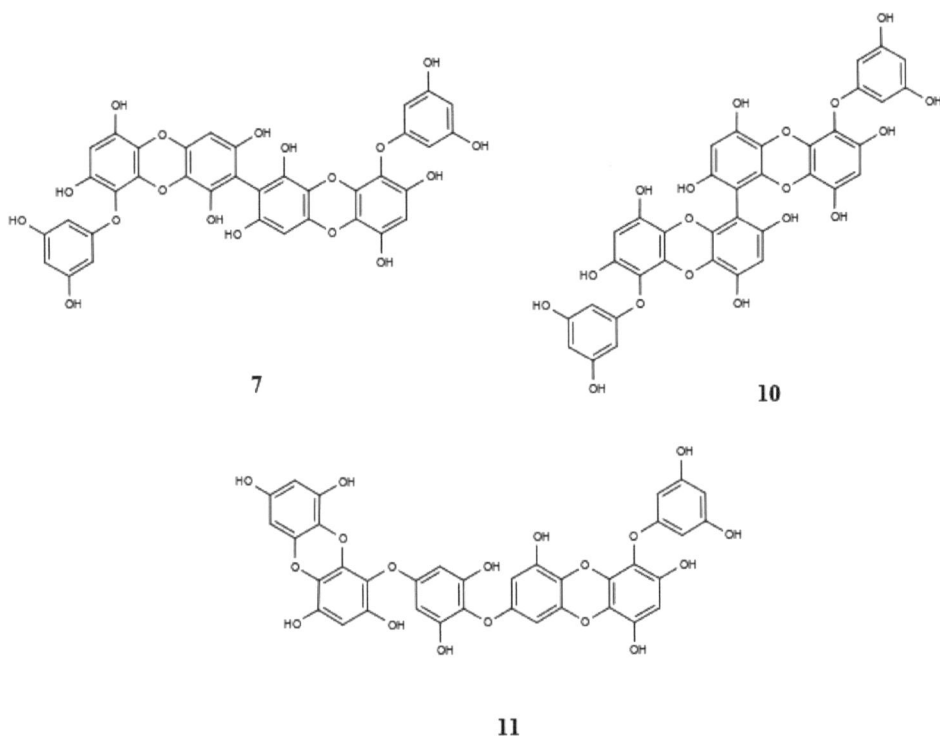

Fig. (15). 2d structures of the potential molecules 7 (8,8'-Bieckol), 10 (6,6'-Bieckol) and 11 (Dieckol).

In view of this, molecular dynamics and re-docking further confirmed the results obtained by structure-based techniques. 17 potential inhibitors of SARS-CoV-2 M^{pro} have been identified among natural substances of marine origin, with a focus on 3 that showed the best results. In addition, the selected compounds showed a better energy score than lopinavir (one of the drugs currently used to treat COVID-19), stimulating further research and testing involving these promising drug candidates.

CONCLUSION

In view of the above, the present study addressed the main characteristics of SARS, as well as the main targets and compounds that have achieved excellent results in *in silico*, *in vitro* and *in vivo* tests. Through the countless compounds evaluated by the most diverse fields of research, the present study addressed the most promising ever reported in the literature, in view of the imminent threat that SARS has been demonstrating, mainly by SARS-CoV-2, justifying the urgent need to develop effective antiviral agents for prevention and treatment.

With this, it is highlighted the paramount importance of studies, which, like this one, seeks to demonstrate the main results of compounds that have potential antivirals for the virus in question, motivating future studies in order to develop antiviral drugs.

LIST OF ABBREVIATIONS

2019-nCoV	new Coronavirus
3CLpro	3-chymotrypsin cysteine protease
ACE2	Angiotensin-Converting Enzyme 2
AZT	zidovudine
BCoV	Bovine Coronavirus
CCoV	Canine Coronavirus
COVID-19	Coronavirus disease-2019
CoVs	Coronaviruses
COX-2	Cyclooxygenase 2
CRS	Cytokine release syndrome
ECoV	Equine Coronavirus
ER	Endoplasmic reticulum
FCoV	Feline Coronavirus
HEV	Hemagglutinating Encephalomyelitis Virus
HR1	Heptal repeat region 1
HR2	Heptal repeat 2
IBV	Infectious Bronchitis Virus
ICTV	International Committee on Virus Taxonomy
IL-6	Interleukin 6
MCP1	Monocyte a chemoattractive protein 1
MERS-CoV	Middle East coronavirus respiratory syndrome
MHV	Murine Hepatitis Virus
MNP	Natural Marine Product
M^{pro}	Main protease
ORFs	Open Read Frame
PEDV	Porcine Epidemic Diarrhea Virus
PP1a	Polyprotein1a
PP1ab	Polyprotein1ab
RBD	Receptor-binding domain

RdRp	RNA-dependent RNA polymerase
RtCoV	Rat Coronavirus
SARS	Severe acute respiratory syndrome
SARS-CoV	Severe acute respiratory syndrome coronavirus
SRD	SR -rich domain
TCoV	Turkey Coronavirus
TGEV	Porcine Transmissible Gastroenteritis Virus
TLR	Toll-Like Receptor
TMI	TM domain
TNF-α	Tumor necrosis factor α
VLPs	Virus-like particles
WHO	World Health Organization
α-CoV	Alphacoronavirus
β-CoV	Betacoronavirus
γ-CoV	Gammacoronavirus
δ-CoV	Deltacoronavirus

CONSENT FOR PUBLICATION

Not applicable.

CONFLICT OF INTEREST

The authors declare no conflict of interest, financial or otherwise.

ACKNOWLEDGEMENTS

The present work was carried out with the support of the Coordination of Improvement of Higher Education Personnel - Brazil (CAPES) - Financing Code 001.

REFERENCES

[1] Forni D, Cagliani R, Clerici M, Sironi M. Molecular evolution of human coronavirus genomes. Trends Microbiol 2017; 25(1): 35-48.
[http://dx.doi.org/10.1016/j.tim.2016.09.001] [PMID: 27743750]

[2] Latinne A, Hu B, Olival KJ, *et al.* Origin and cross-species transmission of bat coronaviruses in China. Nat Commun 2020; 11(1): 4235.
[http://dx.doi.org/10.1038/s41467-020-17687-3] [PMID: 32843626]

[3] Chen B, Tian EK, He B, *et al.* Overview of lethal human coronaviruses. Signal Transduct Target Ther 2020; 5(1): 89.
[http://dx.doi.org/10.1038/s41392-020-0190-2] [PMID: 32533062]

[4]　Jin Y, Lei C, Hu D, Dimitrov DS. Human monoclonal antibodies as candidate therapeutics against emerging viruses. 2017; 11(4): 462-70.
[http://dx.doi.org/10.1007/s11684-017-0596-6]

[5]　Gralinski LE, Sheahan TP, Morrison TE, *et al.* Complement activation contributes to severe acute respiratory syndrome coronavirus pathogenesis. MBio 2018; 9(5): 1-15.
[http://dx.doi.org/10.1128/mBio.01753-18] [PMID: 30301856]

[6]　Wang X, Zou P, Wu F, Lu L. Development of small-molecule viral inhibitors targeting various stages of the life cycle of emerging and re-emerging viruses 2017; 11(4): 449-61.
[http://dx.doi.org/10.1007/s11684-017-0589-5]

[7]　Viroporins E, Castaño-rodriguez C, Honrubia JM, Gutiérrez-álvarez J, Dediego ML, Nieto-torres JL, *et al.* crossm Role of Severe Acute Respiratory Syndrome Coronavirus. 2018; 9(3): 1-23.

[8]　Fouchier RAM, Ph D, Berger A, Ph D, Burguière A, Ph D, *et al.* Identification of a Novel Coronavirus in Patients with Severe Acute Respiratory Syndrome. 2003; 1967-76.

[9]　Nicholls JM, Poon LLM, Lee KC, Ng WF, Lai ST, Leung CY, *et al.* Lung pathology of fatal severe acute respiratory syndrome. 2003; 361: 1773-8.
[http://dx.doi.org/10.1016/S0140-6736(03)13413-7]

[10]　Ding Y, Wang H, Shen H, *et al.* The clinical pathology of severe acute respiratory syndrome (SARS): a report from China. J Pathol 2003; 200(3): 282-9.
[http://dx.doi.org/10.1002/path.1440] [PMID: 12845623]

[11]　Gu J, Gong E, Zhang B, Zheng J, Gao Z, Zhong Y, *et al.* Multiple organ infection and the pathogenesis of SARS. 2005; 202(3): 415-24.
[http://dx.doi.org/10.1084/jem.20050828]

[12]　Helmy YA, Fawzy M, Elaswad A, Sobieh A. The COVID-19 pandemic : a comprehensive review of taxonomy. genetics, epidemiology, diagnosis, treatment, and control 2020.

[13]　Shang J, Ye G, Shi K, *et al.* Structural basis of receptor recognition by SARS-CoV-2. Nature 2020; 581(7807): 221-4.
[http://dx.doi.org/10.1038/s41586-020-2179-y] [PMID: 32225175]

[14]　Chan JFW, Yuan S, Kok KH, *et al.* A familial cluster of pneumonia associated with the 2019 novel coronavirus indicating person-to-person transmission: a study of a family cluster. Lancet 2020; 395(10223): 514-23.
[http://dx.doi.org/10.1016/S0140-6736(20)30154-9] [PMID: 31986261]

[15]　Paraskevisa D, Kostakia EG, Magiorkinisa G, Panayiotakopoulosb G, Sourvinosc G, Tsiodrasd S. Full Genome Evolutionary Analysis of Corona. 2020.

[16]　World Health Organization. Weekly Epidemiological Update on COVID-19 2020.

[17]　Cui J, Li F, Shi ZL. Origin and evolution of pathogenic coronaviruses. Nat Rev Microbiol 2019; 17(3): 181-92.
[http://dx.doi.org/10.1038/s41579-018-0118-9] [PMID: 30531947]

[18]　Guan Y, Zheng BJ, He YQ, Liu XL, Zhuang ZX, Cheung CL, *et al.* Isolation and characterization of viruses related to the SARS coronavirus from animals in Southern China. Science (80-) 2003; 302(5643): 276-8.
[http://dx.doi.org/10.1126/science.1087139]

[19]　Song H-D, Tu C-C, Zhang G-W, *et al.* Cross-host evolution of severe acute respiratory syndrome coronavirus in palm civet and human. Proc Natl Acad Sci USA 2005; 102(7): 2430-5.
[http://dx.doi.org/10.1073/pnas.0409608102] [PMID: 15695582]

[20]　Su S, Wong G, Shi W, *et al.* Epidemiology, genetic recombination, and pathogenesis of coronaviruses. Trends microbiol 2016; 24(6): 490-502.
[http://dx.doi.org/10.1016/j.tim.2016.03.003] [PMID: 27012512]

[21]   Kan B, Wang M, Jing H, *et al.* Molecular evolution analysis and geographic investigation of severe acute respiratory syndrome coronavirus-like virus in palm civets at an animal market and on farms. J Virol 2005; 79(18): 11892-900.
[http://dx.doi.org/10.1128/JVI.79.18.11892-11900.2005] [PMID: 16140765]

[22]   Tu C, Crameri G, Kong X, *et al.* Antibodies to SARS coronavirus in civets. Emerg Infect Dis 2004; 10(12): 2244-8.
[http://dx.doi.org/10.3201/eid1012.040520] [PMID: 15663874]

[23]   Lau SKP, Woo PCY, Li KSM, *et al.* Severe acute respiratory syndrome coronavirus-like virus in Chinese horseshoe bats. Proc Natl Acad Sci USA 2005; 102(39): 14040-5.
[http://dx.doi.org/10.1073/pnas.0506735102] [PMID: 16169905]

[24]   Ge XY, Li JL, Yang XL, *et al.* Isolation and characterization of a bat SARS-like coronavirus that uses the ACE2 receptor. Nature 2013; 503(7477): 535-8.
[http://dx.doi.org/10.1038/nature12711] [PMID: 24172901]

[25]   Wu Z, Yang L, Ren X, Zhang J, Yang F. ORF8-related genetic evidence for chinese horseshoe bats as the source of human severe acute respiratory syndrome coronavirus. 2016; 213: 579-83.

[26]   Alluwaimi AM, Alshubaith IH, Al-ali AM, Abohelaika S. The coronaviruses of animals and birds : their zoonosis , vaccines , and models for SARS-CoV and. 2020; 1-12.

[27]   Lu R, Zhao X, Li J, *et al.* Genomic characterisation and epidemiology of 2019 novel coronavirus: implications for virus origins and receptor binding. Lancet 2020; 395(10224): 565-74.
[http://dx.doi.org/10.1016/S0140-6736(20)30251-8] [PMID: 32007145]

[28]   Hadi A, Kadhom M, Hairunisa N, Trisakti U, Yousif E. A Review on COVID-19 : Origin , Spread , Symptoms , Treatment , and Prevention. 2020.

[29]   Tang X, Wu C, Li X, Song Y, Yao X, Wu X, *et al.* On the origin and continuing evolution of SARS-CoV-2. 2020; 1012-23.
[http://dx.doi.org/10.1093/nsr/nwaa036]

[30]   Hafeez A, Ahmad S, Siddqui SA, Ahmad M. Treatments and prevention 2020; 4(2): 116-25.

[31]   Cascella M, Rajnik M, Cuomo A, Dulebohn SC, Di Napoli R. Features, evaluation and treatment coronavirus (COVID-19). Statpearls.: StatPearls Publishing 2020.

[32]   Angeletti S, Benvenuto D, Bianchi M, Giovanetti M, Pascarella S, Ciccozzi M. RESEARCH ARTICLE COVID □ 2019 : The role of the nsp2 and nsp3 in its pathogenesis. 2020; 1-5.

[33]   Gu J. Christine Korteweg. Pathology and Pathogenesis of Severe Acute 2007; pp. 1136-47.

[34]   ZHEN-WEI LANG, SHI-JIE ZHANG, XINMENG , JUN QIANGLI, CHEN ZHAOSONG, LINGSUN Y-SDD. Special report a clinicopathological study of three cases of severe acute respiratory syndrome (SARS). 2003; 35(December): 526-31.

[35]   Poutanen SM, Low DE, Henry B, *et al.* identification of severe acute respiratory syndrome in canada. N Engl J Med 2003; 348(20): 1995-2005.
[http://dx.doi.org/10.1056/NEJMoa030634] [PMID: 12671061]

[36]   McDermott JE, Mitchell HD, Gralinski LE, *et al.* The effect of inhibition of PP1 and TNFα signaling on pathogenesis of SARS coronavirus. BMC Syst Biol 2016; 10(1): 93.
[http://dx.doi.org/10.1186/s12918-016-0336-6] [PMID: 27663205]

[37]   Tsui PT, Kwok ML, Yuen H, Lai ST. Severe acute respiratory syndrome: clinical outcome and prognostic correlates. Emerg Infect Dis 2003; 9(9): 1064-9.
[http://dx.doi.org/10.3201/eid0909.030362] [PMID: 14519241]

[38]   Weiss SR, Navas-Martin S. Coronavirus pathogenesis and the emerging pathogen severe acute respiratory syndrome coronavirus. Microbiol Mol Biol Rev 2005; 69(4): 635-64.
[http://dx.doi.org/10.1128/MMBR.69.4.635-664.2005] [PMID: 16339739]

[39]   Cheung CY, Poon LLM, Ng IHY, *et al.* Cytokine responses in severe acute respiratory syndrome coronavirus-infected macrophages *in vitro*: possible relevance to pathogenesis. J Virol 2005; 79(12): 7819-26.
        [http://dx.doi.org/10.1128/JVI.79.12.7819-7826.2005] [PMID: 15919935]

[40]   Liu J, Zheng X, Tong Q, *et al.* Overlapping and discrete aspects of the pathology and pathogenesis of the emerging human pathogenic coronaviruses SARS-CoV, MERS-CoV, and 2019-nCoV. J Med Virol 2020; 92(5): 491-4.
        [http://dx.doi.org/10.1002/jmv.25709] [PMID: 32056249]

[41]   Nicholls JM, Poon LLM, Lee KC, *et al.* Since january 2020 elsevier has created a COVID-19 resource centre with free information in english and mandarin on the novel coronavirus COVID- 19 . The COVID-19 resource centre is hosted on Elsevier Connect, the company's public news and information 2020.

[42]   Wong CK, Lam CWK, Wu AKL, *et al.* Plasma inflammatory cytokines and chemokines in severe acute respiratory syndrome. Clin Exp Immunol 2004; 136(1): 95-103.
        [http://dx.doi.org/10.1111/j.1365-2249.2004.02415.x] [PMID: 15030519]

[43]   Chien JY, Hsueh PR, Cheng WC, Yu CJ, Yang PC. Temporal changes in cytokine/chemokine profiles and pulmonary involvement in severe acute respiratory syndrome. Respirology 2006; 11(6): 715-22.
        [http://dx.doi.org/10.1111/j.1440-1843.2006.00942.x] [PMID: 17052299]

[44]   Duggal NK, Emerman M. Evolutionary conflicts between viruses and restriction factors shape immunity. Nat Rev Immunol 2012; 12(10): 687-95.
        [http://dx.doi.org/10.1038/nri3295] [PMID: 22976433]

[45]   Chan PKSJJYS. Tears and conjunctival scrapings for coronavirus in patients with SARS. 2004; 0(0): 968-77.
        [http://dx.doi.org/10.1136/bjo.2003.039461]

[46]   Christian MD, Loutfy M, Mcdonald LC, *et al.* Possible SARS Coronavirus Transmission during Cardiopulmonary Resuscitation. 2004; 10(2).
        [http://dx.doi.org/10.3201/eid1002.030700]

[47]   Cheng VCC, Lau SKP, Woo PCY, Yuen KY. Severe Acute Respiratory Syndrome Coronavirus as an Agent of Emerging and Reemerging Infection 2007; 20(4): 660-94.

[48]   Fraction RE, Function VS. C or r e sp ondence Transmission of 2019-nCoV Infection from an Asymptomatic Contact in Germany. 2020; 2019-.

[49]   Phelan A. L, Rebecca Katz LG. The Novel Coronavirus Originating in Wuhan, China Challenges for Global Health Governance 2020; pp. 2019-20.

[50]   Gorbalenya AE, Baker SC, Baric RS, *et al.* The species and its viruses – a statement of the Coronavirus Study Group. 2020.

[51]   Zhou P, Yang XL, Wang XG, *et al.* A pneumonia outbreak associated with a new coronavirus of probable bat origin. Nature 2020; 579(7798): 270-3.
        [http://dx.doi.org/10.1038/s41586-020-2012-7] [PMID: 32015507]

[52]   Xue L, Li J, Wei L, Ma C. A quick look at the latest developments in the COVID-19 pandemic. J Int Med Res 2020; 48(9)
        [http://dx.doi.org/10.1177/0300060520943802]

[53]   Yao M, Zhang L, Ma J, Zhou L. On airborne transmission and control of SARS-CoV-2. Sci Total Environ 2020; 731: 139178.
        [http://dx.doi.org/10.1016/j.scitotenv.2020.139178] [PMID: 32388162]

[54]   Wang J, Zhao S, Liu M, *et al.* ACE2 expression by colonic epithelial cells is associated with viral infection, immunity and energy metabolism. 2020; 1-13.

[55]   Feng W, Zong W, Wang F, Ju S. Severe acute respiratory syndrome coronavirus 2 (SARS-CoV-2): a

review. 2020; 1-14.

[56]   Li YC. The neuroinvasive potential of SARS-CoV2 may play a role in the respiratory failure of COVID - 19 patients. 2020; 24-7.

[57]   Zochios V, Brodie D, Charlesworth M, Parhar KK. Delivering extracorporeal membrane oxygenation for patients with COVID-19 : what, who, when and how? 2020; 997-1001.
[http://dx.doi.org/10.1111/anae.15099]

[58]   Iwasaki M, Saito J, Zhao H, Sakamoto A, Hirota K, Ma D. Inflammation Triggered by SARS-CoV-2 and ACE2 Augment Drives Multiple Organ Failure of Severe COVID-19: Molecular Mechanisms and Implications. Inflammation 2020.
[PMID: 33029758]

[59]   Hallaj S, Ghorbani A, Mousavi-Aghdas SA, Mirza-Aghazadeh-Attari M, Sevbitov A, Hashemi V, *et al.* Angiotensin-converting enzyme as a new immunologic target for the new SARS-CoV-2. Immunol Cell Biol 2020; 1-14.
[PMID: 32864784]

[60]   Conti P, Ronconi G, Caraffa A, *et al.* Induction of pro-inflammatory cytokines (IL-1 and IL-6) and lung inflammation by Coronavirus-19 (COVI-19 or SARS-CoV-2): anti-inflammatory strategies. J Biol Regul Homeost Agents 2020; 34(2): 327-31.
[PMID: 32171193]

[61]   Tyrrell DAJ, Almeida JD, Cunningham CH, *et al.* Coronaviridae. Intervirology 1975; 5(1-2): 76-82.
[http://dx.doi.org/10.1159/000149883] [PMID: 1184350]

[62]   Chan JFW, To KKW, Chen H, Yuen KY. Cross-species transmission and emergence of novel viruses from birds. Curr Opin Virol 2015; 10(January): 63-9.
[http://dx.doi.org/10.1016/j.coviro.2015.01.006] [PMID: 25644327]

[63]   Cowley JA, Dimmock CM, Spann KM, Walker PJ. Gill-associated virus of penaeus monodon prawns: an invertebrate virus with ORF1a and ORF1b genes related to arteri- and coronaviruses. J Gen Virol 2000; 81(Pt 6): 1473-84.
[http://dx.doi.org/10.1099/0022-1317-81-6-1473] [PMID: 10811931]

[64]   Erles K, Toomey C, Brooks HW, Brownlie J. Detection of a group 2 coronavirus in dogs with canine infectious respiratory disease. Virology 2003; 310(2): 216-23.
[http://dx.doi.org/10.1016/S0042-6822(03)00160-0] [PMID: 12781709]

[65]   Sewda A, Dutt Gupta S. Genetics of severe acute respiratory syndrome coronavirus-2 and diagnosis of coronavirus disease-2019: An overview. J Health Manag 2020; 22(2): 236-47.
[http://dx.doi.org/10.1177/0972063420935548]

[66]   Boni MF, Lemey P, Jiang X, *et al.* Evolutionary origins of the SARS-CoV-2 sarbecovirus lineage responsible for the COVID-19 pandemic. Nat Microbiol 2020; 5(11): 1408-17.
[http://dx.doi.org/10.1038/s41564-020-0771-4] [PMID: 32724171]

[67]   Schwartz DA, Graham AL. Potential maternal and infant outcomes from coronavirus 2019-NCOV (SARS-CoV-2) infecting pregnant women: Lessons from SARS, MERS, and other human coronavirus infections. Viruses 2020; 12(2): 1-16.
[http://dx.doi.org/10.3390/v12020194] [PMID: 32050635]

[68]   Schwartz DA, Dhaliwal A. Infections in pregnancy with COVID-19 and other respiratory RNA virus diseases are rarely, if ever, transmitted to the fetus: Experiences with coronaviruses, parainfluenza, metapneumovirus respiratory syncytial virus, and influenza. Arch Pathol Lab Med 2020; 144(8): 920-8.
[http://dx.doi.org/10.5858/arpa.2020-0211-SA]

[69]   Chen Y, Liu Q, Guo D. Emerging coronaviruses: Genome structure, replication, and pathogenesis. J Med Virol 2020; 92(4): 418-23.
[http://dx.doi.org/10.1002/jmv.25681] [PMID: 31967327]

[70]   Lau SKP, Fan RYY, Luk HKH, *et al.* Replication of MERS and SARS coronaviruses in bat cells offers insights to their ancestral origins. Emerg Microbes Infect 2018; 7(1): 209.
[http://dx.doi.org/10.1038/s41426-018-0208-9] [PMID: 30531999]

[71]   Prajapat M, Sarma P, Shekhar N, *et al.* Drug targets for corona virus: A systematic review. Indian J Pharmacol 2020; 52(1): 56-65.
[http://dx.doi.org/10.4103/ijp.IJP_115_20] [PMID: 32201449]

[72]   Joshi T, Sharma P, Joshi T, Pundir H, Mathpal S, Chandra S. Structure-based screening of novel lichen compounds against SARS Coronavirus main protease (Mpro) as potentials inhibitors of COVID-19. Mol Divers 2020; 0123456789.

[73]   Goyal B, Goyal D. Targeting the Dimerization of the main protease of coronaviruses: A potential broad-spectrum therapeutic strategy. ACS Comb Sci 2020; 22(6): 297-305.
[http://dx.doi.org/10.1021/acscombsci.0c00058] [PMID: 32402186]

[74]   Voss D, Pfefferle S, Drosten C, *et al.* Studies on membrane topology, N-glycosylation and functionality of SARS-CoV membrane protein. Virol J 2009; 6(M): 79.
[http://dx.doi.org/10.1186/1743-422X-6-79] [PMID: 19534833]

[75]   Gui M, Song W, Zhou H, *et al.* Cryo-electron microscopy structures of the SARS-CoV spike glycoprotein reveal a prerequisite conformational state for receptor binding. Cell Res 2017; 27(1): 119-29.
[http://dx.doi.org/10.1038/cr.2016.152] [PMID: 28008928]

[76]   Walls AC, Park YJ, Tortorici MA, Wall A, McGuire AT, Veesler D. Structure, function, and antigenicity of the SARS-CoV-2 spike glycoprotein. Cell 2020; 181(2): 281-292.e6.
[http://dx.doi.org/10.1016/j.cell.2020.02.058] [PMID: 32155444]

[77]   Song W, Gui M, Wang X, Xiang Y. Cryo-EM structure of the SARS coronavirus spike glycoprotein in complex with its host cell receptor ACE2. PLoS Pathog 2018; 14(8): e1007236.
[http://dx.doi.org/10.1371/journal.ppat.1007236] [PMID: 30102747]

[78]   Pak JE, Sharon C, Satkunarajah M, *et al.* Structural insights into immune recognition of the severe acute respiratory syndrome coronavirus S protein receptor binding domain. J Mol Biol 2009; 388(4): 815-23.
[http://dx.doi.org/10.1016/j.jmb.2009.03.042] [PMID: 19324051]

[79]   Wang Q, Zhang Y, Wu L, *et al.* Structural and Functional Basis of SARS-CoV-2 Entry by Using Human ACE2. Cell 2020; 181(4): 894-904.e9.
[http://dx.doi.org/10.1016/j.cell.2020.03.045] [PMID: 32275855]

[80]   Ou X, Liu Y, Lei X, *et al.* Characterization of spike glycoprotein of SARS-CoV-2 on virus entry and its immune cross-reactivity with SARS-CoV. Nat Commun 2020; 11(1): 1620.
[http://dx.doi.org/10.1038/s41467-020-15562-9] [PMID: 32221306]

[81]   Lan J, Ge J, Yu J, *et al.* Structure of the SARS-CoV-2 spike receptor-binding domain bound to the ACE2 receptor. Nature 2020; 581(7807): 215-20.
[http://dx.doi.org/10.1038/s41586-020-2180-5] [PMID: 32225176]

[82]   Liu Z, Xiao X, Wei X, *et al.* Composition and divergence of coronavirus spike proteins and host ACE2 receptors predict potential intermediate hosts of SARS-CoV-2. J Med Virol 2020; 92(6): 595-601.
[http://dx.doi.org/10.1002/jmv.25726] [PMID: 32100877]

[83]   Shang J, Wan Y, Luo C, *et al.* Cell entry mechanisms of SARS-CoV-2. Proc Natl Acad Sci USA 2020; 117(21): 11727-34.
[http://dx.doi.org/10.1073/pnas.2003138117] [PMID: 32376634]

[84]   Xia S, Liu M, Wang C, *et al.* Inhibition of SARS-CoV-2 (previously 2019-nCoV) infection by a highly potent pan-coronavirus fusion inhibitor targeting its spike protein that harbors a high capacity to mediate membrane fusion. Cell Res 2020; 30(4): 343-55.

[http://dx.doi.org/10.1038/s41422-020-0305-x] [PMID: 32231345]

[85]   Pinto D, Park YJ, Beltramello M, *et al.* Cross-neutralization of SARS-CoV-2 by a human monoclonal SARS-CoV antibody. Nature 2020; 583(7815): 290-5.
[http://dx.doi.org/10.1038/s41586-020-2349-y] [PMID: 32422645]

[86]   Tian X, Li C, Huang A, *et al.* Potent binding of 2019 novel coronavirus spike protein by a SARS coronavirus-specific human monoclonal antibody. Emerg Microbes Infect 2020; 9(1): 382-5.
[http://dx.doi.org/10.1080/22221751.2020.1729069] [PMID: 32065055]

[87]   Tseng YT, Chang CH, Wang SM, Huang KJ, Wang CT. Identifying SARS-CoV membrane protein amino acid residues linked to virus-like particle assembly. PLoS One 2013; 8(5): e64013.
[http://dx.doi.org/10.1371/journal.pone.0064013] [PMID: 23700447]

[88]   Hu Y, Wen J, Tang L, *et al.* The M protein of SARS-CoV: basic structural and immunological properties. Genomics, proteomics Bioinforma / Beijing Genomics Inst 2003; 1(2): 118-30.

[89]   Tseng YT, Wang SM, Huang KJ, Lee AI, Chiang CC, Wang CT. Self-assembly of severe acute respiratory syndrome coronavirus membrane protein. J Biol Chem 2010; 285(17): 12862-72.
[http://dx.doi.org/10.1074/jbc.M109.030270] [PMID: 20154085]

[90]   Wang Y, Liu L. The membrane protein of severe acute respiratory syndrome coronavirus functions as a novel cytosolic pathogen-associated molecular pattern to promote beta interferon induction *via* a toll-like-receptor-related TRAF3-independent mechanism. MBio 2016; 7(1): e01872-15.
[http://dx.doi.org/10.1128/mBio.01872-15] [PMID: 26861016]

[91]   Fang X, Gao J, Zheng H, *et al.* The membrane protein of SARS-CoV suppresses NF-kappaB activation. J Med Virol 2007; 79(10): 1431-9.
[http://dx.doi.org/10.1002/jmv.20953] [PMID: 17705188]

[92]   Ghafouri F, Cohan RA, Noorbakhsh F, Samimi H, Haghpanah V. An in-silico approach to develop of a multi-epitope vaccine candidate against SARS-CoV-2 envelope (E) protein. 2020.

[93]   Tilocca B, Soggiu A, Sanguinetti M, Babini G. Immunoinformatic analysis of the SARS-CoV-2 envelope protein as a strategy to assess cross-protection against COVID-19. 2020.
[http://dx.doi.org/10.1016/j.micinf.2020.05.013]

[94]   Duart G, García-Murria MJ, Grau B, Acosta-Cáceres JM, Martínez-Gil L, Mingarro I. SARS-CoV-2 envelope protein topology in eukaryotic membranes. Open Biol 2020; 10(9): 200209.
[http://dx.doi.org/10.1098/rsob.200209] [PMID: 32898469]

[95]   Alam I, Kamau AA, Kulmanov M, *et al.* Functional Pangenome Analysis Shows Key Features of E Protein Are Preserved in SARS and SARS-CoV-2. Front Cell Infect Microbiol 2020; 10(July): 405.
[http://dx.doi.org/10.3389/fcimb.2020.00405] [PMID: 32850499]

[96]   Sarkar M, Saha S. Structural insight into the role of novel SARSCoV-2 E protein: A potential target for vaccine development and other therapeutic strategies. PLoS One 2020; 15: 1-25.

[97]   Gupta MK, Vemula S, Donde R, Gouda G, Behera L, Vadde R. In-silico approaches to detect inhibitors of the human severe acute respiratory syndrome coronavirus envelope protein ion channel. J Biomol Struct Dyn 2020; 0(0): 1-11.
[http://dx.doi.org/10.1080/07391102.2020.1837679] [PMID: 32238078]

[98]   Kang S, Yang M, Hong Z, *et al.* Crystal structure of SARS-CoV-2 nucleocapsid protein RNA binding domain reveals potential unique drug targeting sites. Acta Pharm Sin B 2020; 10(7): 1228-38.
[http://dx.doi.org/10.1016/j.apsb.2020.04.009] [PMID: 32363136]

[99]   Cascarina SM, Ross ED. A proposed role for the SARS-CoV-2 nucleocapsid protein in the formation and regulation of biomolecular condensates. FASEB J 2020; 34(8): 9832-42.
[http://dx.doi.org/10.1096/fj.202001351] [PMID: 32562316]

[100] Chang C, Hou M, Chang C, Hsiao C, Huang T. The SARS coronavirus nucleocapsid protein – Forms and functions. 2020.

[101] Zeng W, Liu G, Ma H, Zhao D, Yang Y, Liu M. Biochemical characterization of SARS-CoV-2 nucleocapsid protein. 2020.
[http://dx.doi.org/10.1016/j.bbrc.2020.04.136]

[102] Cubuk J, Alston JJ, Incicco JJ, Singh S, Stuchell-Brereton MD, Ward MD, *et al.* The SARS-CoV-2 nucleocapsid protein is dynamic, disordered, and phase separates with RNA. bioRxiv 2020; 2020.06.17.158121.
[http://dx.doi.org/10.1101/2020.06.17.158121]

[103] Kannan S, Shaik Syed Ali P, Sheeza A, Hemalatha K. COVID-19 (Novel Coronavirus 2019) - recent trends. Africa Res Bull Econ Financ Tech Ser 2020; 24(4): 2006-11.
[PMID: 32141569]

[104] Ye Q, West AMV, Silletti S, Corbett KD. Architecture and self-assembly of the SARS-CoV-2 nucleocapsid protein. Protein Sci 2020; 29(9): 1890-901.
[http://dx.doi.org/10.1002/pro.3909] [PMID: 32654247]

[105] Wang H, He S, Deng W, *et al.* Comprehensive Insights into the Catalytic Mechanism of Middle East Respiratory Syndrome 3C-Like Protease and Severe Acute Respiratory Syndrome 3C-Like Protease. ACS Catal 2020; 10(10): 5871-90.
[http://dx.doi.org/10.1021/acscatal.0c00110] [PMID: 32391184]

[106] He J, Hu L, Huang X, Wang C, Zhang Z, Wang Y. Potential of coronavirus 3C-like protease inhibitors for the development of new anti-SARS-CoV-2 drugs: Insights from structures of protease and inhibitors. Int J Antimicrob Agents 2020; 56(2): 106055.
[http://dx.doi.org/10.1016/j.ijantimicag.2020.106055]

[107] Jin Z, Zhao Y, Sun Y, *et al.* Structural basis for the inhibition of SARS-CoV-2 main protease by antineoplastic drug carmofur. Nat Struct Mol Biol 2020; 27(6): 529-32.
[http://dx.doi.org/10.1038/s41594-020-0440-6] [PMID: 32382072]

[108] Tahir Ul Qamar M, Alqahtani SM, Alamri MA, Chen LL. Structural basis of SARS-CoV-2 3CL^{pro} and anti-COVID-19 drug discovery from medicinal plants. J Pharm Anal 2020; 10(4): 313-9.
[http://dx.doi.org/10.1016/j.jpha.2020.03.009] [PMID: 32296570]

[109] Zhang L, Lin D, Sun X, *et al.* Crystal structure of SARS-CoV-2 main protease provides a basis for design of improved a-ketoamide inhibitors. Science (80-) 2020; 368(6489): 409-12.

[110] Kneller DW, Phillips G, O'Neill HM, *et al.* Structural plasticity of SARS-CoV-2 3CL M^{pro} active site cavity revealed by room temperature X-ray crystallography. Nat Commun 2020; 11(1): 3202.
[http://dx.doi.org/10.1038/s41467-020-16954-7] [PMID: 32581217]

[111] Ma C, Sacco MD, Hurst B, *et al.* Boceprevir, GC-376, and calpain inhibitors II, XII inhibit SARS-CoV-2 viral replication by targeting the viral main protease. Cell Res 2020; 30(8): 678-92.
[http://dx.doi.org/10.1038/s41422-020-0356-z] [PMID: 32541865]

[112] Sacco MD, Ma C, Lagarias P, *et al.* Structure and inhibition of the SARS-CoV-2 main protease reveals strategy for developing dual inhibitors against Mpro and cathepsin L. 2020.
[http://dx.doi.org/10.1101/2020.07.27.223727]

[113] Jin Z, Du X, Xu Y, *et al.* Structure of M^{pro} from SARS-CoV-2 and discovery of its inhibitors. Nature 2020; 582(7811): 289-93.
[http://dx.doi.org/10.1038/s41586-020-2223-y] [PMID: 32272481]

[114] Narkhede RR, Pise AV, Cheke RS, Shinde SD. Recognition of Natural Products as Potential Inhibitors of COVID-19 Main Protease (Mpro): In-Silico Evidences. Nat Prod Bioprospect 2020; 10(5): 297-306.
[http://dx.doi.org/10.1007/s13659-020-00253-1] [PMID: 32557405]

[115] Fischer A, Sellner M, Neranjan S, Smieško M, Lill MA. Potential inhibitors for novel coronavirus protease identified by virtual screening of 606 million compounds. Int J Mol Sci 2020; 21(10): 1-17.
[http://dx.doi.org/10.3390/ijms21103626] [PMID: 32455534]

[116] Dai W, Zhang B, Jiang XM, *et al.* Structure-based design of antiviral drug candidates targeting the SARS-CoV-2 main protease. Science (80-) 2020; 368(6497): 1331-5.

[117] Gupta S, Singh AK, Kushwaha PP, *et al.* Identification of potential natural inhibitors of SARS-CoV2 main protease by molecular docking and simulation studies. J Biomol Struct Dyn 2020; 0(0): 1-12.
[http://dx.doi.org/10.1080/07391102.2020.1837679] [PMID: 32476576]

[118] Abian O, Ortega-alarcon D, Jimenez-alesanco A, Ceballos-laita L. Structural stability of SARS-CoV-2 3CLpro and identification of quercetin as an inhibitor by experimental screening. 2020; (January):

[119] Gimeno A, Mestres-Truyol J, Ojeda-Montes MJ, *et al.* Prediction of novel inhibitors of the main protease (M-pro) of SARS-CoV-2 through consensus docking and drug reposition. Int J Mol Sci 2020; 21(11): E3793.
[http://dx.doi.org/10.3390/ijms21113793] [PMID: 32471205]

[120] Joshi RS, Jagdale SS, Bansode SB, *et al.* Discovery of potential multi-target-directed ligands by targeting host-specific SARS-CoV-2 structurally conserved main protease. J Biomol Struct Dyn 2020; 0(0): 1-16.
[http://dx.doi.org/10.1080/07391102.2020.1760137] [PMID: 32329408]

[121] Ghosh K, Abdul S, Gayen S, Jha T. Chemical-informatics approach to COVID-19 drug discovery: Exploration of important fragments and data mining based prediction of some hits from natural origins as main protease (Mpro) inhibitors. J Mol Struct 2020; 1224: 129026.
[http://dx.doi.org/10.1016/j.molstruc.2020.129026]

[122] Kuba K, Imai Y, Ohto-Nakanishi T, Penninger JM. Trilogy of ACE2: a peptidase in the renin-angiotensin system, a SARS receptor, and a partner for amino acid transporters. Pharmacol Ther 2010; 128(1): 119-28.
[http://dx.doi.org/10.1016/j.pharmthera.2010.06.003] [PMID: 20599443]

[123] Samavati L, Uhal BD. ACE2, Much More Than Just a Receptor for SARS-CoV-2. Front Cell Infect Microbiol 2020; 10(June): 317.
[http://dx.doi.org/10.3389/fcimb.2020.00317] [PMID: 32582574]

[124] Mathewson AC, Bishop A, Yao Y, *et al.* Interaction of severe acute respiratory syndrome-coronavirus and NL63 coronavirus spike proteins with angiotensin converting enzyme-2. J Gen Virol 2008; 89(Pt 11): 2741-5.
[http://dx.doi.org/10.1099/vir.0.2008/003962-0] [PMID: 18931070]

[125] Fu L, Ye F, Feng Y, *et al.* Both Boceprevir and GC376 efficaciously inhibit SARS-CoV-2 by targeting its main protease. Nat Commun 2020; 11(1): 4417.
[http://dx.doi.org/10.1038/s41467-020-18233-x] [PMID: 32887884]

[126] Choy KT, Wong AYL, Kaewpreedee P, *et al.* Remdesivir, lopinavir, emetine, and homoharringtonine inhibit SARS-CoV-2 replication *in vitro*. Antiviral Res 2020; 178(March): 104786.
[http://dx.doi.org/10.1016/j.antiviral.2020.104786] [PMID: 32251767]

[127] Caly L, Druce JD, Catton MG, Jans DA, Wagstaff KM. The FDA-approved drug ivermectin inhibits the replication of SARS-CoV-2 *in vitro*. Antiviral Res 2020; 178(April): 104787.
[http://dx.doi.org/10.1016/j.antiviral.2020.104787] [PMID: 32251768]

[128] Ngo ST, Quynh Anh Pham N, Thi Le L, Pham D-H, Vu VV. Computational Determination of Potential Inhibitors of SARS-CoV-2 Main Protease. J Chem Inf Model 2020; 60(12): 5771-80.
[http://dx.doi.org/10.1021/acs.jcim.0c00491] [PMID: 32530282]

[129] Neto IF da S, Ricardino IEF, Santos ÍT, *et al.* Uma revisão da atividade antiviral do nim indiano e seu potencial frente ao novo coronavírus (SARS-COV-2). J Bio & Pharmacy 2021; 108-26.

[130] Lopes JG de A, Santos DF, Cabral HR, Júnior PR da S, Silva AA, Moura Y da S. Ivermectina como un posible aliado en el tratamiento de COVID-19: perspectivas sobre su acción antiviral. 2020; 2020: 1-12.

[131] Kwon PS, Oh H, Kwon SJ, *et al.* Sulfated polysaccharides effectively inhibit SARS-CoV-2 *in vitro.* Cell Discov 2020; 6(1): 50.
[http://dx.doi.org/10.1038/s41421-020-00192-8] [PMID: 32714563]

[132] Xia S, Yan L, Xu W, *et al.* A pan-coronavirus fusion inhibitor targeting the HR1 domain of human coronavirus spike. Sci Adv 2019; 5(4): eaav4580.
[http://dx.doi.org/10.1126/sciadv.aav4580] [PMID: 30989115]

[133] Chien M, Anderson TK, Jockusch S, *et al.* Nucleotide Analogues as Inhibitors of SARS-CoV-2 Polymerase, a Key Drug Target for COVID-19. J Proteome Res 2020; 19(11): 4690-7.
[http://dx.doi.org/10.1021/acs.jproteome.0c00392] [PMID: 32692185]

[134] Mahmud S, Uddin MAR, Zaman M, *et al.* Molecular docking and dynamics study of natural compound for potential inhibition of main protease of SARS-CoV-2. J Biomol Struct Dyn 2020; 0(0): 1-9.
[PMID: 32705962]

[135] Gentile D, Patamia V, Scala A, Sciortino MT, Piperno A, Rescifina A. Putative inhibitors of SARS-CoV-2 main protease from a library of marine natural products: A virtual screening and molecular modeling study. Mar Drugs 2020; 18(4): E225.
[http://dx.doi.org/10.3390/md18040225] [PMID: 32340389]

CHAPTER 4

Natural Sourced Traditional Indian and Chinese Medicines to Combat COVID-19

Mayank Kumar Khede[1], Anil Kumar Saxena[2,*] and Sisir Nandi[2,*]

[1] *Care Support and Treatment Division, Chhattishgarh State Aids Control Society, Department of Health and Family Welfare, Chhattisgarh, India*

[2] *Global Institute of Pharmaceutical Education and Research, Kashipur-244713, Uttarakhand, India*

Abstract: The corona virus disease (COVID-19) was started in Wuhan, China, in late 2019. It is caused by a novel strain of severe acute respiratory syndrome corona viruses (SARS-CoV-2) that has become pandemic on March 11, 2020 and endangered the existence of human beings on the earth as the infection has been spreading in mass population day by day within a few months with a high killing rate. The COVID-19 pandemic has pushed the modern health care system of developing and developed countries to their limits for its effective management and control since the drug discovery process is a long journey and challenging task and there is no specific small molecule chemotherapeutics to combat this novel coronavirus. Hence, the existence of human life is a great challenge. Mother Nature has played an important role to combat many pandemics that arrived in past centuries in absence of modern medicines. Nature has been a source of many natural drugs derived from plants' secondary metabolites which may be used to combat COVID-19. Natural sourced traditional Indian and Chinese medicines alternative therapy should be prioritized in combination with modern medicines to combat COVID-19. With rising COVID-19 cases globally, it would be too difficult to provide proper treatment even for the severe cases in hospitals. Therefore, the general public is advised to wear the mask, maintain social distancing, and use sanitizers. The COVID-19 mild infected patients may be isolated at home and can be taken care of by natural medicines. In this chapter, an attempt has been made to repurpose all potential natural drugs and natural Ayurvedic formulations that may be beneficial to combat viruses like the SARS-CoV-2, due to their antiviral and immune-modulator properties available under Indian traditional medicine and Chinese traditional medicine system for the effective treatment or prevention of COVID-19.

Keywords: COVID-19, Drug repurposing, Natural formulations, Traditional Chinese medicines (TCM), Traditional Indian medicines (TIM).

---

[*] **Corresponding author Anil Kumar Saxena and Sisir Nandi:** Global Institute of Pharmaceutical Education and Research, Kashipur-244713, India; Tel: +91 7500458478; E-mails: anilsak@gmail.com, sisir.iicb@gmail.com

Luciana Scotti and Marcus T. Scotti (Eds.)

1. INTRODUCTION TO INDIAN AND CHINESE TRADITIONAL MEDICINE

In the current 21st century, when the whole world is fighting a tough and decisive battle against COVID-19 caused by a novel coronavirus, natural products and their derivatives have potential activities to combat this pandemic [1, 2]. Since the beginning of 2020, new anti COVID-19 drug discovery strategies based on natural products and traditional medicines are evolving as an alternative option till specific anti COVID-19 drugs and vaccines are introduced in the global market to eliminate novel coronavirus [3].

According to the World Health Organization (WHO), the traditional medicine system includes a diversity of health practices, approaches, knowledge, and beliefs that incorporates plant, animal, and/or mineral-based medicines, spiritual therapies, manual techniques, and exercises, which are applied singly or in combination to maintain well-being and to treat or prevent the illness [4]. India, one of the ancient civilizations of the world, has the oldest heritage of the traditional medicine system, nurtured between 2500 B.C and 500 BC. The Sanskrit meaning of Ayu is life and Veda is knowledge or science [5]. Medicinal plants play a major role and constitute the backbone of traditional medicine. The Indian materia medica includes about 2000 drugs that are derived from India's different traditional systems, hence, Indian medicinal plants and other traditional medicines can be considered as a new option to overcome the viral transmission of COVID 19 [6]. Similarly, Traditional Chinese medicine (TCM), is one of the oldest continuously surviving traditions. The TCM is a system of healing that developed in China about 3000 years ago and includes natural herbal medicines used for maintaining good health and treating diseases in Chinese communities and has been adopted recently by other countries worldwide. In the year 2020, the use of TCM has become very popular in China and other parts of the world due to its effective utilization in combating COVID-19 [7]. At this time, in the absence of any specific anti COVID drug, all countries, including India, have to join hands together to fight COVID-19 by practicing precautionary measures such as regular hand washing, wearing of masks, and social distancing to prevent the attack of COVID-19 infection. In this study, an effort has been made to review and enlist the antiviral drugs and formulation of natural origin available and reported in Indian and Chinese traditional systems to combat COVID-19.

In December 2019, the sudden emergence of novel coronavirus (2019-nCoV) was observed by the world. It has been erupted in China Wuhan, Hubei Province, and spread across China and beyond [8]. On January 30, 2020, the World Health Organization (WHO) declared the outbreak a Public Health Emergency of International Concern (PHEIC) [9]. On February 12, 2020, WHO named the disease caused by the novel coronavirus Coronavirus Disease 2019, (COVID-19) [10].

The 2019 novel coronavirus (2019-nCoV) or the severe acute respiratory syndrome coronavirus 2 (SARS-CoV-2), as it is now called [11] has its history began back in the late 1960s when virologist Tyrrell and Bynoe found that they could passage a virus named B814 obtained from the respiratory tract of an adult with a common cold [12]. As a leading virologist, Tyrrell worked with the human strains, and several animal viruses like bronchitis virus, hepatitis virus demonstrated their same morphology under an electron microscope [13, 14]. This new group of viruses was named "coronavirus". Coronaviruses are enveloped positive-sense RNA viruses ranging from 60 nm to 140 nm in diameter with spike-like projections on their surface, giving them a crown-like appearance under the electron microscope; hence the name "coronavirus". The main targets of the SARS-CoV-2 are spike, envelope, membrane, nucleocapsid, and viral genome, which are responsible for the virulence while diffusing into the host cell by binding the viral spike with the human ACE 2 receptor [15] (Fig. **1**).

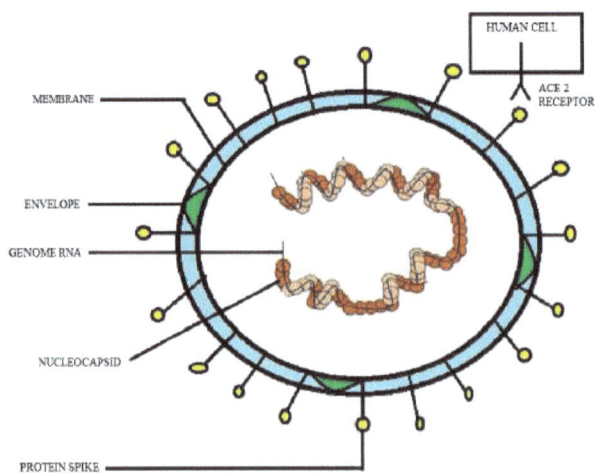

Fig. (1). Structure of novel coronavirus virion and its binding site in human body [15, 16].

Coronaviruses, having a total of 39 species under the broad realm of Riboviria, belong to the family Coronaviridae, suborder Cornidovirineae and order Nidovirales. Human coronavirus (HCoV-HKU1), SARS-CoV, SARS CoV-2, and Middle East respiratory syndrome coronavirus (MERS-CoV), belong to the betacoronavirus genus [16, 17] of them SARS CoV-2 is very dangerous because of its high killing rate of the human population, which directly hit the socioeconomic movement of the world.

Mortality rate, or death rate, is a measure of the number of deaths (in general, or due to a specific cause) in a particular population, scaled to the size of that population, per unit of time. The mortality rate is typically expressed in units of deaths per 1,000 individuals per year. It is distinct from "morbidity", which is either the prevalence or incidence of disease [18]. The COVID-19 pandemic has its epicenter in Wuhan, China infecting the whole world within the last few months. As per World health organization data, COVID-19 is affecting 215 countries and territories around the world, USA, India, and Brazil being the worst affected countries of the world, till 18th October 2020 there were more than 40 million COVID cases reported all over the world, out of which 29.9 million cases recovered and cured of COVID-19 (74.6% recovery rate), and 1.1 Million (2.75% Mortality rate) deaths reported and around 8.97 million are currently active COVID cases globally under treatment [19]. The Table **1** depicts the top five countries of the world worst affected by COVID-19 [19], as per the world health organization (WHO) COVID-19 Dashboard, the USA remains the worst hit country by COVID-19 across the world and has reported 10 million COVID 19 cases till date, out of which 3.3 million are currently active cases having a mortality rate of 2.4% and recovery rate of 63.9%, followed by India with 8.4 million COVID-19 cases out of which 0.5 million currently active cases having a low mortality rate of 1.4% and high recovery rate of 92.3%, Brazil remains in the third position with a total 5.6 million COVID-19 cases with a mortality rate of 2.8% and recovery rate of 89.2%, Russia on the other hand at fourth position reports a total of 1.75 million cases with a mortality rate of 1.72% and recovery rate of 74.8%, last but not the least France at the fifth position as on 7th November 2020, reports a total of 1.66 million cases with a mortality rate of 2.4% and recovery rate of 7.6% [19]. Table **2** depicts the top five countries with the worst COVID-19 mortality rates around the globe [19], Yemen with a total of 2067 COVID-19 cases, out of which 602 deaths, reports the highest mortality rate of 29% in the world, followed up by Mexico having 9.8% mortality rate reporting a total of nine lakh fifty-five thousand COVID-19 Cases, Ecuador remains at third position with a mortality rate of 7.3% followed by Chad and Bolivia reporting a mortality rate of 6.43% and 6.18% respectively [19, 20]. The statistics mentioned above are dynamic and subject to change with time as per the infection, cure, and death rates of countries (Tables **1** and **2**).

Table 1. The top five countries of the world worst affected by COVID-19 (In Millions).

S. No.	Name of Country	Total Cases	Total Deaths	Recovered Cases	Active Cases	Recovery Rate [%]	Mortality Rate [%]
1	U.S.A	10	0.24	6.39	3.39	63.9%	2.4%
2	INDIA	8.46	0.13	7.81	0.52	92.3%	1.5%

(Table 1) cont.....

S. No.	Name of Country	Total Cases	Total Deaths	Recovered Cases	Active Cases	Recovery Rate [%]	Mortality Rate [%]
3	BRAZIL	5.6	0.16	5.06	0.44	89.2%	2.8%
4	RUSSIA	1.75	0.03	1.31	0.44	74.8%	1.7%
5	France	1.66	0.039	0.12	1.5	7.6%	2.4%

Table 2. The top five countries of the world with the worst COVID-19 mortality rate.

S. No.	Name of Country	Total Cases	Total Deaths	Mortality rate [%]
1	Yemen	2067	602	29.0%
2	Mexico	955000	94323	9.8%
3	Ecuador	173000	12761	7.3%
4	Chad	1538	99	6.43%
5	Bolivia	142000	8781	6.18%

2. TRADITIONAL DRUGS AND NATURAL SOURCED FORMULATION FOR TREATMENT OF COVID-19

The COVID-19 is becoming the greatest threat to humanity, posing several challenges to the world's healthcare system and the national integration of each country. Since the outbreak and spread of pandemic all over the world, knowledge of COVID-19 etiology, pathogenesis, and disease management is, however, increasing day by day through the extensive research carried out by the scientists who claimed that COVID-19 spreads from respiratory droplets of the symptomatic person in close contact with a healthy individual or in contact with infected surface or objects [21]. It was found that SARS-CoV-2 negatively affects the immune homeostasis leading to a decrease in the immune response of the body, causing various inflammatory cytokines produced at a much higher rate leading to a cytokine storm also known as hypercytokinemia, which allows more immune cells to be recruited to the site of infection that can lead to organ damage. The damage produced pro-inflammatory cytokines (PIC) and chemokines (CK) which stimulate the host immunological reactions. The coronavirus attacks or invades the human body through human cell surface spike proteins and binds to the angiotensin-converting enzyme-2 (ACE2) receptors of the host cell and hijacks the ACE-2 receptor through its spike protein. The novel coronavirus replicates and produces various pathological symptoms such as diarrhea, high fever, dry cough, severe pneumonia, shortness of breath, and ultimately hypoxia or even death due to multiple organ failure [22, 23]. Currently, in the absence of any specific small molecule chemotherapeutics, to counter-attack COVID-19 by enhancing the body immunity to get prevented from COVID-19 through various immune system modulators remains the only alternative option. Artificial respiration and ventilation have been introduced as a major therapy for the treatment of severe COVID-19 infection cases but the major challenge in treating COVID-19 infection is to counter-attack the over response of the immune system, which damages the respiratory system and other vital body organs leading to the patient transfer to ICU and on ventilators. It ultimately increases the mortality rate [24, 25]. As modern medicine researchers through extensive research are looking for a permanent solution to combat COVID-19, it is also important to look into alternative natural drugs or formulations options available in ancient traditional medicines rich heritage left by our ancestors that may be used to treat or prevent the spread of novel coronavirus infection. The latest study and clinical trials prove that traditional Indian herbs, Crude drugs, or formulations available in Ayurveda and Traditional Chinese medicine (TCM) can be used to alleviate mild to moderate symptoms of COVID-19 along with easing the severe symptoms such as hypoxia or shortness of breath [25].

2.1. Traditional Indian Medicines (TIM) to Combat COVID-19

Ayurveda is one of the renowned written text forms of Indian traditional medicine and the pandemic concept has been explained by Acharya Charaka in Janapadodhwansa Chapter 3rd in Vimana sthana. Acharya Charaka describes that four elements Vayu (air), Jala (water), Desh (soil), and Kala (time) are four responsible factors for the spread of new infections in the society and explained the whole concept of managing pandemic situation [26]. For any pandemic condition Panchakarma (five procedures of purification), Rasayana Chikitsa (immune-modulators therapy), and Sadvritta (good conduct like Mask, personal hygiene, and social distancing) are leading treatments in Ayurveda [26, 27]. Among all the treatments available, the preferred treatment is the Rasayana Chikitsa. Under this treatment, groups of important natural drugs (Rasayana Dravayas) that are supposed to improve defense mechanisms and enhance the immune system, response are administered either as a prophylactic medicine or as a preventive therapy in healthy people mainly as an oral and liquid dosage form either in the form of a tablet, churna or solution [28, 29]. Thus an attempt has been made to focus all potential natural drugs and natural ayurvedic formulations that may be beneficial to combat diseases caused by viruses like the SARS-Co--2, due to their antiviral and immune-modulatory properties available under Indian traditional medicine for the effective treatment or prevention of COVID-19 (Tables 3 and 4).

Withanone of ashwagandha (Indian Ginseng) blocks the binding of 2019-nCoV spike protein with ACE-2 receptor restricting entry of the virus into the human body. It provides antiviral immunity by increasing interferon-gamma (IFN gamma responses) and anti-inflammatory activities by decreasing the quantity of interleukin -1, interleukin -6, and tumor necrosis factor, which are the main factors related to COVID-19 (Fig. **2**). Ashwagandha may be an effective agent in the management of COVID-19 infection by modulation of host Th-1/Th-2 immunity [30]. Giloy (Guduchi) has been found to activate macrophages, NFκB translocation, and cytokine production and hence activate the immune system. The active ingredient tinocodiside of giloy blocks the binding of 2019-nCoV spike protein with ACE-2 receptor restricting entry of the virus into the human body and enhancing immune activity against COVID-19, similar to withanone[31,32]. Scutellarein, a natural flavone found in Tulsi (Indian Basil), is a strong inhibitor of the SARS-CoV helicase enzyme and also inhibits the RdRp enzyme, which is the central enzyme needed by SARS CoV-2 multiplication, and it restricts the replication of the virus in the human body [33].

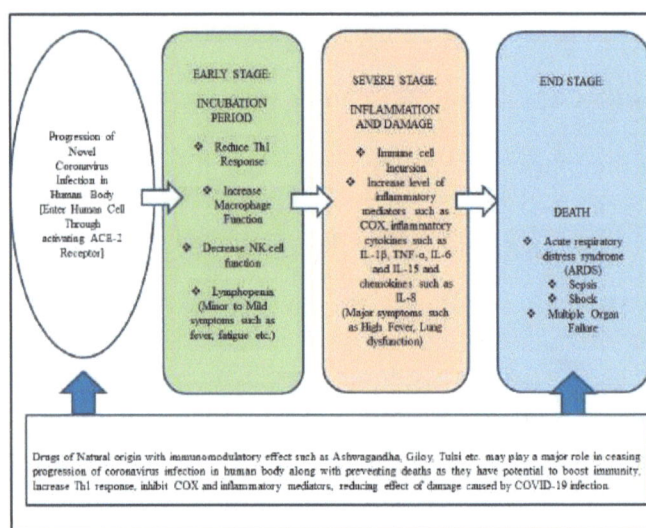

Fig. (2). Progression of Novel Coronavirus infection in the human body and potential role of drugs of natural origin with immune-modulatory property can play to prevent COVID-19 infection [30 - 33].

Table 3. Recommended Drugs of Natural origin under Indian traditional medicine for treatment or prevention of COVID-19.

S.No.	Name of Natural Drug	Botanical Name	Form of Extract	Preparation	Dosage	Common Usage in Ayurveda	References
1.	Ashwagandha (Indian Ginseng, Winter Cherry)	Withania somnifera	Pure Aqueous extract	Aswagandha Dried root Extract or Vati with warm water	500 mg B.D 15 days	As an immune booster and for relieving stress and anxiety	[30]

(Table 3) cont.....

S.No.	Name of Natural Drug	Botanical Name	Form of Extract	Preparation	Dosage	Common Usage in Ayurveda	References
2.	Giloy (Guduchi)	Tinospora cordifolia	Aqueous	Samshamani Vati 500g with warm water	500 mg B.D 15 days	For Blood purifying, immunity enhancer, analgesic, and anti-inflammatory and antipyretic	[31, 32]
3.	Tulsi (Indian Basil)	Ocimum Sanctum	Pure Aqueous extract or Tablet	Tulsi leaf Extract or Vati with warm water	500 mg B.D 15 days	In Respiratory illness, Boost immunity, and digestive stimulant	[33]
4.	Mulethi (Liquorice root)	Glycyrrhiza Glabra	Pure Root Extract of Mulethi	Mulethi Root Extract with Warm water	As directed by the physician (Available in Indian market as Swasari Ras Tablet in combination with other herbal drugs)	As an expectorant and mucolytic. It is also regarded as detoxicant, anti-inflammatory, anti-pyretic, diuretic, immune empowering, and a nerve stimulant	[34]
5.	Kalmegha (Green Chiretta)	Andrograhis Paniculata	Aqueous extract	Kalmegha leaf extract	Kalmegha leaf decoction 50 to 60 ml with water twice a day for 14 days	As a digestive stimulant, hepatoprotective & improves liver functions, Rakta shodhak (blood purifier), reduced inflammation, laxative, a part of this Kalmegh acts on respiratory and metabolic disorders.	[35, 36]
6.	Cinchona bark (Jesuit's bark)	Cinchona officinalis	Pure Bark extract or powder	Cinchona Bark Powder or Tablet	Cinchona bark powder decoction with 50 to 60 ml of warm water or Tablet	As an appetite enhancer; and in stomach problems. It is also used for blood vessel disorders like hemorrhoids and the treatment of malaria	[37, 38]

(Table 3) cont.....

S.No.	Name of Natural Drug	Botanical Name	Form of Extract	Preparation	Dosage	Common Usage in Ayurveda	References
7	Garlic (Lehsun)	Allium sativum	Aqueous extract or tablets	Garlic bulb extract or Tablets	Can be taken in raw form alone or mixed with other drugs[2 to 3gm daily]	For Cardiac Diseases, and anti-inflammatory and antipyretic along with in conditions like hyperlipidemia	[39, 40]
8.	Kalonji (Black Cummin)	Nigella sativa	Kalonji seeds extract or powder	Kalonji Seed Powder or Dried seeds	2 to 5gm Kalonji seed powder decoction with warm water or powder can be directly inhaled through the nose	As anti-inflammatory, Antioxidant and in respiratory disorders	[41, 42]
9.	Sunthi (Ardraka, Dried Ginger)	Zingiber Officinale	Pure Aqueous extract of Ginger Rhizomes	Dried Ginger Rhizomes extract or Powder	Shunthi decoction with 50 ml warm water or Powder [1 to 1.5 gm daily]	Relives Cough, Nausea Vomiting, sore Throat, and as a flavoring agent	[43 - 45]
10.	Turmeric (Haldi)	Curcuma Longa	Aqueous Extract	Turmeric Yellow Dried rhizomes extract or Powder	Turmeric can be utilized in the form of decoction or powder with a daily dosage of 1-3 gm	As an antibacterial agent and in skin disorders, an immunity booster	[46 - 49]
11.	Amla (Indian gooseberry)	Emblica Officinalis	Aqueous extract	Pure Amla Aqueous extract or Amla Dried Powder	Amla extract daily 10 to 20 ml will 50 ml warm water or Tablets or can be taken directly (5 to 10 gm dose)	Thirst Quencher, for Hair fall, Digestion stimulants, skin disorders, respiratory infections, and premature aging.	[50, 51]

(Table 3) cont.....

S.No.	Name of Natural Drug	Botanical Name	Form of Extract	Preparation	Dosage	Common Usage in Ayurveda	References
12.	Black Pepper (Siya mirch,Kaali Mirch)	Piper nigrum	Black Pepper Aqueous Extract or Powder	Black pepper powder decoction or powder	The recommended dosage of black pepper is 0.4-1.25 gm in the form of powder or decoction	For asthma, upset stomach, bronchitis, diarrhea, gas, headache, menstrual pain, stuffy nose, sinus infection, dizziness,	[52, 53]

Table 4. Recommended Ayurvedic Natural drug formulation under Indian traditional medicine for treatment or prevention of COVID-19.

S.No.	Formulation Name	Ingredient	Dose	Usage	Market Formulation	References
1	**Anu Taila (Nasya Therapy)**	A mixture of various oils Jivanti, Jala Sugandha bala, Devadaru, Jalada. Twak,Sevya (Ushira),Gopi (Sariva),Hima (Shweta Chandana) And Darvi (Daruharidra) *etc*	5 to 10 drops for Nasya, as Nasal Drops	For Respiratory infection treatment and prevention	Baidyanath Anu tail and Divya Pharmacy Anu Tail	[54]
2	**Swasari Ras Tablet**	Tablet Swasari Ras is a unique combination of various plant parts, namely, it consists of fruit of Mulethi), Cloves, bark of Cinnamomum, the fruit of Rudanti, a rhizome of Ginger, the fruit of Black pepper *Etc*.	One tablet B.D	For Respiratory infection treatment related to COVID 19, mild to moderate infection	Divya Pharmacy, Swasari Ras Tablet (Coronil Kit)	[55]
3	**Sanjveeni Vati**	It contains ten ingredients - Vidanga, Sunthi, Pippali, Haritaki, Vibitaki, Amalaki, Vacha, Guduchi, Shudha Bhallataka and Shudha Vatsnabha in equal quantity with Gomutra and then mixed well.	One tablet B.D	Upper Respiratory tract infection due to mild covid19 infection	Dabur and Baidyanath, Divya Pharmacy Sanjeevani Vati	[17, 25]

(Table 4) cont.....

S.No.	Formulation Name	Ingredient	Dose	Usage	Market Formulation	References
4.	Samshamani Vati	Tablet of Tinospora Cordifolia(Giloy)	One tablet B.D	Mild to moderate COVID-19 infection	Dabur and Baidyanath, Divya Pharmacy	[17, 25]

Glycyrrhizin, the active constituent of Mulethi (liquorice root) can inhibit the replication of SARS-associated virus along with the inhibition of its penetration into human cells. It also relives mucus production and thus makes it a potential candidate to combat COVID-19 [34]. Andrographolides, the main ingredient of Kalmegha (green chiretta), enhance the immune system by increasing the production of white blood cells, the release of interferon, and the activity of the lymph system. Lymph carries away the by-products of cellular metabolism and act as a shuttle for invading viruses. The research also shows that it may suppress the replication of the SARS-COV thus, it has been taken as a potent candidate for the prevention of COVID-19 [35, 36]. Cinchona bark (Jesuit's bark) produces many phytoactive chinoline derivatives such as cinchonine, quinine, cinchonidine, and quinidine. Recently antimalarial drugs derived from cinchona such as chloroquine and hydroxychloroquine have been found effective against SARS-CoV-2. The research has shown that herbal derivatives; sesquiterpenoids, diterpenoids, triterpenoids, curcumin, and lignoids inhibit SARS-CoV-2, thus making cinchona bark a potential drug that can be used for the treatment of COVID-19 [37, 38]. Garlic (Lehsun) contains active ingredients, including alliin, allicin, ajoene, vinyldithin, S-allylcycsteine, and diallyl sulphides . Hence Garlic has been used as an antioxidant, anti-inflammatory, immune-modulating, antibiotic, bacteriostatic, antifungal, antiviral agent in Ayurveda. It has proteolytic and hemagglutinating activity and can inhibit the viral replication of SARS-CO--2. It has been investigated that garlic modulates cytokine expression in lipopolysacharide activated human blood. It inhibits NF-κB, from which its immune-modulatory effect is evident and helpful in the treatment of COVID 19 [39, 40]. Kalonji (Black Cummin) contains important phytochemicals such as thymoquinone, dithymoquinone, p-cymene, alfa-pinene, thymohydroquinone, sesquiterpene, carvacrol, pentacyclic triterpene, terpineol, and saponins. It exerts immunomodulatory, anti-inflammatory, antibacterial, analgesic, antioxidant, antiasthmatic, bronchodilator in the body. Current research suggests that thymoquinone, the main essential oil constituent of kalonji and other active compounds, has inhibitory effects against SARS-CoV-2 [41, 42]. Sunthi (Ardraka, Dried Ginger), contains N-gingerol, which prevents Th2-mediated immune responses and respiratory airways inflammation. The 6-gingerol was shown to suppress eosinophilia and inhibit the production of TNF-α, IL-1β, and IL-12. Sunthi has antiviral activity against respiratory syncytial virus, Ginger provides bronchodilatory effect and prevents severe alveoli damage caused by inflammatory responses, and ameliorates allergic asthma. Thus it can be a useful drug in the prevention and ceasing of novel coronavirus infection progression and treatment of COVID-19 symptoms [43 - 45]. Turmeric (Haldi), contains important phytochemicals such as curcumin, dihydrocurcumin, and hexahydrocurcumin. Some volatile compounds like cinol, α-phellandrene, borneol, zingiberine are also present. Many research papers suggest that turmeric is extremely effective in acute respiratory distress syndrome (ARDS), COPD, acute lung injury (ALI), and pulmonary fibrosis as it suppresses TNF-α and inhibits NF-κB. In this way, it acts as a potent anti-inflammatory agent and can be used in the prevention of the onset of COVID-19 [46 - 49]. Amla is the richest source of vitamin C, its major chemical constituents are ascorbic acid, iron, calcium, and other bioactive compounds like gallic acid, ellagic acid, norsesquiterpenoids, gearaniin, and prodelphinidin. Studies suggest that amla acts as a potent antioxidant, anti-inflammatory, immune enhancer, free radical scavenger, antipyretic, antitussive, and hematinic agent. Because of its extreme immune empowering property, it is believed to be effective against viral infections, common cold, bronchitis, and influenza. Currently, vitamin C is prescribed for the treatment of COVID 19 mild to moderate symptoms, therefore, Amla being a rich source of natural vitamin C may be used as an alternative to Combat COVID 19 [50, 51]. Black Pepper (Siya mirch, Kaali Mirch), is a rich source of alkaloids and amides viz pipericide, piperine, piperlonguminine, piplartine, and aristolactams. Researchers have demonstrated the antiviral and anti-proliferative action of piperamide derived from black pepper. Besides black pepper has been shown to inhibit the release of Th-2-mediated cytokines, eosinophil infiltration in the lungs, leading to the inhibition of allergic inflammation. Thus, it can be a potential candidate for the prevention of COVID-19 [52, 53].

Repurposing the formulations prepared from natural medicines can be a good strategy to manage acute and mild COVID-19 cases. Table 4 represents ayurvedic formulations prepared under Indian traditional medicines that can be used in the prevention and treatment of COVID-19. Nasya therapy (*Anu taila as nasal drops*) described by Maharishi Charak is recommended to help in mucus discharge, nasal decongestion, respiratory inflammation, and other COVID-19 related disease symptoms. Anu tail is prepared from the mixture of various oils extracted from medicinal plants like Jivanti (*Leptadenia reticulata*), Jala (*Pavonia odorata*), Devdaru (*Cedrus deodara*), Nagarmotha (*Cyperus scariosus*), Dalacini (*Cinn amomum verum*), Sevya (*Chrysopogon zizanioides*), Anantmula (*Hemidesmus indicus*), Sweta candana (*Santalum album*), Daruharidra (*Berberis aristata*), Mulethi (*Glycyrrhiza glabra*), Plawa (*Cyperus platyphyllus*), Agaru (*Aquilaria agallocha*), Satavari (*Asparagus racemosus*), Bela (*Aegle marmelos*), Utpala

(*Nymphaeanouchali*), Bṛhati (*Solanum indicum*), Kaṇṭakari (*Solanum surattense*), Surbhi (*Pluchea lanceolata*), Salaparṇi (*Desmodium gangeticum*),Pṛsniparṇi (*Uraria picta*), Viḍanga (*Embelia ribes*), Tejpatra (*Cinnamomum tamala*), Truṭi (*Elettaria cardamomum*), Reṇuka (*Vitex agnus-castus*), Kamala keṣara (*Nelumbo nucifera*), Ajadugdha (*Goat milk*), and Tila Taila (*Sesamum indicum*). The recommended dose of anu tailam is 5 to 10 drops daily through nasal route [54]. Swasari ras is a tablet prepared from natural drugs and mineral mentioned in ancient Ayurveda and above described natural plant products such as Mulethi, Lavanga, Dalchini, Karkatashringi, Rudanti, Ardraka, Maricha, Pippali, Akarkara (Table **3**) and calcium mineral components such as Kapardak bhasma, Abhraka bhasma, Godanti bhasma and Mukta shukti bhasma responsible for producing immune-modulatory and anti-inflammatory activity in respiratory diseases. It also has high efficacy in the treatment of cough, asthma, inflammation and other lung disorders, therefore can be used to treat mild to moderate COVID-19 infection [55]. Apart from this sanjeevani vati and giloy tablet (*Shamshmani vatika*) mentioned in ayurveda for use in respiratory disorders is also recommended for COVID-19 because of their immuno modulatory property [17,25].

2.2. Traditional Chinese Medicine (TCM) To Combat COVID-19

During the outbreak of SARS coronavirus (SARS-CoV) in late 2002 in the Guangdong Province of China, more than three thousand, Traditional Chinese medicine (TCM) practitioners were sent to Wuhan Hubei for giving treatment as per TCM guidelines and regimen of the Health Ministry of China. Again the COVID-19 treatment protocol has been strictly followed in China in the prevention and control of COVID-19 [56 - 59]. Traditional Chinese medicine is based on the theory that Qi is the basic substance that the human body constitutes and is divided into two Qi, namely healthy Qi refers to elements in the body for its normal functioning and the pathogenic Qi refers to substances that can harm the health of our body. Traditional Chinese medicine can be divided into three categories: clearing heat, eliminating dampness, and detoxification. As per the symptoms caused by COVID-19, it can be classified as a disease related to "wet, heat, congestion", in the lungs due to the presence of pathogenic Qi. In TCM, it is assumed that the lungs are delicate, so the disease first affects the lungs' function. "Wet" refers to the factor with sticky and heavy turbidity that can cause long multiple damages to the body organ. "Hot" refers to the factor with hot, dry, and rising turbidity that can cause alleviated body temperate. "Congestion" is a causative factor that can congest blood circulation and cause symptoms such as pain. So it was suggested to use such TCM herbs during COVID-19 infection, which maintains the proper level of lung Qi by "clearing lung heat and dampness" [60, 61]. Table **5** represents and enlists some of the important TCM herbs and formulations that can be used in the prevention and treatment of COVID-19 infection. Based on the symptoms of COVID-19 pneumonia patients, the most preferred TCM formulation prescribed and suggested to most of the patients in China was Qingfei paidu decoction (QPD). It consists of decoction prepared from herbs like Ephedrae Herba, Glycyrrhizae Radix. Rhizoma Praeprata, Armeniacae Semen Amarum, Gypsum Fibrosum, Cinnamomi Ramulus, Alismatis Rhizoma, Polyporus, Atractylodis Macrocephalae Rhizoma, Poria, Bupleuri Radix, Scutellariae Radix, Pinelliae Rhizoma Praepratum, Zingiberis Rhizoma Recens, Asteris Radix, Belamcandae Rhizoma, Rhizoma, Aurantii Fructus Immaturus, Citri Reticulatae Pericarpium, and Pogostemonis Herba . The QPD acts by inhibiting and alleviating excessive immune response and eliminates inflammation by regulating immune-related and cytokine action-related pathways [59]. Glycyrrhizin, a major active constituent of liquorice root, is the most frequently used Chinese herb in TCM [62] and has been of preference for the prevention and treatment of COVID-19 as research showed potently glycyrrhizin inhibited the replication of clinical isolates of SARS virus [34]. Other than QPD, Yin Qiao San decoction, as per TCM theory, acts by dispersing wind-heat, clears heat, and relieves toxicity. It consists of the extract prepared from Fructus Forsythiae, Flos Lonicerae, Radix Platycodonis, Herba Menthae, Herba Lophatheri, Radix Glycyrrhizae, Herba Schizonepetae, Fermented soybean, Fructus arctii, Rhizoma Phragmitis and can also be used to prevent novel coronavirus infection [63, 64]. The Ma Xin Gan Shi Tang decoction prepared from Ephedrae herba, Armeniacae semenamarum, Glycyrrhizae radix et rhizome, Gypsum fibrosum, and Da Yuan Yin acts by facilitating the flow of the lung "qi" and clears away heat, thus preventing lungs from harmful pathogenic Qi cause of COVID-19 as per TCM theory. As per the research, it shows anti-SARS-CoV activity [62, 65, 66]. Currently, there is no high-quality evidence for the safety of some herbs used under TCM, but also there are no reports of serious adverse reactions when used in optimum dose [67]. TCM can effectively prevent the disease from transforming into severe and critical disease and has been widely adopted in China during the COVID-19 pandemic [68].

Table 5. Important TCM formulation that can be used in the prevention and treatment of COVID-19 infection.

S.No.	Name of TCM Formulation	Therapeutic Use	References
1.	**Qingfei Paidu decoction**	Anti-inflammatory, Treatment of upper respiratory tract infection. Immune system enhancer	[59]
2.	**Yin Qiao San decoction**	Improvement of the function of upper respiratory mucosal immune system.	[67, 68]
3.	**Ma Xin Gan Shi Tang Decoction**	Antiviral effect and respiratory disorders	[67, 68]

CONCLUSION

Under the threat of the COVID-19 pandemic situation, the modern health care system of developing and developed countries has been pushed to their limits for effective management of COVID-19, and as second wave threat is arising in many countries around the world, the traditional natural source drugs to combat COVID-19 as an alternative therapy should be prioritized in combination with modern medicines. More thorough and extensive research will be required by scientists all over the world as it would be a bit too early to depend completely on drugs of natural origin to eliminate the spread of novel coronavirus. However, remembering the most important concept of medicine *i.e.* "prevention is better than cure" and advantages possessed by traditional medicine systems such as fewer side effects, minimum toxicity, simplicity, affordability, and large acceptability by the public, especially in countries like India where drugs of natural origin mentioned above can be highly promoted to maintain and enhance immune system response of the body to prevent effect and damage caused by COVID-19. The evidence and review presented here should draw the attention of healthcare professionals public health specialists around the world, including the World Health Organization and health ministries of various countries, to the unexplored potential of traditional medicine systems for adopting the integrative approaches in the search for solutions to end the COVID-19 pandemic. It is high time to embrace integration with an open mind, especially in countries like India, where Ayurveda is originated, nurtured, and practiced since ancient times. The SARS-COV-2 has been spreading in mass population day by day. It would become too difficult to control even severe cases in hospitals. Therefore, the general public should be careful to maintain social distancing, using masks and sanitizers. The COVID-19 patients with mild symptoms could be controlled at home isolation by repurposing natural medicines.

CONSENT FOR PUBLICATION

Not applicable.

CONFLICT OF INTEREST

The authors declare no conflict of interest, financial or otherwise.

ACKNOWLEDGEMENTS

Declared none.

REFERENCES

[1]   Denaro M, Smeriglio A, Barreca D, *et al.* Antiviral activity of plants and their isolated bioactive compounds: An update. Phytother Res 2020; 34(4): 742-68.

[http://dx.doi.org/10.1002/ptr.6575] [PMID: 31858645]

[2]   Oyero OG, Toyama M, Mitsuhiro N, *et al.* Selective inhibition of hepatitis c virus replication by Alpha-zam, a *Nigella sativa* seed formulation. Afr J Tradit Complement Altern Med 2016; 13(6): 144-8.
[http://dx.doi.org/10.21010/ajtcam.v13i6.20] [PMID: 28480371]

[3]   Mirzaie A, Halaji M, Dehkordi FS, Ranjbar R, Noorbazargan H. A narrative literature review on traditional medicine options for treatment of corona virus disease 2019 (COVID-19). Complement Ther Clin Pract 2020; 40: 101214.
[http://dx.doi.org/10.1016/j.ctcp.2020.101214] [PMID: 32891290]

[4]   World Health Organization. Legal status of traditional medicine and complementary/alternative medicine: a worldwide review 2001; 1-159.

[5]   Mukherjee PK. Evaluation of Indian traditional medicine. Drug Inf J 2001; 35(2): 623-32.
[http://dx.doi.org/10.1177/009286150103500235]

[6]   Balachandar V, Mahalaxmi I, Kaavya J, *et al.* COVID-19: emerging protective measures. Eur Rev Med Pharmacol Sci 2020; 24(6): 3422-5.
[PMID: 32271461]

[7]   Chan K. Chinese medicinal materials and their interface with Western medical concepts. J Ethnopharmacol 2005; 96(1-2): 1-18.
[http://dx.doi.org/10.1016/j.jep.2004.09.019] [PMID: 15588645]

[8]   Li Q, Guan X, Wu P, *et al.* Early transmission dynamics in Wuhan, China, of novel coronavirus-Infected pneumonia. N Engl J Med 2020; 382(13): 1199-207.
[http://dx.doi.org/10.1056/NEJMoa2001316] [PMID: 31995857]

[9]   World Health Organization. Statement on the second meeting of the International Health Regulations. Emergency Committee regarding the outbreak of novel coronavirus January. 2020. Available from: https://www.who.int/news-room/detail/30-01-2020-statement-onthe-second-meeti-g-of-the-international-health-regulations-(2005)

[10]   World Health Organization. WHO Director-General's remarks at the media briefing on 2019-nCoV February 2020. 2020. Available from: https://www.who.int/dg/speeches/detail/whodirector-general-s-remarks-at-the-media-briefing-on-2019-ncov-on-11-february-2020

[11]   Wang C, Horby PW, Hayden FG, Gao GF. A novel coronavirus outbreak of global health concern. Lancet 2020; 395(10223): 470-3.
[http://dx.doi.org/10.1016/S0140-6736(20)30185-9] [PMID: 31986257]

[12]   Tyrrell DA, Bynoe ML. Cultivation of viruses from a high proportion of patients with colds. Lancet 1966; 1(7428): 76-7.
[http://dx.doi.org/10.1016/S0140-6736(66)92364-6] [PMID: 4158999]

[13]   McIntosh K, Becker WB, Chanock RM. Growth in suckling mouse brain of "IBV-like" viruses from patients with upper respiratory tract disease. Proc Natl Acad Sci USA 1967; 58(6): 2268-73.
[http://dx.doi.org/10.1073/pnas.58.6.2268] [PMID: 4298953]

[14]   Witte KH, Tajima M, Easterday BC. Morphologic characteristics and nucleic acid type of transmissible gastroenteritis virus of pigs. Arch Gesamte Virusforsch 1968; 23(1): 53-70.
[http://dx.doi.org/10.1007/BF01242114] [PMID: 4300586]

[15]   Richman DD, Whitley RJ, Hayden FG. Clinical Virology. Washington: ASM Press 2016.
[http://dx.doi.org/10.1128/9781555819439]

[16]   Gorbalenya AE, Baker S. C, Baric R S, *et al.* Severe acute respiratory syndrome-related coronavirus–the species and its viruses, a statement of the coronavirus study group. BioRxiv 2020.

[17]   Vellingiri B, Jayaramayya K, Iyer M, *et al.* COVID-19: A promising cure for the global panic. Sci Total Environ 2020; 725: 138277.

[http://dx.doi.org/10.1016/j.scitotenv.2020.138277] [PMID: 32278175]

[18]   Prospects World Population. the 2010 Revision 2011.

[19]   World Health Organization. COVID Tracker. Retrieved 7th November 2020. Available from: https://covid19.who.int/table

[20]   Johns Hopkins University. COVID-19 Dashboard by the Center for Systems Science and Engineering. Retrieved 7th November 2020. Available from: https://coronavirus.jhu.edu/

[21]   Lu R, Zhao X, Li J, *et al.* Genomic characterisation and epidemiology of 2019 novel coronavirus: implications for virus origins and receptor binding. Lancet 2020; 395(10224): 565-74. [http://dx.doi.org/10.1016/S0140-6736(20)30251-8] [PMID: 32007145]

[22]   Zhou P, Yang XL, Wang XG, *et al.* A pneumonia outbreak associated with a new coronavirus of probable bat origin. Nature 2020; 579(7798): 270-3. [http://dx.doi.org/10.1038/s41586-020-2012-7] [PMID: 32015507]

[23]   Jaimes JA, Millet JK, Stout AE, André NM, Whittaker GR. A tale of two Viruses: the distinct spike glycoproteins of feline coronaviruses. Viruses 2020; 12(1): 1-14. [http://dx.doi.org/10.3390/v12010083] [PMID: 31936749]

[24]   Wang M, Cao R, Zhang L, *et al.* Remdesivir and chloroquine effectively inhibit the recently emerged novel coronavirus (2019-nCoV) in vitro. Cell Res 2020; 30(3): 269-71. [http://dx.doi.org/10.1038/s41422-020-0282-0] [PMID: 32020029]

[25]   Panda AK, Dixit AK, Rout S, *et al.* Ayurvedic practitioner consensus to develop strategies for COVID-19. Jou Ayu Int Med Sci 2020; 1(5): 98-106.

[26]   Pandey G. Hindi commentarator of Charaka Samhita of Agnivesha. Viman Sthan chapter 3 verse 8'. 1st. Chaukumba Sanskrit Sansthan Varanasi 2006; p. 445.

[27]   Niraj S, Varsha S. A review on scope of immuno-modulatory drugs in Ayurveda for prevention and treatment of COVID-19. Plant Sci Today 2020; 7(3): 417-23. [http://dx.doi.org/10.14719/pst.2020.7.3.831]

[28]   Singh S, Byadgi PS, Tripathi JS, *et al.* Clinical appraisal of immunomodulators in Ayurveda in the light of recent pharmacological advances. World J Pharm Res 2015; 4(4): 678-92.

[29]   Chauhan VP, Dutt B, Vyas M, Gupta SK. Effect of immunemodulators (Rasayana Dravya) in Janapadodhwansa WSR to COVID-19. J Ayu Herb 2020; 6(1): 26-9. [http://dx.doi.org/10.31254/jahm.2020.6107]

[30]   Balkrishna A, Pokhrel S, Singh J, *et al.* Coronavirus (COVID-19) entry by disrupting interactions between viral S-Protein receptor binding domain and host ACE2 receptor. Vir Jour 2020; pp. 1-26.

[31]   Sinha K, Mishra NP, Singh J, *et al.* Tinosporacordifolia (Guduchi), a reservoir plant for therapeutic applications: A review. Ind Jour Trad Know 2004; 3(3): 257-70.

[32]   Gupta PK, Chakraborty P, Kumar S, *et al.* G1-4A, a Polysaccharide from Tinospora cordifolia inhibits the survival of Mycobacterium tuberculosis by Modulating host immune responses in TLR4 dependent manner. PLoS One 2016; 11(5): e0154725. [http://dx.doi.org/10.1371/journal.pone.0154725] [PMID: 27148868]

[33]   Pandey R, Chandra P, Srivastava M, Mishra DK, Kumar B. Simultaneous quantitative determination of multiple bioactive markers in Ocimum sanctum obtained from different locations and its marketed herbal formulations using UPLC-ESI-MS/MS combined with principal component analysis. Phytochem Anal 2015; 26(6): 383-94. [http://dx.doi.org/10.1002/pca.2551] [PMID: 26268610]

[34]   Cinatl J, Morgenstern B, Bauer G, Chandra P, Rabenau H, Doerr HW. Glycyrrhizin, an active component of liquorice roots, and replication of SARS-associated coronavirus. Lancet 2003; 361(9374): 2045-6. [http://dx.doi.org/10.1016/S0140-6736(03)13615-X] [PMID: 12814717]

[35]   Liu YT, Chen HW, Lii CK, *et al.* A diterpenoid, 14-deoxy-11, 12-didehydroandrographolide, in Andrographis paniculata reduces steatohepatitis and liver injury in mice fed a high-fat and highcholesterol diet. Nutrients 2020; 12(2): 523.
        [http://dx.doi.org/10.3390/nu12020523]

[36]   Liu Z, Xiao X, Wei X, *et al.* Composition and divergence of coronavirus spike proteins and host ACE2 receptors predict potential intermediate hosts of SARS-CoV-2. J Med Virol 2020; 92(6): 595-601.
        [http://dx.doi.org/10.1002/jmv.25726] [PMID: 32100877]

[37]   Murauer A, Ganzera M. Quantitative determination of major alkaloids in Cinchona bark by Supercritical Fluid Chromatography. J Chromatogr A 2018; 1554: 117-22.
        [http://dx.doi.org/10.1016/j.chroma.2018.04.038] [PMID: 29699870]

[38]   Wen CC, Kuo YH, Jan JT, *et al.* Specific plant terpenoids and lignoids possess potent antiviral activities against severe acute respiratory syndrome coronavirus. J Med Chem 2007; 50(17): 4087-95.
        [http://dx.doi.org/10.1021/jm070295s] [PMID: 17663539]

[39]   Shang A, Cao SY, Xu XY, *et al.* Bioactive compounds and biological functions of garlic (*Allium sativum* L). Foods 2019; 8(7): 246.
        [http://dx.doi.org/10.3390/foods8070246] [PMID: 31284512]

[40]   Schäfer G, Kaschula CH. The immunomodulation and anti-inflammatory effects of garlic organosulfur compounds in cancer chemoprevention. Anticancer Agents Med Chem 2014; 14(2): 233-40.
        [http://dx.doi.org/10.2174/18715206113136660370] [PMID: 24237225]

[41]   Al-Jassi MS. Chemical composition and microflora of black cumin (*Nigella sativa* L.) seeds growing in Saudi Arabia. Food Chem 1992; 45(4): 239-42.
        [http://dx.doi.org/10.1016/0308-8146(92)90153-S]

[42]   Koshak DAE, Koshak PEA. *Nigella sativa* L as a potential phytotherapy for coronavirus disease 2019: A mini review of in silico studies. Curr Ther Res Clin Exp 2020; 93: 100602.
        [http://dx.doi.org/10.1016/j.curtheres.2020.100602] [PMID: 32863400]

[43]   Tripathi S, Maier KG, Bruch D, Kittur DS. Effect of 6-gingerol on pro-inflammatory cytokine production and costimulatory molecule expression in murine peritoneal macrophages. J Surg Res 2007; 138(2): 209-13.
        [http://dx.doi.org/10.1016/j.jss.2006.07.051] [PMID: 17291534]

[44]   Ahui MLB, Champy P, Ramadan A, *et al.* Ginger prevents Th2-mediated immune responses in a mouse model of airway inflammation. Int Immunopharmacol 2008; 8(12): 1626-32.
        [http://dx.doi.org/10.1016/j.intimp.2008.07.009] [PMID: 18692598]

[45]   Çifci A, Tayman C, Yakut Hİ, *et al.* Ginger (*Zingiber officinale*) prevents severe damage to the lungs due to hyperoxia and inflammation. Turk J Med Sci 2018; 48(4): 892-900.
        [PMID: 30121057]

[46]   Shakibaei M, John T, Schulze-Tanzil G, Lehmann I, Mobasheri A. Suppression of NF-kappaB activation by curcumin leads to inhibition of expression of cyclo-oxygenase-2 and matrix metalloproteinase-9 in human articular chondrocytes: Implications for the treatment of osteoarthritis. Biochem Pharmacol 2007; 73(9): 1434-45.
        [http://dx.doi.org/10.1016/j.bcp.2007.01.005] [PMID: 17291458]

[47]   Prasad S, Aggarwal BB. Turmeric, 'the golden spice: From traditional medicine to modern medicine' Herbal Medicine: Biomolecular and Clinical Aspects, Oxidative Stress & Disease Series. U.S.A: CRC Press 2011; pp. 259-84.

[48]   Lelli D, Sahebkar A, Johnston TP, Pedone C. Curcumin use in pulmonary diseases: State of the art and future perspectives. Pharm Res 2017; 115: 133-48.
        [http://dx.doi.org/10.1016/j.phrs.2016.11.017] [PMID: 27888157]

[49]   Bhat AS, Rather SA, Iqbal A, Qureshi HA, Islam N. Immunomodulators for Curtailing COVID-19: a

Positive Approach. J Drug Deliv Ther 2020; 10(3-s) (Suppl. 3): 286-94.
[http://dx.doi.org/10.22270/jddt.v10i3-s.4085]

[50]   Hemilä H. Vitamin C and SARS coronavirus. J Antimicrob Chemother 2003; 52(6): 1049-50.
[http://dx.doi.org/10.1093/jac/dkh002] [PMID: 14613951]

[51]   Saini A, Sharma S, Chhibber S. Protective efficacy of *Emblica officinalis* against *Klebsiella pneumoniae* induced pneumonia in mice. Indian J Med Res 2008; 128(2): 188-93.
[PMID: 19001683]

[52]   Kim SH, Lee YC. Piperine inhibits eosinophil infiltration and airway hyperresponsiveness by suppressing T cell activity and Th2 cytokine production in the ovalbumin-induced asthma model. J Pharm Pharmacol 2009; 61(3): 353-9.
[http://dx.doi.org/10.1211/jpp.61.03.0010] [PMID: 19222908]

[53]   Mair EM, Liu R, Atanasov AG, Schmidtke M, Dirsch VM, Rollinger JM. Antiviral and anti-proliferative *in vitro* activities of piperamides from black pepper. Planta Med 2016; 81(S 01) (Suppl. 1): S1-S381.
[http://dx.doi.org/10.1055/s-0036-1596830]

[54]   Shukla V, Tripathi RD. Charaka Saṁhita. 2nd ed., New Delhi, India: Chaukhambha Sanskrit Pratishthan 2017.

[55]   Balkrishna A, Solleti SK, Singh H, Tomer M, Sharma N, Varshney A. Calcio-herbal formulation, Divya-Swasari-Ras, alleviates chronic inflammation and suppresses airway remodelling in mouse model of allergic asthma by modulating pro-inflammatory cytokine response. Biomed Pharmacother 2020; 126(11006): 110063.
[http://dx.doi.org/10.1016/j.biopha.2020.110063] [PMID: 32145582]

[56]   Peiris JSM, Yuen KY, Osterhaus AD, Stöhr K. The severe acute respiratory syndrome. N Engl J Med 2003; 349(25): 2431-41.
[http://dx.doi.org/10.1056/NEJMra032498] [PMID: 14681510]

[57]   Zhong N, May RM, McLean AR, *et al.* Management and prevention of SARS in China. Philos Trans R Soc Lond B Biol Sci 2004; 359(1447): 1115-6.
[http://dx.doi.org/10.1098/rstb.2004.1491] [PMID: 15306397]

[58]   Jin YH, Cai L, Cheng ZS, *et al.* A rapid advice guideline for the diagnosis and treatment of 2019 novel coronavirus (2019-nCoV) infected pneumonia (standard version). Mil Med Res 2020; 7(1): 4.
[http://dx.doi.org/10.1186/s40779-020-0233-6] [PMID: 32029004]

[59]   Ren JR, Zhang A, Wang X. Traditional Chinese Medicine for COVID-19 Treatment. Pharm Res 2020; 155: 1-2.

[60]   Wang WY, Yang J. An overview of the thoughts and methods of epidemic prevention in ancient Chinese Medicine. Jil Jour Trad Chin Med 2020; 31: 197-9.

[61]   Xu J, Zhang Y. Traditional Chinese Medicine treatment of COVID-19. Comp Ther Clin Prac 2020; 39(101165): 101165.
[http://dx.doi.org/10.1016/j.ctcp.2020.101165] [PMID: 32379692]

[62]   Yang Y, Islam S, Wang J, *et al.* Traditional Chinese Medicine in the Treatment of Patients Infected with 2019-New Coronavirus (SARS-CoV-2): A Review and Perspective'. Int J Med Sci 2020; 17(18): 3125-45.
[PMID: 33173434]

[63]   Liu LS, Lei N, Lin Q, *et al.* The Effects and Mechanism of Yinqiao Powder on Upper Respiratory Tract Infection. Int J Biotechnol Wellness Ind 2015; 4(2): 57-60.
[http://dx.doi.org/10.6000/1927-3037.2015.04.02.2]

[64]   Fu YJ, Yan YQ, Qin HQ, *et al.* Effects of different principles of Traditional Chinese Medicine treatment on TLR7/NF-κB signaling pathway in influenza virus infected mice. Chin Med 2018; 13(42): 42.

[http://dx.doi.org/10.1186/s13020-018-0199-4] [PMID: 30151032]

[65]   Bao L. Research progress of Da Yuan Yin on the treatment of infectious diseases. Jour Emer Trad Chin Med 2010; 2: 263-87.

[66]   Cui HT, Li YT, Guo LY, *et al.* Traditional Chinese medicine for treatment of coronavirus disease 2019: a review. Trad Chin Med 2020; 5(2): 65-73.
        [http://dx.doi.org/10.53388/TMR20200222165]

[67]   Luo H, Li Q, Flower A, Lewith G, Liu J. Comparison of effectiveness and safety between granules and decoction of Chinese herbal medicine: a systematic review of randomized clinical trials. J Ethnopharmacol 2012; 140(3): 555-67.
        [http://dx.doi.org/10.1016/j.jep.2012.01.031] [PMID: 22343092]

[68]   Luo H, Tang QL, Shang YX, *et al.* Can Chinese Medicine Be Used for Prevention of Corona Virus Disease 2019 (COVID-19)? A Review of Historical Classics, Research Evidence and Current Prevention Programs. Chin J Integr Med 2020; 26(4): 243-50.
        [http://dx.doi.org/10.1007/s11655-020-3192-6] [PMID: 32065348]

CHAPTER 5

Peptidomimetic and Peptide-Derived Against 3CL^{pro} from Coronaviruses

Paulo Fernando da Silva Santos-Júnior[1], João Xavier de Araújo-Júnior[2] and Edeildo Ferreira da Silva-Júnior[1,2,*]

[1] *Chemistry and Biotechnology Institute, Federal University of Alagoas, Maceió, Brazil*

[2] *Laboratory of Medicinal Chemistry, Pharmaceutical Sciences Institute, Federal University of Alagoas, Maceió, Brazil*

Abstract: SARS-CoV-2 is an RNA virus responsible for causing pandemic COVID-19, which has taken on unprecedented proportions so far in global health and economic aspects. In this context, the search for effective drugs against SARS-CoV-2 has become a priority for the global scientific community, where the chymotrypsin-like picornavirus 3C-like protease (3CL^{pro}, which is also named as main protease (M^{pro}), or only 3C) is a promising druggable target since it is crucial for the process of viral replication. Several 3CL^{pro} inhibitors have been recently reported in the literature. Thus, peptidomimetics have emerged as a potential class for designing new effective drugs against COVID-19, in addition to lopinavir/ritonavir, in which these drugs are currently being investigated in clinical trials. In this chapter, we describe peptidomimetic and peptide-derived inhibitors of 3CL^{pro} from SARS-CoV-2, and also SARS- and MERS-CoV viruses, summarizing all relevant studies based on warhead groups utilization and SAR analysis for all of them in order to contribute to the development of compounds more selective, effective, and low-costs to combat these emerging viruses.

Keywords: 3CL^{pro} inhibitors, Drug Design, MERS-CoV, Peptidomimetics, SARS-CoV, SARS-CoV-2.

1. INTRODUCTION

Coronavirus (CoV) refers to enveloped viruses belonging to the family *Coronaviridae* (subfamily: *Coronavirinae*; order: *Nidovirales*), which is responsible for causing potential severe infectious processes in the human respiratory tract [1, 2].

* **Corresponding author Edeildo Ferreira da Silva-Júnior:** Chemistry and Biotechnology Institute, Federal University of Alagoas, Maceió, Brazil and Laboratory of Medicinal Chemistry, Pharmaceutical Sciences Institute, Federal University of Alagoas, Maceió, Brazil; Tel: +55-87-9-9610-8311; E-mail: edeildo.junior@iqb.ufal.br

Luciana Scotti and Marcus T. Scotti (Eds.)

Two serious epidemics were caused by CoV, being *Middle East Respiratory Syndrome-coronavirus* (MERS-CoV), Arabian Peninsula, causing a total of 740 deaths, and 2,123 cases, in 2014. Besides, *Severe Acute Respiratory Syndrome-coronavirus* (SARS-CoV) was responsible for infecting 8,500 individuals, leading to 800 deaths in Guangdong province of China, between 2002-2003 [3 - 5].

Recently declared a pandemic by WHO (March 11th, 2020), COVID-19 is caused by the SARS-CoV-2 (previously called 2019-nCoV) [6]. Initially, it was reported on December 8th, 2019, in Wuhan, Huabei, China [7 - 9], causing severe respiratory complications. So far, this new-CoV has infected more than 246 million individuals worldwide, causing more than 5 million deaths, up to November 3rd 2021 [10].

Even in the third outbreak caused by a coronavirus, there is still no approved treatment or selective antiviral agents to combat this virus, nor approved vaccines [11 - 14]. Thus, current therapy involves treating symptoms, as well as providing oxygenation to the affected individuals, in addition to protective methods to avoid viral transmissions, such as wearing masks, hand hygiene, and social distancing [15, 16].

Medicinal chemistry has concentrated strategies for the development of bioactive compounds against the new coronavirus targeting enzymes [17, 18], in special the chymotrypsin-like picornavirus 3C-like protease (3CL^{pro}, also called main protease (M^{pro}), or only 3C), which emerges as the main druggable target from SARS-, MERS-CoV, and SARS-CoV-2 [17 - 22].

This protease (corresponding to nsP5) is directly responsible for the cleavage of the pp1a and pp1ab proteins, thus exercising a primordial function for controlling the viral cycle of replication [23 - 25]. Moreover, the genome sequence of SARS-CoV-2 3CL^{pro} is closely similar to the same protein from SARS-CoV [26, 27].

The utilization of peptide-based drugs (also named peptidomimetics) has been widely related to the design of bioactive compounds since this chemical class is involved in several regulatory processes in the human organism [28, 29]. Furthermore, endogenous peptides tend to demonstrate a strong binding with enzymatically active sites [30, 31].

In this context, this chapter summarizes strategies for developing peptidomimetics against 3CL^{pro} from MERS-, SARS-CoV, and SARS-CoV-2. We aim to demonstrate some warhead groups used in the design of these inhibitors, as well as discuss SAR analysis involving the most promising compounds, thus providing valuable information to assist in the development of new anti-virus drugs against this global emergency.

2. CHEMISTRY ASPECTS OF PEPTIDOMIMETICS

Peptides are intrinsically related to several physiological mechanisms in humans, in order to promote regulation of functions in the immune, digestive, defense, reproductive, respiratory, circulatory systems, in addition to metabolism and reproduction. Thus, at least 60 peptides have been described in the literature for therapeutic use in different clinical stages, being reported as inhibitors against HIV protease, hepatitis C virus (HCV), antimicrobial, treatment of dry eye syndrome (DED), among other activities, as described in Fig. (**1**) [31 - 35].

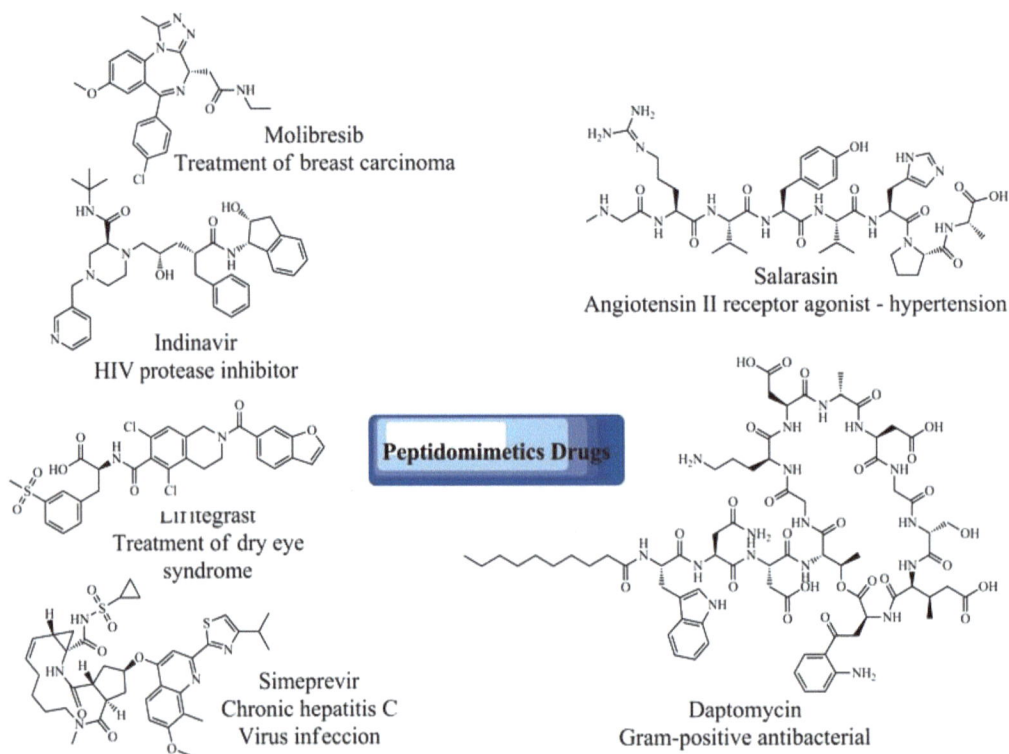

Fig. (1). Peptide-based drugs and their biological applications.

In 2010, four peptide drugs were responsible for US$ 1 billion in global sales, demonstrating the therapeutic potential from this drug design approach [36]. However, the peptide-based drug design still has a significant disadvantage in some pharmacokinetic aspects due to their high molecular mass can result in deficient absorption since there is no specific transport system for them. Also, these compounds present limited stability in toward proteolysis from the gastrointestinal system and serum [30, 33, 37].

Chemically, peptidomimetic compounds were classified by Pelay-Gimeno and coworkers (2015) according to their degree of peptide character [38], as shown in Table **1**.

Table 1. Chemical classification of peptidomimetic compounds.

Type	Structural Feature
Class A	Modified peptides
Class B	Modified peptides / foldamers
Class C	Structural mimetics
Class D	Mechanistic mimetics

Class A is characterized by analogs that follow the sequence of amino acids involved in the precursor peptide (pp), as well as its bioactive conformation. Then, their structural modifications are limited to a restricted number of amino acids; in Class B the derivatives are similar to the topological alignment of side chains with their corresponding pp. So, their modifications include unnatural amino acids small molecules, in addition to foldamers, such as β and α/β peptides/peptoids; On other hand, Class C is characterized by having the central scaffold of derivatives based on the orientation of key residues from the bioactive conformation of the respective pp, where several structural modifications can be performed in order to modify the peptide backbone; Finally, Class D mimics the pp's mode of action, without necessarily having a structural relationship with it, where such molecules could be designed based on Class C, considering the affinity optimization, or even designed by using virtual screening of large compounds' libraries.

Based on these chemical aspects mentioned above, the design strategy of peptide-based molecules is directly related to the knowledge involving the target protein in the sense of structure and sequence, function, and binding modes at the active site [39, 40].

Thus, structure-activity relationship (SAR) studies involving a group of peptides allow the definition of the minimum sequence fundamental to the activity, defining key residues inherent to the activity, as well as the main pharmacophore groups [39, 40].

Once fundamental residues, pharmacophore groups, sequence, and structural features are defined, peptide-based compounds tend to have great structural diversity as well as natural products, unlike synthetic drugs that normally target heteroaromatic groups and have few or no stereogenic centers [31 - 33].

From this perspective, the synthesis of these compounds encompasses the coupling between two amino acids or peptide fragments, forming an amide bond. It can basically occur in two different ways, being in solution (classic synthesis), where the carboxyl group of the acyl receptor is then amidated or esterified; on polymeric support (solid-phase) so that the carboxyl group is covalently bonded to resin or polymeric support [41 - 44].

Finally, classical synthesis can take place in the $N{\to}C$-terminal direction or the other way around, where solid-phase synthesis normally occurs in the $C{\to}N$-terminal direction [31, 45, 46].

3. BIOCHEMISTRY ASPECTS AND MOLECULAR HOMOLOGY OF 3CL[PRO] FROM MERS-COV, SARS-COV, AND SARS-COV-2

3.1. Structure, Function, and Druggability of 3CL[pro] from Coronaviruses

Homology studies indicate meaningful similarity between 3CL[pro] from the SARS-CoV-2 genome and the same protein from other coronaviruses responsible for causing the severe respiratory syndrome. Interestingly, the similarity of the amino acid sequence to SARS-CoV 3CL[pro] is approximately 96%, while the MERS-CoV 3CL[pro] presents only about 50% [47, 48].

In this context, it is observed that there is a great similarity between the 3CL[pro] active sites from the three main human coronaviruses, which makes this a potential druggable target in the search for effective inhibitors against this severe disease, being able to use it as a starting material for studies involving anti-CoV agents [49, 50].

This protease is essential to the proteolytic processing of polyproteins, acting in at least 11 cleavage sites at the polyprotein 1ab (replicase 1ab, ~790 kDa). Then, its inhibition would reflect the blocking of viral replication [27, 51, 52]. Considering that there are no human proteases with similar cleavage specificity, inhibitors targeting this enzyme do not constitute considerable toxicity [53, 54].

3.2. Catalytic Site of 3CL[pro] from Coronaviruses

The catalytic dyad (Fig. **2**) of this cysteine protease involves cysteine and histidine amino acids in its active center (in this case, Cys[141] and His[41] residues). Although other cysteines and serine proteases have a third catalytic residue, this region of the active site is occupied by a water molecule, exhibiting hydrogen-bonding interactions with His[41] and Asp[187] residues [55, 56].

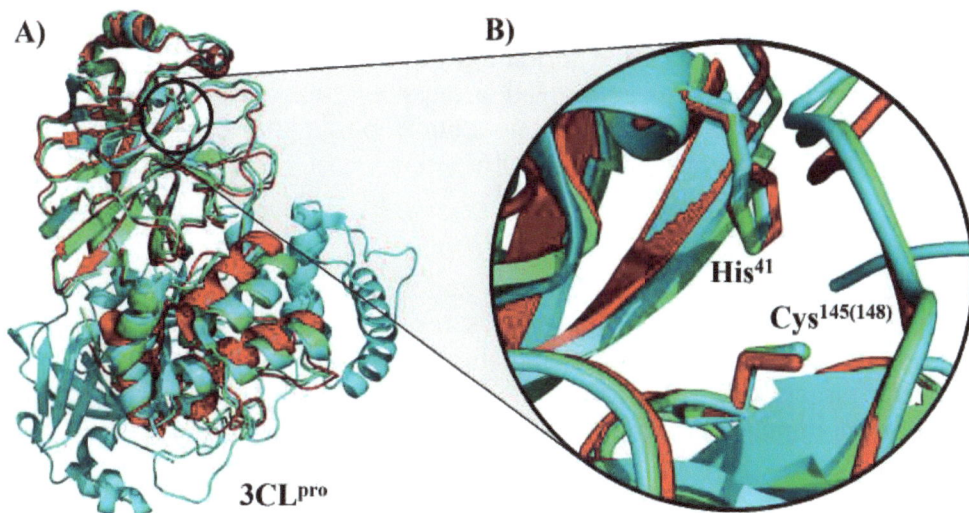

Fig. (2). Structural alignment (A) showing the similar conformation for catalytic dyad (B) from 3CL^pro in Coronavirus. In red: MERS-CoV, cyan: SARS-CoV; and green: SARS-CoV-2. Finally, "Cys^145(148) residue" means Cys^145 from SARS- and SARS-CoV-2, and Cys^148 from MERS-CoV.

However, the catalytic dyad from MERS-CoV 3CL^pro is constituted of Cys^{148} and His^{41} residues, along with an extended binding site. Comparatively, studies suggest that SARS- and SARS-CoV-2 have the residues of Cys^{145} and His^{41} conserved (although the position of Cys residue may vary in some PDB crystallographic structures), indicating the continued investigation of inhibitors already studied for the 2002-2003 outbreak (Fig. **2**) [18, 50, 51].

Moreover, it is believed that the catalytic mechanism follows several steps. Initially, the proton from the cysteine residue (-SH) is abstracted by the imidazole ring at the histidine residue (NH_2^+), resulting in a nucleophilic thiolate (-S$^-$). Thus, this species attacks the amide bond of substrates, where the *N*-terminal peptide product is released due to the abstraction of histidine protons prior to the thioester is hydrolyzed to release the *C*-terminal product, causing it to restore the catalytic dyad [57 - 59].

4. CORONAVIRUSES 3CL^PRO AND THEIR INHIBITORS

From the crystallized structure of 3CL^pro from Coronaviruses, a variety of enzyme inhibitors have been reported in the literature in recent years. In view of the potential of this target, peptidomimetic compounds stand out in the drug design as promising inhibitors [34, 57, 60].

With this, the mechanism of action of these analogs that mimic natural peptide substrates initially involves the formation of a non-covalent complex with the 3CL[pro] enzyme. In contrast, warhead groups are normally spatially directed towards the catalytic residues, suffering a nucleophilic attack and thus forming a covalent complex with cysteine residue [61 - 63].

4.1. *Warhead Groups*

Covalent drugs have a mechanism of action involving the formation of an irreversible bond with 3CL[pro]. Nonetheless, the scientific community was "afraid" to develop this class of inhibitors since they could target other enzymes that are not initial targets (off-target) to confer undesirable toxicity or even the over-activation of immune responses [64 - 66].

Nowadays, there is a great interest in medicinal chemistry for the development of irreversible inhibitors since these tend to demonstrate advantages, such as prolonged duration of action with a molecular target when compared to reversible inhibitors, which can reduce the dosage/concentration of the drug, increasing the selectivity [67 - 69] considerably.

Recently, the reactivity of some warhead groups toward cysteine amino acid residue (pKa = 9) was investigated at pH 9.8, using kinetics assay by NMR [70]. In this context, the authors suggested that trifluoroketone, oxaborole, and nitrile groups correspond to "reversible" covalent inhibitors. In contrast, Michael acceptors are likely to be reversible, although the authors report that due to the rate of the reverse reaction is slow, these could be irreversible in many cases. Additionally, the authors reported that Michael acceptors are soft electrophiles and could react more quickly with cysteine (soft nucleophile), when compared to serine (hard nucleophile)) [67, 71].

Several irreversible inhibitors are found in the literature (Fig. **3**), although many of them have been developed without this intention, demonstrating this mechanism for serendipity [72 - 74].

In this context, warhead groups generally involve chemotypes of fragments such as Michael acceptors, aldehyde, keto groups, nitrile, nitroanilide, and aza-epoxide/aziridine (Fig. **4**), and these may perform a covalent bond with the Cys[145] residue from the 3CL[pro] S1' pocket [63, 65, 66].

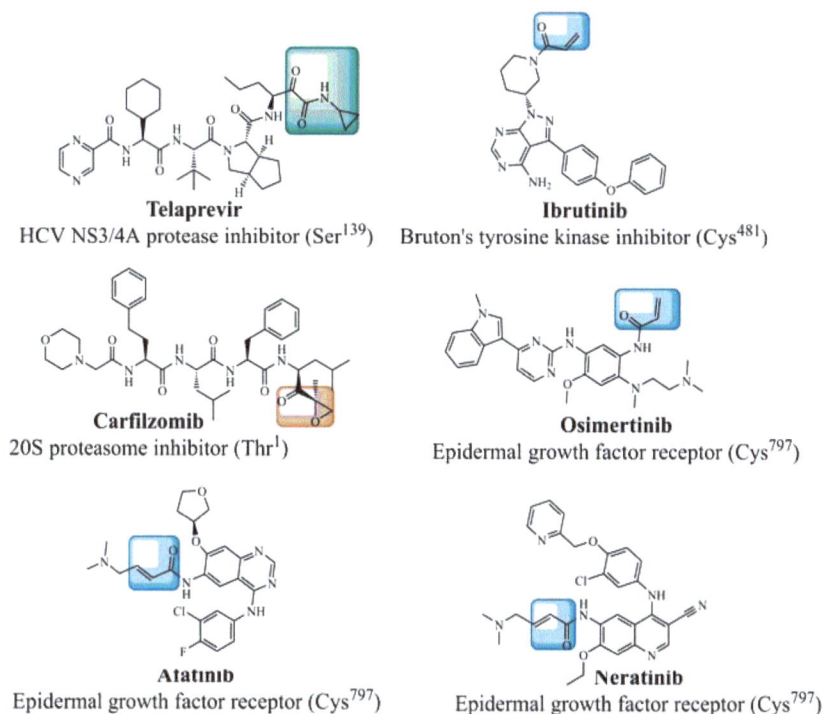

Fig. (3). FDA-approved drugs that covalently bind to their respective targets. Warhead groups are highlighted, being Michael acceptor (blue), *a*-ketoamide (green), and epoxide (orange).

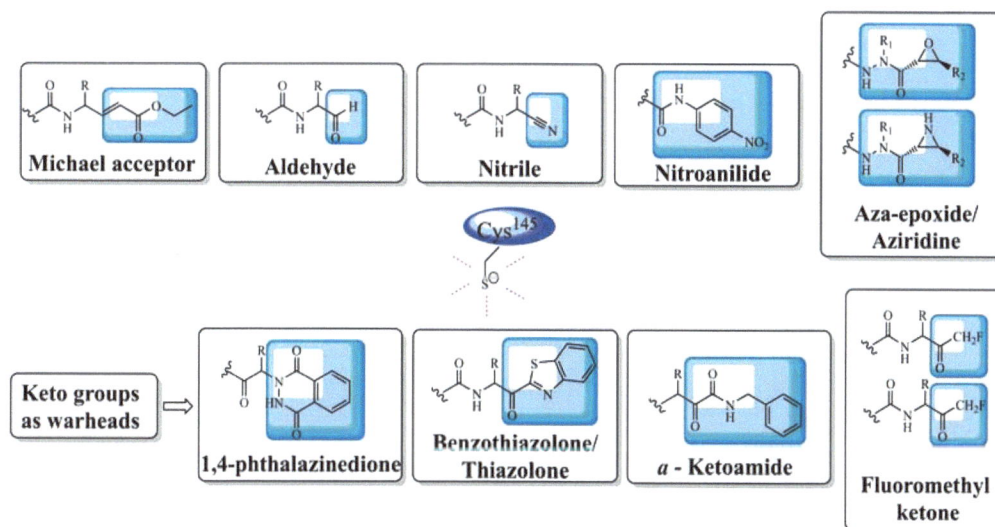

Fig. (4). The most common warhead groups present in 3CL^{pro} inhibitors from Coronaviruses.

4.2. Peptidomimetics Containing Michael Acceptors as Warhead Groups

Several studies involving the design of peptidomimetics containing Michael acceptor groups as warheads are reported in the literature. Ghosh and coworkers (2005) [77] designed and evaluated three peptides as inhibitors of SARS-CoV $3CL^{pro}$, where this study was one of the first involving such a chemical approach.

The authors analyzed the structure of the superimposed X-ray crystal of $3CL^{pro}$ from Transmissible gastroenteritis coronavirus (TGEV), using hexapeptidyl chloromethyl ketone CMK (1) and AG-7088 (2) as substrate-analog initiating structures, and a powerful inhibitor of $3CL^{pro}$ from human rhinovirus (HRV), culminating in the derivative (3) (Fig. 5).

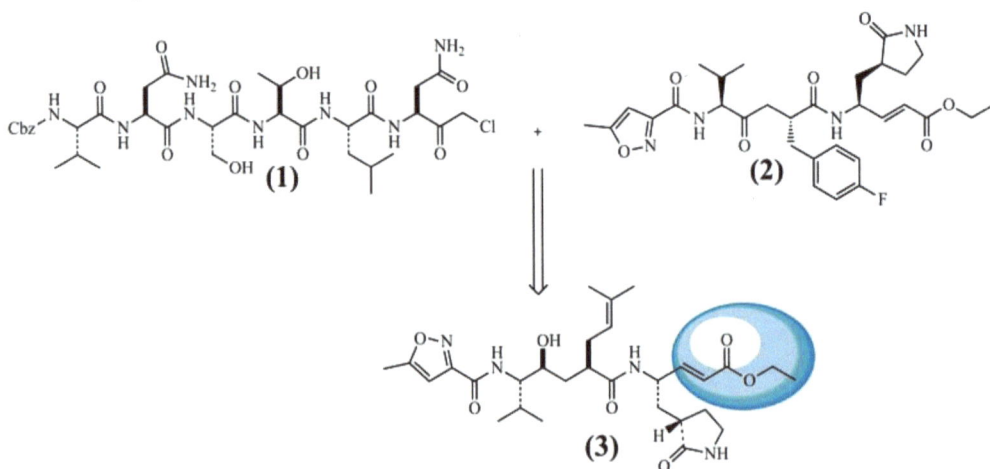

Fig. (5). Peptidomimetic inhibitor derived from CMK and AG-7088 inhibitors.

The compound (3), which corresponds to a bioisoster of analog (2), presented a K_{inact} (min^{-1}) value of 0.045, with IC$_{50}$= 70 μM upon SARS-CoV infected cells, in addition to no toxicity in concentrations up to 100 μM. Additionally, compound (3) performs hydrogen-bonding interactions with Glu^{166} and Cys^{145} residues, confirmed by X-ray crystallography data.

Designing active compounds from fragments containing Michael acceptors, Shie and coworkers (2005) [78] described the obtainment of analog (4), where it was designed by using the bioisosterism technique, based on the compound AG-7088 (2).

Derivative (4) presented IC$_{50}$= 1 μM against SARS-CoV $3CL^{pro}$, in addition to EC$_{50}$ = 0.18 μM against infected cells (Figure 6). Molecular docking analyzes demonstrated that it performs hydrogen-bonding interactions with Gln^{192}, Glu^{166}, and Gln[189] residues, where the authors suggest that it is crucial for inhibitory activity. Furthermore, this compound did not present cytotoxicity (until 200 μM concentration). In contrast, it presented a SI value higher than 1000, constituting a promising compound in the development of anti-viral inhibitors.

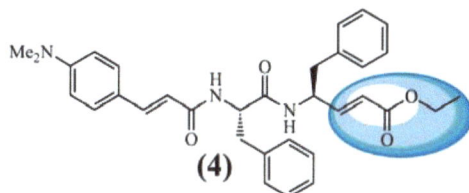

Fig. (6). Bioisoster-derived from AG-7088 (2) inhibitor.

Still following the design of derivatives of the inhibitor AG-7088 (**2**) through the technique of bioisosterism, Yang and coworkers (2006) [79] reported the potent inhibitor (**5**) against 3CL^pro from SARS-CoV, so that it presented $K_i = 0.0058$ μM, besides $IC_{50} = 0.88$ μM of antiviral activity in front of 229E cell, corroborating the potential of this drug design technique (Fig. 7).

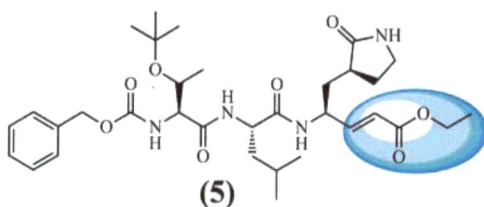

Fig. (7). New bioisoster from AG-7088 inhibitor with anti-SARS-CoV 3CL^pro activity.

The development of peptidomimetics as inhibitors of SARS-CoV 3CL^pro initially focused on producing bio-derived compounds based on the inhibitor AG-7088 (**2**), which, although inactive upon this target, it was a precursor for several potent analogs. Other bio-derivatives were described by Ghosh and colleagues (2007) [80], where analog (**6**) showed promising 3CL^pro inhibition (Fig. **8**), exhibiting an IC_{50} value of 10 μM. On the other hand, it was not successful when tested against infected cells with SARS-CoV.

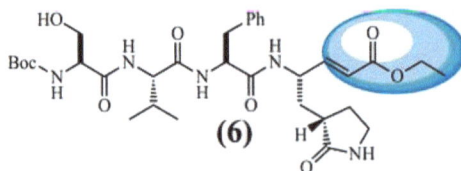

Fig. (8). Peptidomimetic inhibitors of 3CL^{pro} from SARS-CoV.

Finally, the most potent peptide-inhibitor of 3CL^{pro} from MERS-CoV **(7)** was reported by Yang and coworkers (2005) [81], where it was designed to act on the catalytic dyad by using a Michael acceptor as warhead group (Fig. **9**).

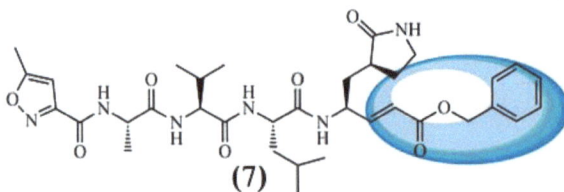

Fig. (9). The most promising inhibitor against MERS-CoV 3CL^{pro} was found in the literature.

In this context, this compound was designed considering that the S1, S2, and S4 subsites are crucial for the recognition of the substrate, in order to mimic the side chains of the substrate from the P4-P1 residues, and interact with the subsites aforementioned.

The most promising inhibitor **(7)** showed IC$_{50}$= 0.28 µM upon MERS-CoV 3CL^{pro}, being also explored in SARS-CoV 3CL^{pro} (EC$_{50}$= 16.77 µM) [56] and modified proteases GS-WT$_{12}$ (K$_i$= 9.0 ± 0.8 µM), WT-GPH$_6$ (K$_i$= 2.3 ± 0.1 µM), and WT (K$_i$= 1.9 ± 0.1 µM) [82].

4.3. Peptidomimetics Containing Aldehydes as Warhead Groups

One of the first series of peptidomimetics containing an aldehyde function as a warhead group was described by Al-Gharabli and coworkers (2006) [83], in which these compounds were designed to inhibit the SARS-CoV 3CL^{pro}.

The authors started from the structure of the irreversible inhibitor of 3CL^{pro}, TGEV CMK **(1),** which was found to be canonically bound to this target (PDB ID: 1P9U). On the other hand, the authors observed that CMK **(1)** presents a binding mode on a different side chain from the SARS-CoV 3CL^{pro}, which is non-canonical (PDB ID: 1UK4). Finally, this work describes that the sequential variations in the P1 site produced the most potent inhibitors **(8)** and **(9),** with IC$_{50}$ = 7.5 µM for both (Fig. **10**).

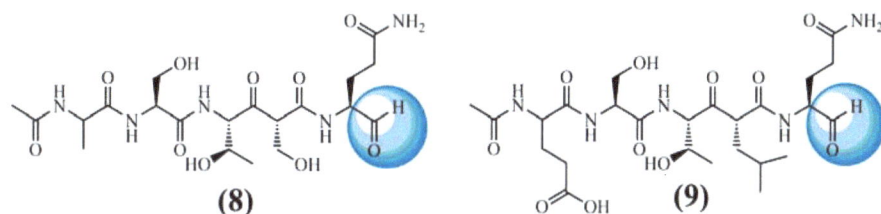

Fig. (10). CMK-based inhibitors containing an aldehyde function as a warhead group (in blue).

Following the analysis of peptidomimetics compounds containing aldehydes as a warhead group, Kumar and coworkers (2017) [84] published a study containing a series of 4 new derivatives designed as inhibitors of SARS- and MERS-CoV 3CL^{pro}, where the results obtained are summarized in Table **2**.

Table 2. Results of inhibitory analysis enzymatic and antiviral assays for compounds 10-13.

-	IC$_{50}$ for 3CL^{pro} (µM)		-		
Compound	**MERS-CoV**	**SARS-CoV**	**CC$_{50}$ (µM)^a**	**EC$_{50}$ (µM)^b**	**SI^c**
(10)	>25	>25	>100	>100	N.D.^{d}
(11)	2.4 ± 0.3	0.7±0.2	>100	1.4 ± 0.0	>71.4
(12)	4.7 ± 0.6	0.5±0.1	>100	1.2 ± 0.6	>83.3
(13)	1.7 ± 0.3	0.2±0.07	58.6±1.2	1.2 ± 0.6	97.9
GEM^d	N.D.	N.D.	>100	8.3 ± 0.9	>12.1

^{a}50% cytotoxic concentration in MDCK cells. ^{b}for MERS-CoV. ^{c}Selectivity index. ^{d}Not determined. ^{d}Gemcitabine hydrochloride.

Structure-activity relationship (SAR) revealed that the inactive derivative **(10)** was the only one that did not have a halogenated or nitrogenated substituent at the phenyl group. Nevertheless, the most active derivative **(13)** constitutes the only derivative doubly substituted with halogens (containing fluorine and chlorine at positions 2 and 4, respectively) **(11)**, concluding that such electron-withdrawing groups are of great importance for the inhibitory activity of both activities on SARS- and MERS-CoV 3CL^{pro}. By using *in silico* molecular docking simulations, the authors observed that the most promising derivative **(13)**, suffers a nucleophilic attack from the catalytic residue Cys[148] at the aldehyde (warhead group), forming a stable tetrahedral species, in which the resulting oxyanion species is stabilized by His[41].

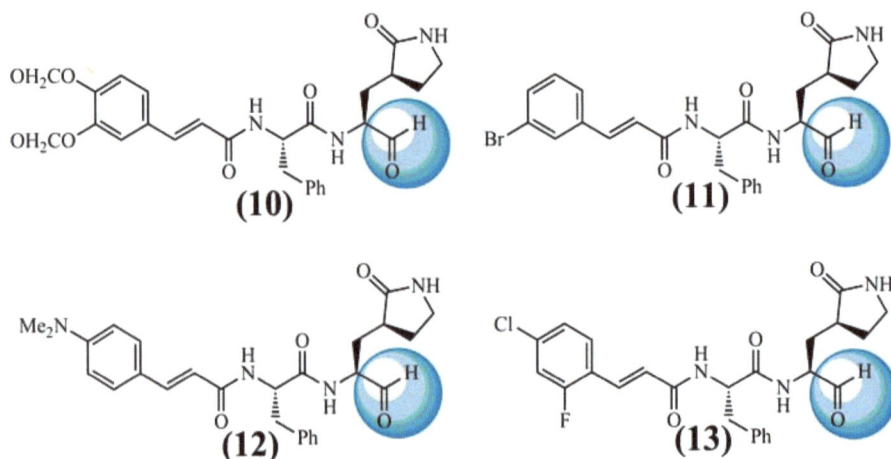

Fig. (11). Promising peptidomimetic compounds containing aldehyde as a warhead group (in blue).

Akagi and colleagues (2011) [85] reported a study demonstrating that the selection of the amino acid sequence Acyl-Ser-Ala-Val-Leu-His-CHO corresponds to a promising scaffold for the development of peptidomimetic inhibitors, in which it was selected by screening of P1 site residue. This study resulted in the derivative **(14)** as the most promising in terms of inhibition upon SARS-CoV 3CL^{pro}, with IC$_{50}$= 5.7 μM. Fig. **(12)** demonstrates how this inhibitor interacts with the protease. In addition, all these interactions were observed by using X-ray crystallographic analysis, resulting in PDB ID: 3AW0.

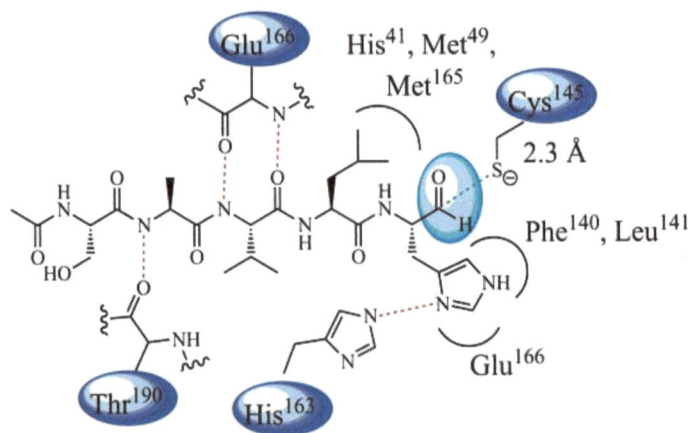

Fig. (12). Interactions of the most promising inhibitor (14) at the active site from the 3CL^{pro} from SARS-CoV (PDB ID: 3AW0). H-bonding interactions are shown as red dotted lines. Nucleophilic attack by the Cys^{145} residue is shown in a green dotted line.

Recently, Dai and coworkers (2020) [86] designed and synthesized 2 peptidomimetic derivatives containing the aldehyde as a warhead group. These compounds were designed based on the natural substrate of SARS-CoV-2 3CL^{pro} (MCA-AVLQ↓SGFR-Lys (Dnp)-Lys-NH$_2$). In this context, the dashed fragments in Fig. (13) (the cyclohexyl (15) and 3-fluorophenyl (16) rings) were inserted to fill the S2 pocket, this pocket has the possibility of promoting hydrophobic and π-π stacking interactions. In addition, these analogs interact with the catalytic dyad Cys^{145} and His^{41}, confirmed by X-ray crystallographic analysis.

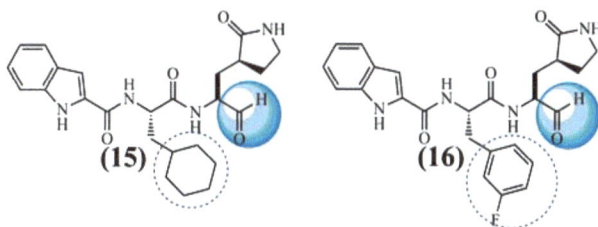

Fig. (13). Promising SARS-CoV-2 3CL^{pro} inhibitors.

Finally, derivatives (15) and (16) presented IC$_{50}$= 0.05 μM and 0.04 μM, respectively. Additionally, these analogs were tested against infected cells, exhibiting EC$_{50}$ values of 0.42 and 0.33 μM, respectively. Furthermore, both compounds were non-cytotoxic up to 100 μM concentration, resulting in SI values higher than 238 and 303 for compounds (15) and (16), respectively.

4.4. Peptidomimetics Containing Keto Groups as Warheads

4.4.1. Fluoromethyl Ketone Group

Compounds containing the fluoromethyl ketone group (17) are promising protease inhibitors, since the halomethyl group thermodynamically stabilizes the hemiacetal form over the ketone form, in which it can suffer a nucleophilic attack by a water molecule to the carbonyl group (19) or, still, by the thiol group from the cysteine residue present at the catalytic site (18) [61, 62, 87] (Fig. 14).

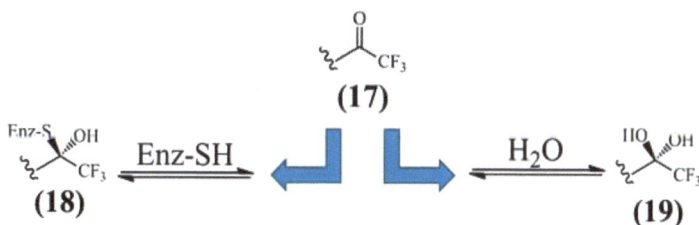

Fig. (14). Adducts formed by the nucleophilic addition of water and Cys thiol on a halogenated α-halogenated carbonyl.

In this context, due to the tetrahedral intermediate formed by the thiol attack to the α-halogenated carbonyl (18) is relatively more stable [61, 62, 87].

Based on this information, a series of peptidomimetic compounds containing a fragment of trifluoromethyl ketone was described by Sydnes and colleagues (2006) [87], where a total of 11 new compounds were obtained, culminating in the development of two moderate SARS-CoV 3CL^{pro} inhibitors, compounds (20) and (21) (Fig. 15). Still, derivatives (20) and (21) were assessed for inhibitory activity toward the aforementioned target, in which analogs (20) and (21) presented K_i values of 116.1 and 134.5 μM, respectively.

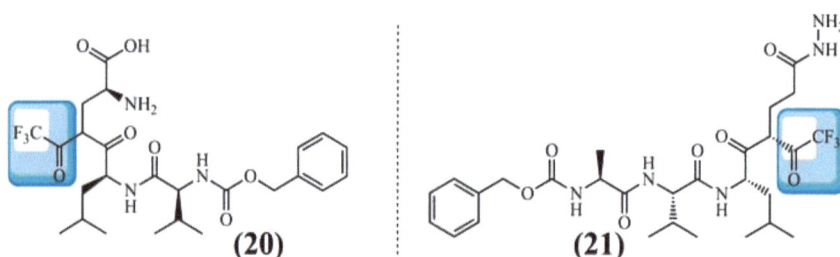

Fig. (15). Inhibitors of SARS-CoV 3CL^{pro} containing the trifluoromethyl ketone groups.

Following the development studies of 3CL^{pro} inhibitors containing the trifluoromethyl ketone group, Shao and colleagues (2008) [88] reported a study showing the synthesis and biological evaluation of eight new peptidomimetic derivatives. Then, the derivative (22) (Fig. 16) exhibited an IC$_{50}$ value of 10 μM against the SARS-CoV 3CL^{pro}. X-ray crystallography data revealed that such a compound is covalently connected with the Cys^{145} residue from the catalytic triad.

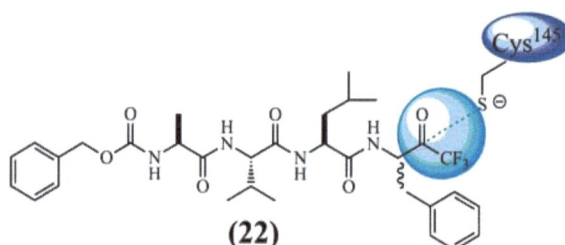

Fig. (16). Trifluoromethyl ketone inhibitor of SARS-CoV 3CL^{pro} reported by Shao *et al.* (2008). Nucleophilic attack by the Cys^{145} residue is shown in a green dotted line.

Finally, Regnier and colleagues (2009) [89] described a study involving the synthesis of seven new peptidomimetics, in which the design involved the conservation of the trifluoromethyl ketone. In addition, the authors performed structural modifications at the Glu side chain or Gln residue around the P1 position in order to prevent a possible formation of a cyclic structure by intramolecular nucleophilic attack on α-halogenated carbonyl, modulating possible hydrogen-bonding interactions at the active site (Fig. **17**). Thus, the derivative **(26)** proved to be the most promising of the idealized series, where it presented $K_i = 21$ μM against SARS-CoV 3CL^{pro}, constituting yet another promising peptidomimetic containing the warhead group trifluoromethyl ketone, contributing to further studies aimed at the search for bioactive compounds against the coronavirus.

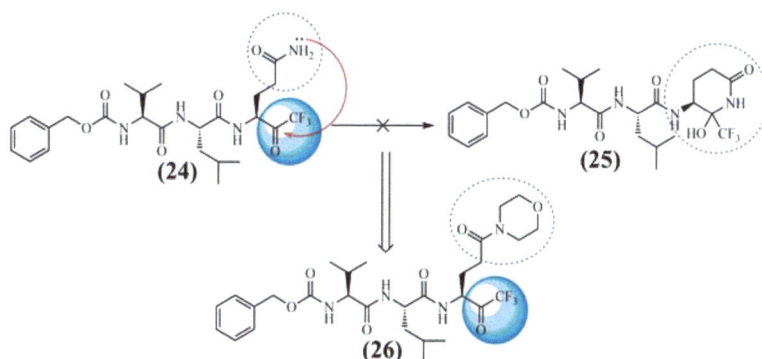

Fig. (17). Design involving the 3CL^{pro} inhibitor (26).

4.4.2. 1,4-Peptidomimetics Containing Phthalazinediones as Warhead Groups

1,4-Phthalazinedione warhead group can be used for designing protease inhibitors. The mechanism of the reaction of this fragment towards the catalytic cysteine residues involves the formation of an intramolecular bond between the carbonyl and -NH from the ring in the compound **(27)**, making the carbonyl group more susceptible to a nucleophilic attack by increasing its acidic character (Fig. **18**) [20, 27, 49, 90].

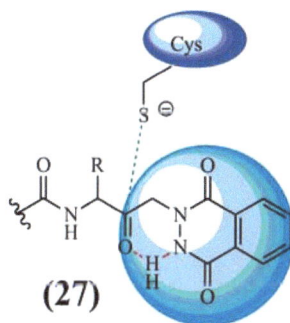

Fig. (18). Intramolecular hydrogen-bonding interaction is favored by the presence of a 1,4-Phthalazinedione warhead group. H-bonding interactions are shown as red dotted lines. Nucleophilic attack by the Cys[145] residue is shown in a green dotted line.

Based on this, Jain and coworkers (2004) [90] developed four new peptidomimetic derivatives containing 1,4-Phthalazinedione group, in which the authors designed their compounds deeming the chemical structures from inhibitors of Hepatitis A virus (HAV) 3CL^{pro}, yielding the compounds **(28)** and **(29)**, exhibiting IC$_{50}$ values of 13 µM and 1.6 µM, respectively (Fig. **19**).

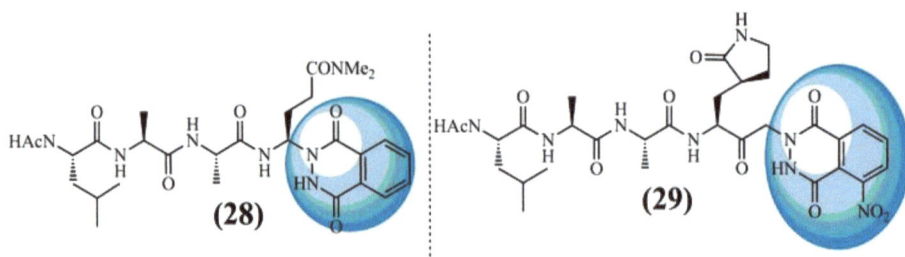

Fig. (19). Potential inhibitors of 3CL^{pro} designed by Jain *et al.* (2004).

Derivatives **(30-33)** showed promising inhibitory activity against SARS-CoV 3CL^{pro}, with values of IC$_{50}$ of 0.6, 2.7, 2.9, and 3.4, respectively (Fig. **20**). In this context, the aforementioned analogs contribute to the development of new inhibitory compounds in the face of this severe disease.

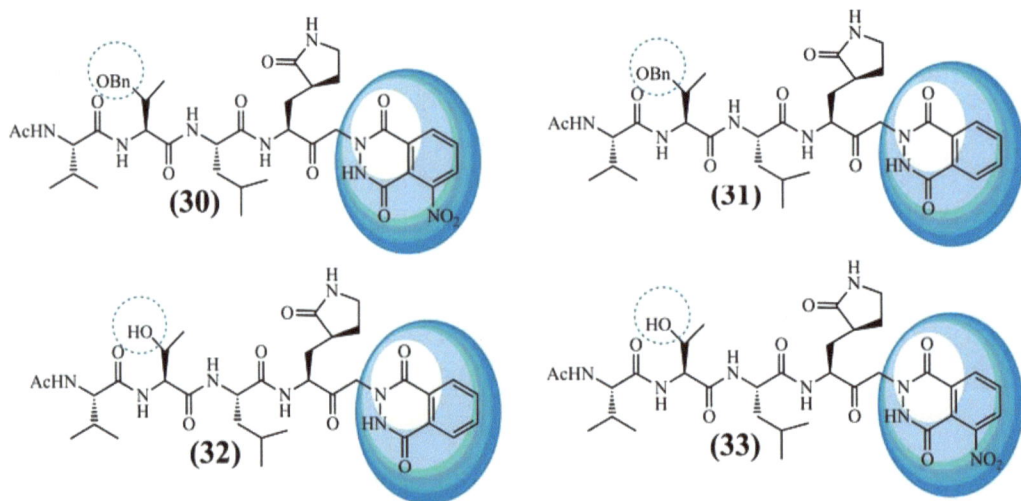

Fig. (20). Promising SARS-CoV 3CL^{pro} inhibitors.

Still, it was observed that the most promising derivative **(30)** has a nitro (NO$_2$) group at the 1,4-Phthalazinedione moiety, in addition to having the benzylether (BnO) substituent at the dashed region, as shown in Fig. **(20)**.

4.4.3. Peptidomimetics Containing Benzothiazolones/thiazolones as Warhead Groups

One of the first studies reporting the utilization of benzothiazolones/thiazolones as warhead groups on the development of peptidomimetics as inhibitors of 3CL^{pro} from SARS-CoV was performed by Regnier, and colleagues (2009) [89], in which the authors described a study involving the synthesis of eight new peptidomimetics derivatives. The compounds' design involved the conservation of benzothiazolone/thiazolone rings as warheads in order to promote chemical modifications at the Glu side chain or Gln residue around the P1 position (Fig. **17**). Then, analog (**34**) was found to be the most promising among the synthesized series of molecules, exhibiting a K_i value of 2.20 μM upon SARS-CoV 3CL^{pro}. Furthermore, it was observed by using molecular docking (PDB ID: 1WOF) that this compound performs hydrogen-bonding interactions with Gln[189], Glu[166], His[41], His[164], His[163], Gly[143], and Ser[144] residues, and also it interacts with Cys[145] residue (Fig. **21**).

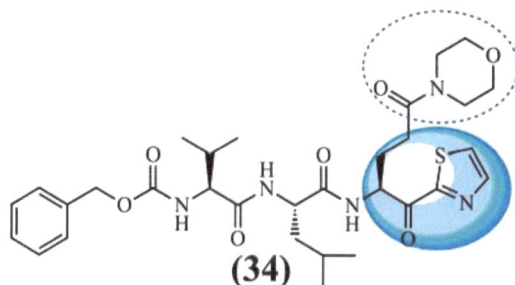

(34)

Fig. (21). The best analog containing a thiazolone ring as a warhead group.

Posteriorly, Thanigaimalai and coworkers (2013) [91], as well as Konno and coworkers (2013) [92] reported in three studies the design of new peptidomimetics, exploring the benzothiazole ring as a warhead group. Then, the authors synthesized derivatives based on the peptide sequence Z-Val-Leu-Ala(pyrrolidone-3-yl)-2-thiazoles previously reported [89], in order to interact with the catalytic residue (Cys-S$^-$).

Among all the active compounds in the aforementioned works, analogs (**35 and 36**) exhibited K_i values of 0.0063 and 0.65 μM, respectively. Besides, analog (**37**) demonstrated a K_i value of 0.46 μM. Lastly, the authors analyzed molecular docking results and concluded that all these inhibitors primarily interact with the catalytic cysteine (Cys[145]), corroborating with their experimental assays (Fig. **22**).

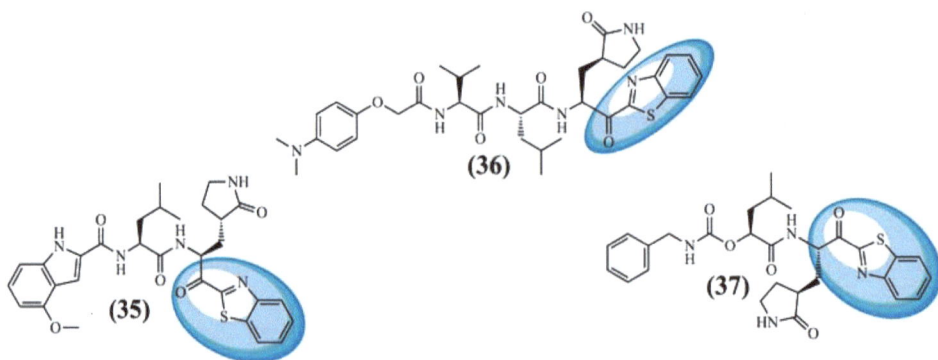

Fig. (22). Most promising 3CL^pro inhibitors containing benzothiazolone rings as warhead groups.

4.4.4. Peptidomimetics Containing α-ketoamides as Warhead Groups

The development of peptidomimetic inhibitors of 3CL^pro containing α-ketoamides as warhead groups were recently reported by Zhang and coworkers (2020) [75, 76], analyzing cocrystallized compounds with a broad antiviral spectrum into the crystallographic 3CL^pro structures, with the following PDB entries: 1UJ1, 2BX3, and 2BX4.

Posteriorly, it was decided to use a 5-member ring (γ-lactam), a glutamine derivative, as P1 residue, since this protease specifically cleaves the peptide bond after a P1-glutamine residue. The probable explanation for that is may because the more rigid lactam ring leads to a reduction in the loss of entropy directly after the binding complex formation, in comparison to the more flexible glutamine side chain.

Among the series of 11 final compounds, derivatives (**38** and **39**) were demonstrated to be the most promising SARS-CoV 3CL^pro inhibitors, with IC_{50} values of 0.24 and 0.33 µM, respectively. In addition, these compounds also showed promising activity against infected cells with SARS-CoV, displaying EC_{50} values of 1.9 and 7.2 µM, respectively (Fig. **23**).

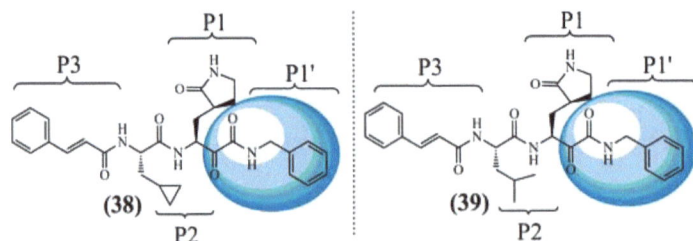

Fig. (23). Promising peptidomimetics containing α-ketoamide warheads.

4.4.5. Peptidomimetics Containing Nitroanilides as Warhead Groups

Shie and coworkers (2005) [93] reported a study demonstrating the design and synthesis of peptide derivatives in order to evaluate the nitroanilide group as a substrate fragment of the 3CL^pro enzyme from SARS-CoV. According to the authors, the evaluation of peptide compounds started by analyzing compounds containing a *p*-nitroaniline substituent **(40)** at the *C*-terminal glutamine, culminating in the most promising derivative of the synthesized series (Fig. **24**).

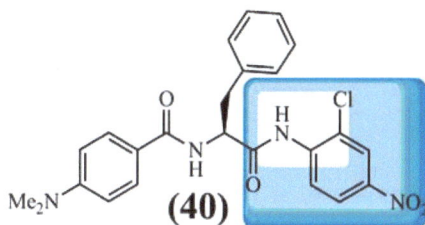

Fig. (24). Peptidomimetic compound containing a nitroanilide group as a warhead.

For this purpose, this promising derivative **(40)** exhibited IC_{50}= 0.06 μM (K_i= 0.03 μM) against 3CL^pro SARS-CoV. Then, this promising inhibitor was analyzed *in silico* by means of molecular docking in order to observe possible interactions with the target (PDB ID: 1UK4). Finally, the aforementioned compound is found in the pocket formed by Thr[25], His[41], Cys[44], Thr[45], and Ala[46] residues, where the nitro group is responsible for the formation of hydrogen-bonding interactions with the amine group (NH) of this last residue. Also, the chlorine atom interacts with γ-S atom at the Cys[145] and ε-N2 atom of His[41], thus being able to interact with the catalytic dyad.

4.5. Peptidomimetics Containing Nitriles as Warhead Groups

Nitriles as warhead groups toward SARS-CoV 3CL^pro were described by Chuck and coworkers (2013) [94], in which the authors, based on the auto-cleavage sequence of this target (TSAVLQ) designed a series of four new derivatives. In addition, it was verified that the best compound **(41)** containing a nitrile group as a warhead remains covalently bound to the thiol group from the Cys[145] residue, confirmed by X-ray crystallography of the inhibitor-enzyme complex [71, 95]. Finally, the derivative **(41)** presented an IC_{50} value of 4.6 against SARS-CoV 3CL^pro (Fig. **25**).

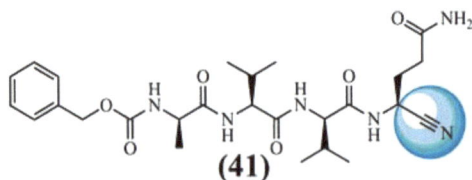

Fig. (25). Peptidomimetic containing a nitrile as a warhead group.

4.6. Peptidomimetics Containing Aza-epoxides and Aziridines as Warhead Groups

Aza-epoxide/aziridine peptides were described in the literature as a class of irreversible and selective inhibitors for cysteine proteases since these chemical groups resemble an extended peptide substrate, with the insertion of an epoxide group at the susceptible region to a nucleophilic attack, likely as observed for carbonyl-containing analogs (Fig. **26**) [96, 97].

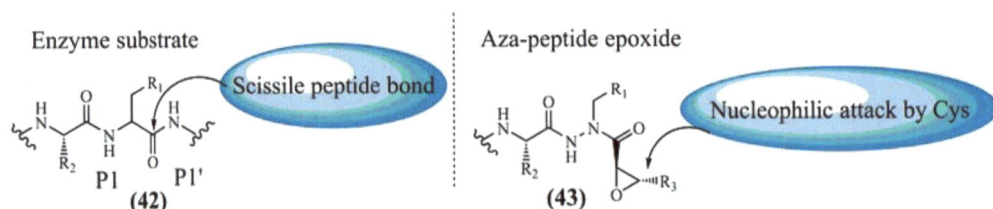

Fig. (26). Design of an aza-peptide epoxide as an inhibitor of cysteine proteases.

Deeming these facts, Martina and coworkers (2005) [98] designed and synthesized a new series of 27 peptide compounds containing the aziridine ring as a warhead group, which is a bioisoster with an electrophilic center and susceptible to nucleophilic attacks by amino acid residues from the active protease site. With this, the best compound **(44)** showed 54% inhibition at 100 μM concentration upon SARS-CoV 3CL[pro], obtained in the FRET-based assay. In addition, molecular docking studies (PDB ID: 1UK4) suggested that **(40)** is found to be placed into the S1 pocket, close to the Cys[145] residue. Furthermore, the authors reported that this compound interacts through hydrogen-bonding interactions with Ser[144], Ser[1], His[163], and His[172] (Fig. **27**).

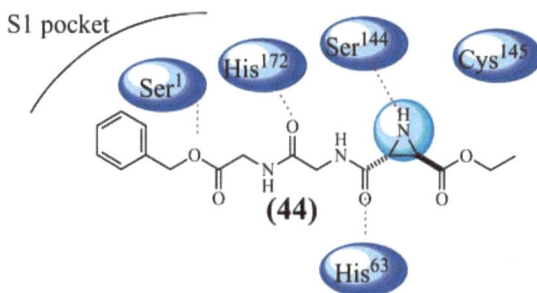

Fig. (27). Interactions between the *trans*-aziridine (43) and SARS-CoV 3CL^{pro} (PDB ID: 1UK4). H-bonding interactions are shown as red dotted lines.

Thereafter, Lee and colleagues (2006) [99] reported that compound **(45)**, an aza-epoxide peptidomimetic analog, presented a *Ki* value of $1,900 \pm 400 \text{ M}^{-1} \text{ s}^{-1}$ against SARS-CoV 3CL^{pro} (Fig. **28**).

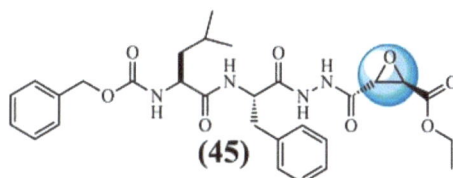

Fig. (28). Compound (2*S*, 2*S*)-aza-epoxide an irreversible inhibitor of SARS-CoV 3CL^{pro}.

Additionally, the authors reported an analysis by X-ray crystallography that it was possible to observe the irreversible mode of inhibition for it. Finally, data from kinect assays demonstrated that only *S, S*-diastereomer covalently interacts with the enzyme and leads to the inhibition of the target. In contrast, this fact does not occur in its *R, R*-diastereomer.

5. DRUG REPURPOSING FOR PEPTIDOMIMETICS

The technique of drug repurposing consists of a new therapeutic indication, different from the initial ones, for drugs that are already on the market or even compounds that have failed in clinical trials. Thus, it constitutes a fast and efficient strategy for *"discovering new drugs"*, especially during a pandemic situation [100, 101].

In this context, the strategy is basically based on two pathways: (*i*) virtual screening approaches (cheminformatics, bioinformatics, and biological systems) based on described targets, molecular mechanisms, ligands' structures; or, (*ii*) experimental (phenotypic screening, high-throughput screening) based on a large screening of several compounds' libraries at the same time [21, 102, 103]. During a pandemic situation, it is well-known that following the (*i*) path is the most viable, fast, and low-cost to obtain effective pharmacotherapy against a specific disease. Considering the COVID-19 pandemic, the repurposing of anti-HIV peptidomimetic drugs emerged as a promising alternative to select inhibitor of SARS-CoV-2 3CL^{pro} (Fig. **29**), in which the drugs lopinavir (**46**), ritonavir (**47**) [104], darunavir (**48**), and saquinavir (**49**) were identified as the most promising candidates in clinical trials [105].

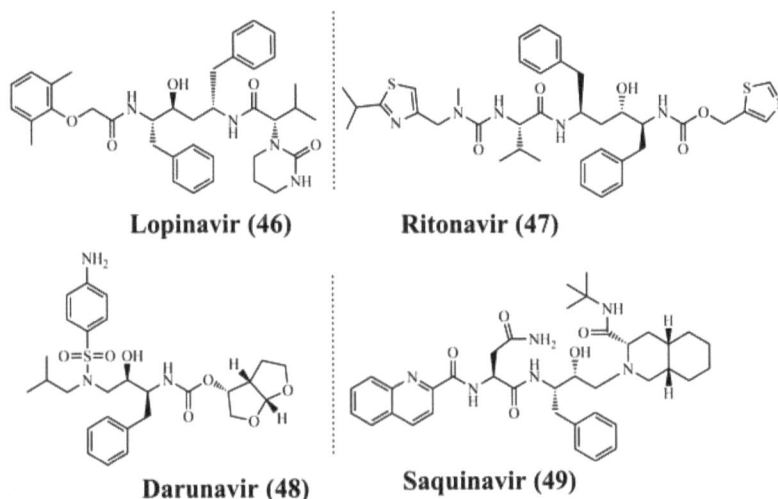

Lopinavir (46)   **Ritonavir (47)**

Darunavir (48)   **Saquinavir (49)**

Fig. (29). Anti-HIV peptidomimetic drugs with anti-SARS-CoV-2 activity.

Therefore, in a systematic review performed by Yao and coworkers [104], Lopinavir (**46**) has been reported as effective *in vitro* test, as well as its association with Ritonavir (**47**) demonstrated to be essential in clinical management, especially in the initial stages COVID-19. Finally, these peptidomimetic drugs are potential compounds in the search for an effective and safe treatment against COVID-19.

6. FINAL CONSIDERATIONS AND FUTURE OUTLOOK

The pandemic caused by the new coronavirus (also named COVID-19) has represented the biggest global health emergency in the last 100 years, with serious clinical consequences for infected individuals, where the prognosis is still unclear. In addition, the severe recession in the world economy demonstrates that efforts in the search for an effective and safe pharmacological treatment should aim a greater speed, combined with the reliability and safety of clinical data obtained from several research groups worldwide.

3CL^{pro}, the main protease from SARS-CoV-2, constitutes a promising druggable target for designing potential antiviral peptidomimetic compounds, having as examples peptidomimetic drugs FDA-approved against HIV and HCV. In addition, the chemical structure conserved in MERS-CoV and, especially in SARS-CoV, is highlighted, confirmed by tridimensional models by using genetic homology, in which studies searching for new inhibitors against these two previous outbreaks-responsible Coronaviruses could be reused and redirected to find alternatives for combating SARS-CoV-2.

Although the clinical approval of drugs seems slow, the search for protease inhibitors against SARS-CoV-2 shows to be a promising alternative for the obtainment of compounds, considering the specificity of this target since it differs significantly from other human proteases.

Deeming that the COVID-19 outbreak will not be the last one to emerge from animals (based on human history), we believe that this review is (and also it will be) essential to design and develop peptidomimetic compounds by utilizing different warhead groups, which could be effective, selective, safe, and low-cost.

CONSENT FOR PUBLICATION

Not applicable.

CONFLICT OF INTEREST

The authors declare no conflict of interest, financial or otherwise.

ACKNOWLEDGEMENTS

The authors thank the Coordenação de Aperfeiçoamento de Pessoal de Nível Superior (CAPES), Fundação de Amparo à Pesquisa de Alagoas (FAPEAL,) and the National Council for Scientific and Technological Development (CNPq) for their support to the Brazilian Post-Graduate Programs. Moreover, the authors also thank the Research Collaboratory for Structural Bioinformatics-Protein Data Bank to provide access to crystallographic structures of targets (available at: https://www.rcsb.org/), which allowed us to elaborate some illustrations for this article.

REFERENCES

[1] Azhar EI, Hui DSC, Memish ZA, Drosten C, Zumla A. The Middle East Respiratory Syndrome (MERS). Infect Dis Clin North Am 2019; 33(4): 891-905.
[http://dx.doi.org/10.1016/j.idc.2019.08.001] [PMID: 31668197]

[2] Khan G, Sheek-Hussein M. The Middle East Respiratory Syndrome Coronavirus: An Emerging Virus of Global Threat. Elsevier Inc. 2020.

[3]   Báez-Santos YM, St John SE, Mesecar AD. The SARS-coronavirus papain-like protease: structure, function and inhibition by designed antiviral compounds. Antiviral Res 2015; 115: 21-38.
[http://dx.doi.org/10.1016/j.antiviral.2014.12.015] [PMID: 25554382]

[4]   de Groot RJ, Baker SC, Baric RS, *et al.* Middle East respiratory syndrome coronavirus (MERS-CoV): announcement of the Coronavirus Study Group. J Virol 2013; 87(14): 7790-2.
[http://dx.doi.org/10.1128/JVI.01244-13] [PMID: 23678167]

[5]   Chan JFW, Yuan S, Kok KH, *et al.* A familial cluster of pneumonia associated with the 2019 novel coronavirus indicating person-to-person transmission: a study of a family cluster. Lancet 2020; 395(10223): 514-23.
[http://dx.doi.org/10.1016/S0140-6736(20)30154-9] [PMID: 31986261]

[6]   WHO. WHO Director-General's opening remarks at the media briefing on COVID-19 2020.https://www.who.int/dg/speeches/detail/who-director-general-s-opening-remarks-at-t-e-media-briefing-on-covid-19---11-march-2020

[7]   Gorbalenya AE, Baker SC, Baric RS, *et al.* The species Severe acute respiratory syndrome-related coronavirus: classifying 2019-nCoV and naming it SARS-CoV-2. Nat Microbiol 2020; 5(4): 536-44.
[http://dx.doi.org/10.1038/s41564-020-0695-z] [PMID: 32123347]

[8]   Chen N, Zhou M, Dong X, *et al.* Epidemiological and clinical characteristics of 99 cases of 2019 novel coronavirus pneumonia in Wuhan, China: a descriptive study. Lancet 2020; 395(10223): 507-13.
[http://dx.doi.org/10.1016/S0140-6736(20)30211-7] [PMID: 32007143]

[9]   Kasmi Y, Khataby K, Souiri A, Ennaji MM. Coronaviridae: 100,000 Years of Emergence and Reemergence. Emerg. Reemerging Viral Pathog 2020; pp. 127-49.

[10]   WHO.   Novel   Coronavirus   (COVID-19)   ation.
https://experience.arcgis.com/experience/685d0ace521648f8a5beeeee1b9125cd

[11]   Li H, Liu S-M, Yu X-H, Tang S-L, Tang C-K. Coronavirus disease 2019 (COVID-19): current status and future perspectives. Int J Antimicrob Agents 2020; 55(5): 105951.
[http://dx.doi.org/10.1016/j.ijantimicag.2020.105951] [PMID: 32234466]

[12]   Malik YS, Sircar S, Bhat S, *et al.* Emerging novel coronavirus (2019-nCoV)-current scenario, evolutionary perspective based on genome analysis and recent developments. Vet Q 2020; 40(1): 68-76.
[http://dx.doi.org/10.1080/01652176.2020.1727993] [PMID: 32036774]

[13]   Zhou Y, Hou Y, Shen J, Huang Y, Martin W, Cheng F. Network-Based Drug Repurposing for Human Coronavirus 2020.
[http://dx.doi.org/10.1101/2020.02.03.20020263]

[14]   Liao J, Way G, Madahar V. Target Virus or Target Ourselves for COVID-19 Drugs Discovery?-Lessons Learned from Anti-Influenzas Virus Therapies. Med drug Discov 2020; 100037.

[15]   Li Y, Zhang J, Wang N, *et al.* Therapeutic Drugs Targeting 2019-NCoV Main Protease by High-Throughput Screening bioRxiv 2020.
[http://dx.doi.org/10.1101/2020.01.28.922922]

[16]   Kruse RL. Therapeutic strategies in an outbreak scenario to treat the novel coronavirus originating in Wuhan, China. F1000 Res 2020; 9: 72.
[http://dx.doi.org/10.12688/f1000research.22211.2] [PMID: 32117569]

[17]   Santos-Júnior PF da S, Nascimento IJ dos S, Aquino TM, *et al.* Drug Discovery Strategies Against Emerging Coronaviruses : A Global Threat. 2020; 8: 1-56.

[18]   Silva LR, da Silva Santos-Júnior PF, de Andrade Brandão J, *et al.* Druggable targets from coronaviruses for designing new antiviral drugs. Bioorg Med Chem 2020; 28(22): 115745.
[http://dx.doi.org/10.1016/j.bmc.2020.115745] [PMID: 33007557]

[19]   Chen YW, Yiu CB, Wong K. Prediction of the 2019-NCoV 3C-like protease (3cl pro) structure :

virtual screening reveals velpatasvir. Ledipasvir, and other drug repurposing candidates 2019; pp. 1-15.

[20] Sisay M. 3CL^{pro} inhibitors as a potential therapeutic option for COVID-19: Available evidence and ongoing clinical trials. Pharmacol Res 2020; 156: 104779.
[http://dx.doi.org/10.1016/j.phrs.2020.104779] [PMID: 32247821]

[21] Wu C, Liu Y, Yang Y, *et al.* Analysis of therapeutic targets for SARS-CoV-2 and discovery of potential drugs by computational methods. Acta Pharm Sin B 2020; 10(5): 766-88.
[http://dx.doi.org/10.1016/j.apsb.2020.02.008] [PMID: 32292689]

[22] Nascimento I, De Aquino TM, Santos-Júnior PFS, De Araújo-júnior JX, Silva-júnior EF. Molecular Modeling Applied to Design of Cysteine Protease Inhibitors – A Powerful Tool for the Identification of Hit Compounds Against Neglected Tropical Diseases. Frontiers in computational chemistry 2020; 5: pp. 1-48.

[23] Anand K, Ziebuhr J, Wadhwani P, Mesters JR, Hilgenfeld R. Coronavirus Main Proteinase (3CLpro) Structure: Basis for Design of Anti-SARS Drugs. Science (80-) 2003; 300: 1763-7.

[24] Perlman S, Netland J. Coronaviruses post-SARS: update on replication and pathogenesis. Nat Rev Microbiol 2009; 7(6): 439-50.
[http://dx.doi.org/10.1038/nrmicro2147] [PMID: 19430490]

[25] Tomar S, Johnston ML, St John SE, *et al.* Ligand-induced dimerization of middle east respiratory syndrome (mers) coronavirus nsp5 protease (3clpro): implications for nsp5 regulation and the development of antivirals. J Biol Chem 2015; 290(32): 19403-22.
[http://dx.doi.org/10.1074/jbc.M115.651463] [PMID: 26055715]

[26] Hall DC Jr, Ji HF. A search for medications to treat COVID-19 *via in silico* molecular docking models of the SARS-CoV-2 spike glycoprotein and 3CL protease. Travel Med Infect Dis 2020; 35: 101646.
[http://dx.doi.org/10.1016/j.tmaid.2020.101646] [PMID: 32294562]

[27] Tahir ul Qamar M, Alqahtani SM, Alamri MA, Chen LL. Structural basis of sars-cov-2 3clpro and anti-covid-19 drug discovery from medicinal plants. J Pharm Anal 2020.

[28] Robson B. COVID-19 Coronavirus spike protein analysis for synthetic vaccines, a peptidomimetic antagonist, and therapeutic drugs, and analysis of a proposed achilles' heel conserved region to minimize probability of escape mutations and drug resistance. Comput Biol Med 2020; 121: 103749.
[http://dx.doi.org/10.1016/j.compbiomed.2020.103749] [PMID: 32568687]

[29] Maximova K, Reuter N, Trylska J. Peptidomimetic inhibitors targeting the membrane-binding site of the neutrophil proteinase 3. Biochim Biophys Acta Biomembr 2019; 1861(8): 1502-9.
[http://dx.doi.org/10.1016/j.bbamem.2019.06.009] [PMID: 31229588]

[30] Reese HR, Shanahan CC, Proulx C, Menegatti S. Peptide science: A "rule model" for new generations of peptidomimetics. Acta Biomater 2020; 102: 35-74.
[http://dx.doi.org/10.1016/j.actbio.2019.10.045] [PMID: 31698048]

[31] Qvit N, Rubin SJS, Urban TJ, Mochly-Rosen D, Gross ER. Peptidomimetic therapeutics: scientific approaches and opportunities. Drug Discov Today 2017; 22(2): 454-62.
[http://dx.doi.org/10.1016/j.drudis.2016.11.003] [PMID: 27856346]

[32] Lobo-Ruiz A, Tulla-Puche J. Synthetic approaches of naturally and rationally designed peptides and peptidomimetics. Peptide applications in biomedicine, biotechnology and bioengineering. Elsevier Inc. 2018; pp. 23-49.
[http://dx.doi.org/10.1016/B978-0-08-100736-5.00002-8]

[33] Mabonga L, Paul A. A Synthetic Tool for Inhibiting Protein – Protein Interactions in Cancer. 2020; 225-41.

[34] Pillaiyar T, Meenakshisundaram S, Manickam M. Recent Discovery and Development of Inhibitors Targeting Coronaviruses. Drug Discov Today 2020; 25(4): 668-88.
[http://dx.doi.org/10.1016/j.drudis.2020.01.015]

[35] Molchanova N, Hansen PR, Franzyk H. Advances in development of antimicrobial peptidomimetics as potential drugs. Molecules 2017; 22(9): 22.
[http://dx.doi.org/10.3390/molecules22091430] [PMID: 28850098]

[36] Sachdeva S. Peptides as 'Drugs': The Journey so Far. Int J Pept Res Ther 2017; 23: 49-60.
[http://dx.doi.org/10.1007/s10989-016-9534-8]

[37] Kumar MS. Peptides and peptidomimetics as potential antiobesity agents: overview of current status. Front Nutr 2019; 6: 11.
[http://dx.doi.org/10.3389/fnut.2019.00011] [PMID: 30834248]

[38] Pelay-Gimeno M, Glas A, Koch O, Grossmann TN. Structure-based design of inhibitors of protein-protein interactions: mimicking peptide binding epitopes. Angew Chem Int Ed Engl 2015; 54(31): 8896-927.
[http://dx.doi.org/10.1002/anie.201412070] [PMID: 26119925]

[39] Lenci E, Trabocchi A. Peptidomimetic toolbox for drug discovery. Chem Soc Rev 2020; 49(11): 3262-77.
[http://dx.doi.org/10.1039/D0CS00102C] [PMID: 32255135]

[40] Stone L. Prostate cancer: Peptidomimetics have potential. Nat Rev Urol 2017; 14(6): 328.
[PMID: 28401956]

[41] Beadle JD, Knuhtsen A, Hoose A, Raubo P, Jamieson AG, Shipman M. Solid-phase synthesis of oxetane modified peptides. Org Lett 2017; 19(12): 3303-6.
[http://dx.doi.org/10.1021/acs.orglett.7b01466] [PMID: 28585839]

[42] Roesner S, Saunders GJ, Wilkening I, *et al.* Macrocyclisation of small peptides enabled by oxetane incorporation. Chem Sci (Camb) 2019; 10(8): 2465-72.
[http://dx.doi.org/10.1039/C8SC05474F] [PMID: 30881675]

[43] Reguera L, Rivera DG. Multicomponent reaction toolbox for peptide macrocyclization and stapling. Chem Rev 2019; 119(17): 9836-60.
[http://dx.doi.org/10.1021/acs.chemrev.8b00744] [PMID: 30990310]

[44] Morejón MC, Laub A, Westermann B, Rivera DG, Wessjohann LA. Solution- and solid-phase macrocyclization of peptides by the ugi-smiles multicomponent reaction: synthesis of n-aryl-bridged cyclic lipopeptides. Org Lett 2016; 18(16): 4096-9.
[http://dx.doi.org/10.1021/acs.orglett.6b02001] [PMID: 27505031]

[45] Ricardo MG, Marrrero JF, Valdés O, Rivera DG, Wessjohann LA. A peptide backbone stapling strategy enabled by the multicomponent incorporation of amide N-substituents. Chemistry 2019; 25(3): 769-74.
[http://dx.doi.org/10.1002/chem.201805318] [PMID: 30412333]

[46] Nguyen HT, Guégan JP, Poissonnier A, *et al.* Synthesis of peptidomimetics and chemo-biological tools for CD95/PLCγ1 interaction analysis. Bioorg Med Chem Lett 2019; 29(16): 2094-9.
[http://dx.doi.org/10.1016/j.bmcl.2019.07.006] [PMID: 31301931]

[47] Stoermer M. Homology Models of the Papain-Like Protease PLpro from Coronavirus 2019-NCoV. ChemRxiv. Cambridge: Cambridge Open Engage 2020.

[48] Tilocca B, Soggiu A, Sanguinetti M, *et al.* Comparative computational analysis of SARS-CoV-2 nucleocapsid protein epitopes in taxonomically related coronaviruses. Microbes Infect 2020; 22(4-5): 188-94.
[http://dx.doi.org/10.1016/j.micinf.2020.04.002] [PMID: 32302675]

[49] Ullrich S, Nitsche C. The SARS-CoV-2 main protease as drug target. Bioorg Med Chem Lett 2020; 30(17): 127377.
[http://dx.doi.org/10.1016/j.bmcl.2020.127377] [PMID: 32738988]

[50] Griffin JWD. SARS-CoV and SARS-CoV-2 main protease residue interaction networks change when

bound to inhibitor N3. J Struct Biol 2020; 211(3): 107575.
[http://dx.doi.org/10.1016/j.jsb.2020.107575] [PMID: 32653646]

[51]   Theerawatanasirikul S, Kuo CJ, Phetcharat N, Lekcharoensuk P. *In silico* and *in vitro* analysis of small molecules and natural compounds targeting the 3CL protease of feline infectious peritonitis virus. Antiviral Res 2020; 174: 104697.
[http://dx.doi.org/10.1016/j.antiviral.2019.104697] [PMID: 31863793]

[52]   Muramatsu T, Takemoto C, Kim YT, *et al.* SARS-CoV 3CL protease cleaves its C-terminal autoprocessing site by novel subsite cooperativity. Proc Natl Acad Sci USA 2016; 113(46): 12997-3002.
[http://dx.doi.org/10.1073/pnas.1601327113] [PMID: 27799534]

[53]   Rut W, Groborz K, Zhang L, *et al.* Substrate Specificity Profiling of SARS-CoV-2 Mpro Protease Provides Basis for Anti-COVID-19 Drug. Design bioRxiv 2020.

[54]   Zhang L, Lin D, Sun X, *et al.* Crystal Structure of SARS-CoV-2 Main Protease Provides a Basis for Design of Improved a-Ketoamide Inhibitors. Science (80-) 2020; 368: 409-12.

[55]   Ho BL, Cheng SC, Shi L, Wang TY, Ho KI, Chou CY. Critical Assessment of the Important Residues Involved in the Dimerization and Catalysis of MERS Coronavirus Main Protease. PLoS One 2015; 10(12): e0144865.
[http://dx.doi.org/10.1371/journal.pone.0144865] [PMID: 26658006]

[56]   Jin Z, Du X, Xu Y, *et al.* Structure of M^pro from SARS-CoV-2 and discovery of its inhibitors. Nature 2020; 582(7811): 289-93.
[http://dx.doi.org/10.1038/s41586-020-2223-y] [PMID: 32272481]

[57]   Pillaiyar T, Manickam M, Namasivayam V, Hayashi Y, Jung SH. An Overview of Severe Acute Respiratory Syndrome-Coronavirus (SARS-CoV) 3CL Protease Inhibitors: Peptidomimetics and Small Molecule Chemotherapy. J Med Chem 2016; 59(14): 6595-628.
[http://dx.doi.org/10.1021/acs.jmedchem.5b01461] [PMID: 26878082]

[58]   Muramatsu T, Kim YT, Nishii W, Terada T, Shirouzu M, Yokoyama S. Autoprocessing mechanism of severe acute respiratory syndrome coronavirus 3C-like protease (SARS-CoV 3CLpro) from its polyproteins. FEBS J 2013; 280(9): 2002-13.
[http://dx.doi.org/10.1111/febs.12222] [PMID: 23452147]

[59]   Bzówka M, Mitusińska K, Raczyńska A, Samol A, Tuszyński JA, Góra A. Structural and Evolutionary Analysis Indicate That the SARS-CoV-2 Mpro Is a Challenging Target for Small-Molecule Inhibitor Design. Int J Mol Sci 2020; 21(9): 21.
[http://dx.doi.org/10.3390/ijms21093099] [PMID: 32353978]

[60]   Pillaiyar T, Wendt LL, Manickam M, Easwaran M. The Recent Outbreaks of Human Coronaviruses: A Medicinal Chemistry Perspective. Med Res Rev 2020.
[PMID: 32852058]

[61]   He J, Hu L, Huang X, *et al.* Potential of coronavirus 3C-like protease inhibitors for the development of new anti-SARS-CoV-2 drugs: Insights from structures of protease and inhibitors. Int J Antimicrob Agents 2020; 56(2): 106055.
[http://dx.doi.org/10.1016/j.ijantimicag.2020.106055] [PMID: 32534187]

[62]   Liu Y, Liang C, Xin L, *et al.* The development of Coronavirus 3C-Like protease (3CL^pro) inhibitors from 2010 to 2020. Eur J Med Chem 2020; 206: 112711.
[http://dx.doi.org/10.1016/j.ejmech.2020.112711] [PMID: 32810751]

[63]   Teruya K, Hattori Y, Shimamoto Y, *et al.* Structural basis for the development of SARS 3CL protease inhibitors from a peptide mimic to an aza-decaline scaffold. Biopolymers 2016; 106(4): 391-403.
[http://dx.doi.org/10.1002/bip.22773] [PMID: 26572934]

[64]   Noe MC, Gilbert AM. Targeted Covalent Enzyme Inhibitors. Annual Reports in Medicinal Chemistry. Academic Press Inc. 2012; Vol. 47: pp. 413-39.

[65]   Yver A. Osimertinib (AZD9291)-a science-driven, collaborative approach to rapid drug design and development. Ann Oncol 2016; 27(6): 1165-70.
[http://dx.doi.org/10.1093/annonc/mdw129] [PMID: 26961148]

[66]   Craven GB, Affron DP, Allen CE, *et al.* High-Throughput Kinetic Analysis for Target-Directed Covalent Ligand Discovery. Angew Chem Int Ed Engl 2018; 57(19): 5257-61.
[http://dx.doi.org/10.1002/anie.201711825] [PMID: 29480525]

[67]   Gehringer M. Covalent inhibitors: back on track? Future Med Chem 2020; 12(15): 1363-8.
[http://dx.doi.org/10.4155/fmc-2020-0118] [PMID: 32597212]

[68]   Gehringer M, Laufer SA. Emerging and Re-Emerging Warheads for Targeted Covalent Inhibitors: Applications in Medicinal Chemistry and Chemical Biology. J Med Chem 2019; 62(12): 5673-724.
[http://dx.doi.org/10.1021/acs.jmedchem.8b01153] [PMID: 30565923]

[69]   Copeland RA. The drug-target residence time model: a 10-year retrospective. Nat Rev Drug Discov 2016; 15(2): 87-95.
[http://dx.doi.org/10.1038/nrd.2015.18] [PMID: 26678621]

[70]   Martin JS, MacKenzie CJ, Fletcher D, Gilbert IH. Characterising covalent warhead reactivity. Bioorg Med Chem 2019; 27(10): 2066-74.
[http://dx.doi.org/10.1016/j.bmc.2019.04.002] [PMID: 30975501]

[71]   Ábrányi-Balogh P, Petri L, Imre T, *et al.* A road map for prioritizing warheads for cysteine targeting covalent inhibitors. Eur J Med Chem 2018; 160: 94-107.
[http://dx.doi.org/10.1016/j.ejmech.2018.10.010] [PMID: 30321804]

[72]   Martín-Gago P, Olsen CA. Arylfluorosulfate-Based Electrophiles for Covalent Protein Labeling: A New Addition to the Arsenal. Angew Chem Int Ed Engl 2019; 58(4): 957-66.
[http://dx.doi.org/10.1002/anie.201806037] [PMID: 30024079]

[73]   Sutanto F, Konstantinidou M, Dömling A. Covalent inhibitors: a rational approach to drug discovery. RSC Med Chem 2020; 11(8): 876-84.
[http://dx.doi.org/10.1039/D0MD00154F] [PMID: 33479682]

[74]   Ghosh AK, Samanta I, Mondal A, Liu WR. Covalent Inhibition in Drug Discovery. ChemMedChem 2019; 14(9): 889-906.
[http://dx.doi.org/10.1002/cmdc.201900107] [PMID: 30816012]

[75]   Galasiti Kankanamalage AC, Kim Y, Damalanka VC, *et al.* Structure-guided design of potent and permeable inhibitors of MERS coronavirus 3CL protease that utilize a piperidine moiety as a novel design element. Eur J Med Chem 2018; 150: 334-46.
[http://dx.doi.org/10.1016/j.ejmech.2018.03.004] [PMID: 29544147]

[76]   Zhang L, Lin D, Kusov Y, *et al.* α-ketoamides as broad-spectrum inhibitors of coronavirus and enterovirus replication: structure-based design, synthesis, and activity assessment. J Med Chem 2020; 63(9): 4562-78.
[http://dx.doi.org/10.1021/acs.jmedchem.9b01828] [PMID: 32045235]

[77]   Ghosh AK, Xi K, Ratia K, *et al.* Design and synthesis of peptidomimetic severe acute respiratory syndrome chymotrypsin-like protease inhibitors. J Med Chem 2005; 48(22): 6767-71.
[http://dx.doi.org/10.1021/jm050548m] [PMID: 16250632]

[78]   Shie JJ, Fang JM, Kuo TH, *et al.* Inhibition of the severe acute respiratory syndrome 3CL protease by peptidomimetic α,β-unsaturated esters. Bioorg Med Chem 2005; 13(17): 5240-52.
[http://dx.doi.org/10.1016/j.bmc.2005.05.065] [PMID: 15994085]

[79]   Yang S, Chen S-J, Hsu M-F, *et al.* Synthesis, crystal structure, structure-activity relationships, and antiviral activity of a potent SARS coronavirus 3CL protease inhibitor. J Med Chem 2006; 49(16): 4971-80.
[http://dx.doi.org/10.1021/jm0603926] [PMID: 16884309]

[80]   Ghosh AK, Xi K, Grum-Tokars V, *et al.* Structure-Based Design, Synthesis, and Biological Evaluation of Peptidomimetic SARS-CoV 3CLpro Inhibitors 2007; 5876-80.

[81]   Yang H, Xie W, Xue X, *et al.* Design of wide-spectrum inhibitors targeting coronavirus main proteases. PLoS Biol 2005; 3(10): e324.
[http://dx.doi.org/10.1371/journal.pbio.0030324] [PMID: 16128623]

[82]   Xue X, Yang H, Shen W, *et al.* Production of authentic SARS-CoV M(pro) with enhanced activity: application as a novel tag-cleavage endopeptidase for protein overproduction. J Mol Biol 2007; 366(3): 965-75.
[http://dx.doi.org/10.1016/j.jmb.2006.11.073] [PMID: 17189639]

[83]   Al-Gharabli SI, Shah ST, Weik S, *et al.* An efficient method for the synthesis of peptide aldehyde libraries employed in the discovery of reversible SARS coronavirus main protease (SARS-CoV Mpro) inhibitors. ChemBioChem 2006; 7(7): 1048-55.
[http://dx.doi.org/10.1002/cbic.200500533] [PMID: 16688706]

[84]   Kumar V, Shin JS, Shie JJ, *et al.* Identification and evaluation of potent Middle East respiratory syndrome coronavirus (MERS-CoV) 3CL^Pro inhibitors. Antiviral Res 2017; 141: 101-6.
[http://dx.doi.org/10.1016/j.antiviral.2017.02.007] [PMID: 28216367]

[85]   Akaji K, Konno H, Mitsui H, *et al.* Structure-based design, synthesis, and evaluation of peptide-mimetic SARS 3CL protease inhibitors. J Med Chem 2011; 54(23): 7962-73.
[http://dx.doi.org/10.1021/jm200870n] [PMID: 22014094]

[86]   Dai W, Zhang B, Jiang XM, *et al.* Structure-Based Design of Antiviral Drug Candidates Targeting the SARS-CoV-2 Main Protease. Science (80-) 368: 1331-5.2020;

[87]   Sydnes MO, Hayashi Y, Sharma VK, *et al.* Synthesis of Glutamic Acid and Glutamine Peptides Possessing a Trifluoromethyl Ketone Group as SARS-CoV 3CL Protease Inhibitors. 2006; 62: 8601-9.

[88]   Shao Y-M, Yang W-B, Kuo T-H, *et al.* Design, synthesis, and evaluation of trifluoromethyl ketones as inhibitors of SARS-CoV 3CL protease. Bioorg Med Chem 2008; 16(8): 4652-60.
[http://dx.doi.org/10.1016/j.bmc.2008.02.040] [PMID: 18329272]

[89]   Regnier T, Sarma D, Hidaka K, *et al.* New developments for the design, synthesis and biological evaluation of potent SARS-CoV 3CL(pro) inhibitors. Bioorg Med Chem Lett 2009; 19(10): 2722-7.
[http://dx.doi.org/10.1016/j.bmcl.2009.03.118] [PMID: 19362479]

[90]   Jain RP, Vederas JC. Structural Variations in Keto-Glutamines for Improved Inhibition against Hepatitis A Virus 3C Proteinase. 2004; 14: 3655-8.

[91]   Thanigaimalai P, Konno S, Yamamoto T, *et al.* Design, synthesis, and biological evaluation of novel dipeptide-type SARS-CoV 3CL protease inhibitors: structure-activity relationship study. Eur J Med Chem 2013; 65: 436-47.
[http://dx.doi.org/10.1016/j.ejmech.2013.05.005] [PMID: 23747811]

[92]   Konno S, Thanigaimalai P, Yamamoto T, *et al.* Design and synthesis of new tripeptide-type SARS-CoV 3CL protease inhibitors containing an electrophilic arylketone moiety. Bioorg Med Chem 2013; 21(2): 412-24.
[http://dx.doi.org/10.1016/j.bmc.2012.11.017] [PMID: 23245752]

[93]   Shie J, Fang J, Kuo C, Kuo T, Liang P, Huang H. Discovery of Potent Anilide Inhibitors against the Severe Acute Respiratory Syndrome 3CL Protease. 2005; 4469-73.

[94]   Chuck CP, Chen C, Ke Z, Wan DC, Chow HF, Wong KB. Design, synthesis and crystallographic analysis of nitrile-based broad-spectrum peptidomimetic inhibitors for coronavirus 3C-like proteases. Eur J Med Chem 2013; 59: 1-6.
[http://dx.doi.org/10.1016/j.ejmech.2012.10.053] [PMID: 23202846]

[95]   Silva DG, Ribeiro JFR, De Vita D, *et al.* A comparative study of warheads for design of cysteine protease inhibitors. Bioorg Med Chem Lett 2017; 27(22): 5031-5.

[http://dx.doi.org/10.1016/j.bmcl.2017.10.002] [PMID: 29054358]

[96]   Asgian JL, James KE, Li ZZ, *et al.* Aza-Peptide Epoxides : A New Class of Inhibitors Selective for Clan CD Cysteine Proteases. 2002; 4958-60.
[http://dx.doi.org/10.1021/jm025581c]

[97]   Lee T, Cherney MM, Huitema C, *et al.* Crystal Structures of the Main Peptidase from the SARS Coronavirus Inhibited by a Substrate-like Aza-Peptide Epoxide. 2005; 1137-51.
[http://dx.doi.org/10.1016/j.jmb.2005.09.004]

[98]   Martina E, Stiefl N, Degel B, *et al.* Screening of electrophilic compounds yields an aziridinyl peptide as new active-site directed SARS-CoV main protease inhibitor. Bioorg Med Chem Lett 2005; 15(24): 5365-9.
[http://dx.doi.org/10.1016/j.bmcl.2005.09.012] [PMID: 16216498]

[99]   Lee TW, Cherney MM, Liu J, *et al.* Crystal structures reveal an induced-fit binding of a substrate-like Aza-peptide epoxide to SARS coronavirus main peptidase. J Mol Biol 2007; 366(3): 916-32.
[http://dx.doi.org/10.1016/j.jmb.2006.11.078] [PMID: 17196984]

[100]   dos Santos Nascimento IJ, de Aquino TM, da Silva-Júnior EF. Drug Repurposing: A Strategy for Discovering Inhibitors against Emerging Viral Infections. Curr Med Chem 2020; 27.
[PMID: 32787752]

[101]   Elfiky AA. Ribavirin, Remdesivir, Sofosbuvir, Galidesivir, and Tenofovir against SARS-CoV-2 RNA dependent RNA polymerase (RdRp): A molecular docking study. Life Sci 2020; 253: 117592.
[http://dx.doi.org/10.1016/j.lfs.2020.117592] [PMID: 32222463]

[102]   Pillaiyar T, Meenakshisundaram S, Manickam M, Sankaranarayanan M. A medicinal chemistry perspective of drug repositioning: Recent advances and challenges in drug discovery. Eur J Med Chem 2020; 195: 112275.
[http://dx.doi.org/10.1016/j.ejmech.2020.112275] [PMID: 32283298]

[103]   Momattin H, Al-Ali AY, Al-Tawfiq JA. A Systematic Review of therapeutic agents for the treatment of the Middle East Respiratory Syndrome Coronavirus (MERS-CoV). Travel Med Infect Dis 2019; 30: 9-18.
[http://dx.doi.org/10.1016/j.tmaid.2019.06.012] [PMID: 31252170]

[104]   Yao TT, Qian JD, Zhu WY, Wang Y, Wang GQ. A systematic review of lopinavir therapy for SARS coronavirus and MERS coronavirus-A possible reference for coronavirus disease-19 treatment option. J Med Virol 2020; 92(6): 556-63.
[http://dx.doi.org/10.1002/jmv.25729] [PMID: 32104907]

[105]   Amin SA, Jha T. Fight against novel coronavirus: A perspective of medicinal chemists. Eur J Med Chem 2020; 201: 112559.
[http://dx.doi.org/10.1016/j.ejmech.2020.112559] [PMID: 32563814]

SUBJECT INDEX

www.ingramcontent.com/pod-product-compliance
Lightning Source LLC
Chambersburg PA
CBHW041659210326
41598CB00007B/469